The British Columbia

Atlas of Wellness

1st Edition

Leslie T. Foster

C. Peter Keller

with contributions from Jack Boomer, Diane Braithwaite, John Fowler, Michael Hayes, Perry Hystad, Patti Jensen, Ken Josephson, Perry Kendall, Brian McKee, Gord Miller, Aleck Ostry, David Weicker, and Martin Wright

Canadian Western Geographical Series • Volume 42
Copyright 2007 © Western Geographical Press

Western Geographical Press

Department of Geography, University of Victoria
P.O. Box 3050, Victoria, BC, Canada V8W 3P5
phone: (250) 721-7331 fax: (250) 721-6216

Canadian Western Geographical Series

editorial address
Harold D. Foster, Ph.D.
Department of Geography
University of Victoria
Victoria, British Columbia
Canada

SERIES EDITOR'S ACKNOWLEDGEMENTS

Special thanks are due to two members of the Department of Geography, Diane Braithwaite and Ken Josephson, for their dedication and hard work in ensuring the successful publication of this, the 42nd volume of the Canadian Western Geographical Series.

Library and Archives Canada Cataloguing in Publication

Foster, Leslie T., 1947-
The British Columbia atlas of wellness / Leslie T. Foster, C. Peter
Keller ; with contributions from Jack Boomer ... [et al.]. -- 1st ed.

(Canadian western geographical series, ISSN 1203-1178 ; 42)
Includes bibliographical references.
ISBN 978-0-919838-32-1 (bound)

1. British Columbia--Statistics, Medical--Maps. 2. Health status indicators--
British Columbia--Maps. 3. Public health--British Columbia--Statistics--Maps.
I. Keller, C. Peter, 1959- II. Boomer, Jack III. Title. IV. Title: Atlas of wellness.
V. Series.

RA407.5.C3F68 2007   614.4'2711   C2007-906673-9

Eco Audit

The Western Geographical Press uses environmentally responsible papers. By choosing 100% post-consumer recycled fibre instead of virgin paper for this printed material the following savings to our natural resources were realized:

Trees Saved	Waterbourne waste saved	Saved wastewater	Solid waste not generated	Greenhouse gases saved	Natural gas saved
30	12.1 lbs	18,113 gallons	1,919 lbs	4,214 lbs	4,392 ft³

This is equivalent to .6 American football fields of trees, a shower that lasts 3.8 days and emissions of .4 car(s) for a year.

Above information is based on:
3,553 lbs of Silva Enviro 100% PCW paper

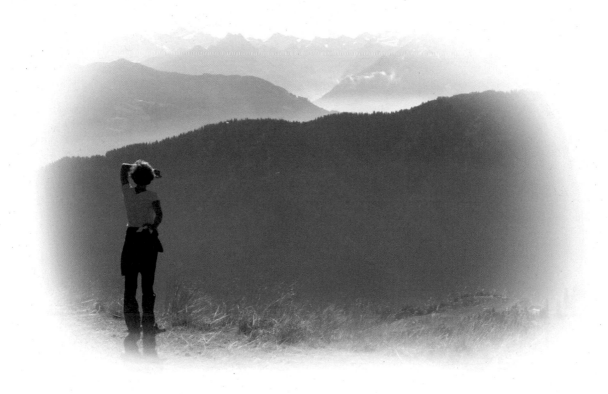

Contents

List of Contributors

The production of this Atlas contains written and cartographic contributions from the following individuals:

Jack Boomer, director of the Clean Air Coalition of BC, which includes the Heart and Stroke Foundation of BC and Yukon and the BC Lung Association, was responsible for Chapter 5, pp. 95-114.

Diane Braithwaite, department secretary, Department of Geography, University of Victoria, was responsible for copy editing and layout.

Leslie T. Foster, adjunct professor in the department of Geography and the School of Child and Youth Care, University of Victoria, was co-editor and responsible for Chapter 1, pp. 1-7; Chapter 3, pp. 21-31; Chapter 4, pp. 33-47; Chapter 5, pp. 49-73, 78-93, 95-114, 137-138, 142-149, 164-165, 173-174, 182-183, 185-208; and Chapter 6, pp. 209-222.

John Fowler, senior laboratory instructor, Department of Geography, University of Victoria, was responsible for maps on pp. 34, 35, 37, 39, 86, 87, 135, 148, 149, 164, 182.

Michael Hayes, associate dean, Faculty of Health Sciences, Simon Fraser University, was responsible for Chapter 2, pp. 17-19.

Perry Hystad, MSc student in the Department of Geography, University of Victoria, and since September of 2007, PhD student in the Department of Health Care and Epidemiology, University of British Columbia, was responsible for Chapter 1, pp. 3-7.

Patti Jensen, co-director, Interdisciplinary Women's Reproductive Health Research Training, Child and Family Research Institute, and associate professor, Department of Health Care and Epidemiology, University of British Columbia, was responsible for Chapter 5, pp. 175-181.

Ken Josephson, cartographer, Department of Geography, University of Victoria, was responsible for design, layout and technical production.

Peter Keller, dean, Faculty of Social Sciences, and professor, Department of Geography, University of Victoria, was co-editor and responsible for Chapter 1, pp. 3-7.

Perry Kendall, provincial health officer, Province of BC, was responsible for the Foreword, p. iv.

Brian McKee, Ashgrove Geographic Services Ltd., was responsible for compilation of all maps and tables, except as noted, and Chapter 3, pp. 30-31; Chapter 6, 209-213.

Gord Miller, Social Science and Humanities Research Council doctoral fellow, Centre for Community Health Promotion Research, University of Victoria, was responsible for Chapter 2, pp. 9-17.

Aleck Ostry, Canada Research Chair in the Social Determinants of Community Health, and associate professor, Department of Geography, University of Victoria, was responsible for Chapter 5, pp. 115-136, 140, 167-172.

David Weicker, athletics and sports consultant, Stellar J Consulting Group, was responsible for Chapter 5, pp. 137-138, 150-163.

Martin Wright, executive director, Strategic Policy and Planning, Ministry of Children and Family Development, was responsible for Chapter 5, pp. 54, 74-77.

Photo credits go to Analisa Blake; Diane Braithwaite; Les Foster; Ken Josephson; Peter Keller; Olaf Niemann and the Spatial Sciences Laboratory, University of Victoria; Dan Smith; Crystal Tremblay; and Chris Virtue.

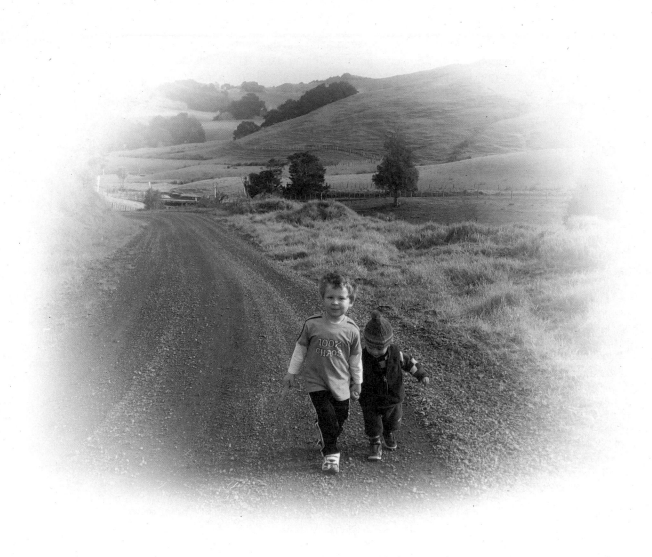

Acknowledgements

As with any publication of this nature, the final product is the result of the efforts of many individuals and groups acting, knowingly or unknowingly, as a formal or informal team. The *BC Atlas of Wellness* is no exception, and many people and organizations, too numerous to mention them all, have had important input to this publication. While we thank all of the writers and cartographers who are mentioned specifically within the book for their contributions, there are several individuals and groups that we would like to acknowledge at this time.

Andrew Hazlewood of the Ministry of Health must be thanked for the original idea for the *BC Atlas of Wellness*. In addition, he arranged for financial assistance so that the Atlas could be produced and distributed throughout the province. Andrew was also the original chair of the interministry ActNow BC Assistant Deputy Ministers' Committee before being joined as co-chair by John Mills of the Ministry of Tourism, Sports and the Arts. John has also been an enthusiastic supporter of the project. The Assistant Deputy Ministers' Committee has been a wonderful group to work with. Members of the committee, who represent every ministry in the provincial government, acted as a sounding board for ideas and enthusiastically joined in debate about the appropriateness of the individual indicators that form the bases for the maps produced in the Atlas. Members gave readily of their own time, and freed up staff for discussion purposes. They also pointed us to other individuals and organizations who had ideas to offer, many of which have been included in some form in the Atlas. Ministries provided access to appropriate data which have been mapped in the Atlas. The Population and Public Health Evidence and Data Expert Group, co-chaired by John Millar of the Provincial Health Services Authority and Martha Burd of the Ministry of Health, provided a forum to discuss the Atlas near the end of the project and provided very useful advice about wellness and its indicators.

Special thanks go to the following: from the Ministry of Health, Richard Mercer, Laurie Woodland, Russell Fairburn, Rosemary Armour, Ron Danderfer, Shelley Canitz, Wayne Mitic, Gayle Downey, Kersteen Johnston, Tom Gregory, Trevor Hancock, and Perry Kendall; from the Ministry of Children and Family Development, Martin Wright, Kim Danderfer, Jeannie Cosgrove, and Thomas Godfrey; from the Ministry of Labour and Citizen's Services, Pat Bluemel, Karen Calderbank, and Dave O'Neil; from the Ministry of Education, Heather Hoult, Helen Myers, Karlic Ho, and Marie Ann Maruca; from the Ministry of Tourism, Sports and the Arts, Sharon White and Del Nyberg; from the Ministry of Environment, Jenny Feick and staff; from the Ministry of Transportation, Mary Koyl and staff; from BC Recreation and Parks Association, Suzanne Allard Strutt, Sharon Meredith, Lisah Hansen, and Trina Sporer; from Sports BC, Gail Donahue and Sandra Stevenson; from 2010 Legacies Now, Patti Hunter and Bryna Kopelow; from the McCreary Centre Society, Minda Chittenden, Elizabeth Saewyc, and Roger Tonkin; from the Heart and Stroke Foundation, Mark Collison; from BC Transit, Mike Davies and Helen Cook; and from Interior Health Authority, Ron Dovell. Ron Duffell of the Ministry of Tourism, Sports and the Arts, as secretary to the Assistant Deputy Ministers' Committee, has enthusiastically provided his support throughout major transition phases of the project, and provided feedback at critical junctures.

The completion of this Atlas would not have been possible without the outstanding contributions of Brian McKee, who was responsible for the initial data preparation and compilation for this Atlas. He stayed the course despite its complicated twists and turns. At the University of Victoria, thanks go to John Fowler who was instrumental in the development of all of the final maps and tables. Ken Josephson and Diane Braithwaite, both working in the Department of Geography and for the Western Geographical Press, undertook the major tasks of design, final copyediting, and layout of the Atlas.

We would also like to thank our colleagues in the Department of Geography and the Human and Social Development Faculty who provided encouragement and support throughout our work on the project.

Last, but far from least, we would like to acknowledge the encouragement and support of our families. For Les, his wife Mary provided so many different kinds of assistance—emotional, research, and secretarial, to mention but a few—and his children, Noëlle, Stefan, Chris, and Dylan, were always supportive of the project, even when it took time away from the family vacation. For Peter, the encouragement, selfless support, and feedback always offered by his wife Eileen, and the understanding by his children Connor and Alison for dad's endless hours at work, accompanied by their humourous teasing, are acknowledged.

Leslie T. Foster and C. Peter Keller,
University of Victoria, August 2007

Preface

In 2005, we completed the BC Mortality Atlas, a web-based update (*www.geog.uvic.ca/mortality*) to an earlier publication titled *The Geography of Death: Mortality Atlas of British Columbia, 1985-1989* (Foster and Edgell, 1992). We were beginning work on a youth atlas and a seniors atlas for BC when Andrew Hazlewood, Assistant Deputy Minister of Population, Health and Wellness in the Ministry of Health, organized a brief meeting to discuss the concept of a wellness approach to mapping health in BC. Mapping health-related data in the province has a tradition over the past two decades, but mapping has tended to look at mortality, morbidity, or system use, not the actual "health" or wellness of British Columbians. To our knowledge, the concept of taking a wellness approach had not been tried before. Hence, the genesis of this Atlas.

The interministry ActNow BC Assistant Deputy Ministers' Committee, co-chaired by Andrew Hazlewood and John Mills, was tasked with providing advice and implementing projects that would support the provincial government's ActNow BC initiative announced in early 2005. The overall goal of ActNow BC was to help make BC the healthiest jurisdiction to host a modern day Olympic and Paralympic games. The Atlas could assist in focusing the attention of diverse ministries on ways to contribute to ActNow BC, and also ensure that actions to support the initiative would recognize the geographical diversity of the province. It was well known that achieving the provincial goals of ActNow BC would require attention to the fact that health, wellness, illness, and health system infrastructure varied substantially throughout the province. As such, it was important to get a geographical base line of these variations so that differences, and anticipated improvements, could be measured over time. This first edition of the *BC Atlas of Wellness* contributes to this process.

Unlike mortality, which is readily defined, measuring and mapping wellness is much more challenging. Like health, wellness is a term that is used in everyday discourse without much thought to what it entails. There is an assumption that everyone knows what it is. Achieving some definition of wellness, and agreement around what influences it, has been one of the major challenges in developing and organizing this Atlas. A second major challenge has been defining an appropriate geographical unit for mapping purposes. Within the province, there are myriad geographical administrative units for which data are collected: municipalities, local health areas, federal and provincial electoral ridings, school districts, regional districts, health service delivery areas, economic development regions, and health authorities, to name but a few. Given the tight timelines for producing this Atlas, our approach has been to use existing data, albeit from a variety of sources. In addition, we use data that are collected periodically so that trends and changes can be mapped over time. Consequently, to the extent possible, we have mapped data at the Health Service Delivery Area (HSDA) level. While a finer scale would have been preferred, the reasons for choosing the HSDA level are of a practical nature. The HSDA is the most detailed level for which key survey data (particularly the 14,000 sample Canadian Community Health Survey) are available. Furthermore, this survey is repeated on a regular basis and also provides an opportunity for comparisons with other parts of the country. As such, changes over time can be measured and mapped. A selected number of indicators are also mapped by other administrative units, most notably School Districts, BC Games Zones, and Economic Development Regions. In addition, there are a limited number of what we refer to as "custom maps," which have a different basis altogether. These are based on the ready availability of unique indicator data.

The Atlas is organized into several chapters that provide background and context, but primarily follow the main "pillars" of the ActNow BC initiative. The first chapter gives an introduction to the Atlas and a brief background of the ActNow BC initiative. In addition, a brief introduction to health-related mapping, particularly for BC, is provided. Chapter two presents a synopsis of the concept of wellness, and an introduction to the determinants of health and wellness. Chapter three provides an overview of the key data sources, and instructions on "how to use and read" the maps provided in the Atlas. Chapter four offers a geographical context for the Atlas, particularly with respect to the demographic and physical aspects of the province. Chapter five is the main chapter and, after a series of maps showing the socio-economic and demographic determinants of, or assets for, health and wellness, follows closely the key pillars of the ActNow BC initiative, providing maps and commentary on indicators related to tobacco smoke-free environments, nutrition and food security, physical activity, healthy weights, healthy pregnancy, and wellness outcomes. Chapter six provides a series of maps and commentary based on a combination of selected indicators contained within the Atlas.

Throughout the Atlas, a "half-full" or asset approach to mapping indicators is taken, rather than a "half-empty" or deficit approach. Put simply, this involves using indicators such as healthy weight rather than overweight status or obesity, non-smoking behaviour rather than smoking behaviour, activity-related indicators rather than those related to inactivity, and good health indicators rather than illness measures. This is our way of using the wellness concept in the Atlas. This approach will not be without its critics. Some will argue that focusing on wellness or positive aspects of health will provide an unfair picture of health and wellness in the province by ignoring or minimizing problem issues and areas that need addressing, and may leave an impression that all is "well" in the province. That is not our intent. Each colour map shows those areas that are doing best as measured by key indicators, and those that are not. As such, the regions requiring improvement in wellness issues are readily apparent. Further, we are aware that problem areas and issues will continue to be pursued by others, as is currently the case.

It is not our intent to explain the variations in the many indicators that we map. The aim of the *BC Atlas of Wellness* is to present data in a useful form that is readily understandable. The maps "speak for themselves," and our job is to describe the key points that emerge from the maps and accompanying tables as a basis for discussion by interested groups and individuals. It is our hope that they will ask questions of themselves, and others in their community, about the "whys and wherefores" of the patterns that emerge.

We anticipate that this novel approach—to mapping the positive, rather than the negative, mapping the assets, rather than the deficits—will result in useful discourse on why variations exist and what can be done about them. This can only help improve the overall health and wellness of the province and its residents.

Leslie T. Foster and C. Peter Keller
University of Victoria, August 2007

Foreword

Geographical mapping has been, and continues to be, an important technique used by a variety of public health-related disciplines to show health and wellness patterns within populations. John Snow, viewed by many as the first modern-day epidemiologist, mapped cholera victims in London in 1854 and was able to identify how the disease was transmitted and thus make recommendations to prevent future outbreaks. The *BC Atlas of Wellness* follows a distinguished tradition in health-related mapping to show variations and inequities in various wellness-related indicators. While many previous health-related atlases have focused on system use and problem areas, this Atlas is unique in that its focus is on assets rather than deficits. In public health, we are accustomed to focusing on problems and finding ways to minimize their impacts or prevent them entirely. By focusing on the concept of wellness, which, like health, is multi-faceted in nature, this Atlas provides a wealth of different types of indicators that reflect many key dimensions of wellness. In all, over 270 separate maps are included, along with supporting tables that provide data related to approximately 120 indicators of the various dimensions of wellness.

While the topics included in the Atlas cover traditional indicators related to the determinants of health and wellness and healthy public policies, there are also many unique indicators. The material is grounded in the physical and demographic diversity of BC, and an important feature of the Atlas is that it uses the ActNow BC health promotion initiative as a framework to present the mapped indicators. This initiative is based on several key areas of public health: smoking; nutrition; physical exercise; weight; and pregnancies. While these areas are all covered in the Atlas, it takes a positive approach to the indicators being mapped: rather than mapping smoking, it looks at non-smoking behaviour and environments, at healthy nutrition and policy adoption rather than poor nutrition, at physical activities rather than sedentary activities, at healthy weights rather than obesity, and at conditions that promote healthy pregnancy rather than potentially damaging behaviour during pregnancy. Furthermore, it provides information on outcomes in terms of how the population views certain components of their health and wellness, and also provides an interesting yet simple approach to determining potential benchmarks for specific wellness features.

The Atlas has contributions from a variety of partners, including scholars from several institutions, graduate students, consultants, health advocacy groups, and public servants. Its aims are to measure and show the level of regional inequities in wellness, and to generate questions and discussions among community groups, public health policy and decision makers, school boards, and local governments on why one region does better than other regions on one or more indicators. Are regional inequalities in wellness indicators important enough to warrant local action? If so, what can be done to improve wellness? What can be learned from the regions that are the best or excel on certain dimensions of wellness?

The material presented here shows regional variations, as well as variations based on gender and age groupings. In some instances, statistical testing shows whether or not differences are significant. As such, the information can be used to help target health promotion initiatives both geographically and demographically. The maps and tables have also been created from a variety of scattered data sources, some of which may not be that well known to policy makers and others interested in wellness. The Atlas, by adding value to raw data so that rates can be compared among regions, and providing them publicly, essentially makes them available to any one who wishes to use the data for their own purposes. Further, the Atlas is available to all who have access to the internet through the website *www.geog.uvic.ca/wellness*, and additional and updated data will be made available through this website in the future.

By focusing on assets and taking a wellness approach, the *BC Atlas of Wellness* provides a unique and most interesting look at health and wellness in the province. It will assist communities and regions to learn more about their health and wellness relative to other parts of the province, and it complements reports that have been produced through my office.

P.R.W. Kendall, OBC, MBBS, MSc, FRCPC
Provincial Health Officer
British Columbia

1

Introduction to the Atlas

The background to the development of the *BC Atlas of Wellness* is described in the following pages. It springs from the ActNow BC initiative, which was introduced by the BC government in early 2005 to encourage British Columbians to make healthy lifestyle choices to improve their quality of life, reduce the incidence of preventable chronic disease, and reduce the burden on the health care system. ActNow BC is an integrated, government-wide approach that engages the contributions of partners in other levels of government (e.g., municipalities), non-government organizations, schools, communities, and the private sector to develop and deliver programs and services to assist individuals to quit or never start smoking, to be more physically active, eat healthier foods, achieve and maintain a healthy weight, and make healthy choices in pregnancy. The key thrusts of ActNow BC are described, as these provide the framework for the maps that follow later in the Atlas. A second part to this chapter provides a discussion on why we have taken the approach of mapping wellness through a variety of indicators, and reviews some of the key literature related to the mapping approach to health and wellness. The final section considers the goals of this Atlas and the reasons behind them.

The Emergence of ActNow BC

In April 2004, the Select Standing Committee on Health was asked, among other things, to investigate successful health promotion campaigns in other jurisdictions with a view to assessing their usefulness for BC. The Committee was also asked to look at how to promote "healthy lifestyles" and to consider savings that might result from the improved fitness of the general population, and children and youth in particular (BC Select Standing Committee on Health, 2004).

The report was delivered 8 months later and indicated that 40% of the most common chronic diseases were a result of one or more of the following preventable factors: smoking, poor diet, physical inactivity, the resulting overweight status or obesity, and irresponsible use of alcohol.

The Committee noted that failure to reduce the occurrence of those diseases that were actually preventable resulted in great human, social, and economic costs. In total, the Committee made no fewer than 29 recommendations and stated that there were no "quick or easy fixes" to achieve savings or improvements in health and wellness. As the Committee noted, "The path to health and wellness for British Columbians will not be an easy road to travel" (Ibid., p. 4), and the greatest concerns were related to the rates of obesity, poor nutrition, and physical inactivity, which had reached epidemic proportions in society.

Touting the 2010 Winter Olympics, which BC had won the opportunity to host, the Committee felt that the entire BC population could respond to the excitement of the games and join the athletes in achieving personal bests and improving their own health. The members noted that "The need to *act now* [emphasis added] is urgent" (Ibid., p. 2) if the health care system is not to be overwhelmed, and suggested that funding for public health should be gradually doubled as a proportion of the total health care budget from 3% to 6%. Community and municipal organizations were seen as crucial to making a difference.

In releasing its strategic plan in 2005, the Province responded to the concerns of the Committee, setting as one of "Five Great Goals" for the next few years to "lead the way in North America in healthy living and physical fitness" (*www.bcbudget.gov.bc.ca/2006/stplan/*).

Key actions to accomplish this goal included:

- making BC the healthiest jurisdiction to ever host a modern Olympic and Paralympic games;

- encouraging British Columbians to reduce tobacco use, increase physical activity and improve nutrition, and make healthier choices during pregnancy (set out by the specific targets of ActNow BC);

- encouraging British Columbians to make healthier living choices that support a sustainable health care system by reducing the burden of chronic disease; and

- closing the gap in health status between Aboriginal and non-Aboriginal British Columbians.

In the discussion of the goal, it was noted that being overweight or obese contributed to many preventable diseases, and resulted in premature death, and that increased levels of physical exercise could combat some of these conditions. It further stated that tobacco was still a major cause of preventable morbidity and premature mortality.

The ActNow BC Framework

ActNow BC was created in 2005, following the release of the province's strategic plan, and assigned the leadership role to the Ministry of Health to make it a comprehensive health promotion initiative. The key was to help ensure that citizens could make positive lifestyle choices and also be active in order to stay well and in good health.

While the goals for improvement were set for 2015/16, the 2010 Olympics were clearly seen as an event that could help to rally the population around the need to achieve the goals suggested by the BC Select Standing Committee on Health. ActNow BC adopted the actions identified by the strategic plan to improve the health and wellness of the province, and added the need to build community capacity to create healthier and sustainable, economically viable communities.

Although the provincial strategic plan had set goals to be achieved by 2015/16, ActNow BC set more ambitious goals to be achieved by 2010, the year the Olympics are to be hosted. The targets included:

- reduce tobacco use by 10%;

- increase the number of people who eat at least five servings of fruits and vegetables every day by 20%;

- increase the number of people who are physically active by 20%;

- reduce the number of BC adults who are overweight by 20%;

- increase the number of women counselled about alcohol use during pregnancy by 50%.

It was recognized that success in achieving these goals needed long term changes in beliefs, values, and behaviours, and while government could be the leader, it could not do it alone. There was a need for influential community partners, and four key partners were singled out: 2010 Legacies Now, BC Recreation and Parks Association (BCRPA), BC Healthy Living Alliance (BCHLA), and the Union of BC Municipalities (UBCM).

2010 Legacies Now was first created in 2000 to assist with the Olympic bid and to help ensure that the benefits of the 2010 Olympics were shared throughout the province. It became an independent society in 2002 with a mandate to ensure "a strong and lasting sport system for the province that increased participation from Playground to Podium and supported safe, healthy, and vibrant communities." Its mandate was expanded in early 2004 to include the arts, volunteerism, and literacy, and to develop a network of community committees throughout the province to support these areas. These are all important initiatives that develop assets for wellness. The organization also administers Action Schools! BC, a program that will be described later in the Atlas (*www.2010legaciesnow.com*).

The BCRPA, like 2010 Legacies Now, is a non-profit society and, as its name suggests, is "dedicated to building and sustaining active healthy lifestyles and communities in BC." It also has a role in helping to increase sports and recreation activity in the province and has responsibility for administering the Active Community program, which will be discussed in greater detail later (*www.bcrpa.bc.ca*).

The BCHLA was formed in response to the ActNow BC initiative. It works to promote physical activity, healthy eating, and smoke-free living, and consists of a variety of key organizations with interests in chronic disease issues (e.g., BC Lung Association, Canadian Diabetes Association, Heart and Stroke Foundation of BC and Yukon, Arthritis Society of BC/Yukon, Canadian Cancer Society–BC/Yukon Chapter, and BC Pediatric Society), and other key organizations such as the Centre on Aging at the University of Victoria, Directorate of Agencies for School Health BC, Public Health Association of BC, BCRPA, Dieticians of Canada, and UBCM. BCHLA produced several important documents in early 2005 that have been significant in terms of giving publicity to ActNow BC goals (BCHLA, 2005a), as well as providing an analysis of the risk factors associated with chronic disease and an effectiveness analysis of interventions (BCHLA, 2005b). This Alliance received approximately $25 million in 2006 to help government achieve its ActNow BC goals (*www.bchealthyliving.ca*).

The fourth key organization is the UBCM, which has represented the interests of municipalities in the province for more than a century. The UBCM has been provided government funding to establish a Community Health Promotion Fund that provides grants, on a competitive basis, to local government to support health promotion focusing on healthy living and chronic disease prevention in support of the ActNow BC goals. The UBCM also supports the BC Healthy Communities initiative, which aims to help improve collective health and wellness at the community level.

At the same time the provincial government recognized it could not achieve its goal to "lead the way in North America in healthy living and physical fitness" without help from many partners, the Ministry of Health also realized that it needed a broad-based alliance within government to marshal a cross-government or horizontal focus on this ambitious health promotion initiative. All ministries within government have the ability to influence the achievement of ActNow BC. To help focus on the ActNow BC initiative, a cross-ministry group of assistant deputy ministers from each ministry in government was created, and $15 million over 3 years was made available from the Ministry of Health for projects brought forward that supported the ActNow BC goal. Ministries, or their funded agencies, needed to match these funds in order to qualify for funding. The development of the *BC Atlas of Wellness* is part of this cross-government initiative and has been supported by the Assistant Deputy Ministers' Committee. In August 2006, government created a Minister of State position, filled by the Honourable Gordon Hogg, who was assigned to lead ActNow BC. The minister is responsible for the government-wide approach of the initiative. Under his direction, all provincial ministries are identifying strategies and actions that support the goals of ActNow BC. The *BC Atlas of Wellness* was developed, in part, to assist ministries to understand how, through the development of indicators, both obvious and novel, they might contribute to the achievement of ActNow BC goals.

This background is important as a context for understanding how the *BC Atlas of Wellness* is put together in terms of its framework and in terms of the indicators included. The next section reviews some of the factors related to health and wellness mapping.

Why Maps and Atlases?

Communication via maps pre-dates written communication and can be traced back to as early as 30,000 BC (Robinson et al., 1995). Today, rarely a day goes by without maps being featured in the media to help locate an issue, to understand geographical relationships, or to explain geographical variation. The common expression that "a picture is worth (or can save) a thousand words" certainly also holds true for a map. But a map also can generate a hundred questions! Why are there geographical patterns? What is causing them? Is it a good thing? If not, what can be done to improve matters?...and so on.

Research has shown that the public wants maps packaged in the form of atlases to allow them to browse their neighbourhood and territory, to understand regional variation, and to allow for relative comparison (i.e., "how am I doing in my neighbourhood compared to other neighbourhoods or regions?") (Keller, 1995). The public also has clear ideas about what it wants such atlases to look like (Hocking and Keller, 1992, 1993; Keller, Hocking, and Wood, 1995), and what purpose and role communication technologies like the Internet should play in facilitating access to such atlases (Harrower, Keller and Hocking, 1997).

The purpose of this Atlas is to communicate data about key wellness indicators for BC, and to highlight patterns that emerge from these data in an interesting and informative way. The objective is not only to help people recognize and understand why certain geographical patterns may occur, but also to encourage questions provincially, regionally, and locally as to why the patterns are the way they are, why wellness varies over space, and what can or should be done about it.

In this chapter, we offer some background by briefly tracing the relationship between mapping and wellness with a focus on Canada and BC.

Maps and Health and Wellness

The use of maps and atlases to understand health and illness patterns has a long and distinguished history. The seminal work in health geography, and the origin of modern epidemiology, was the 1854 mapping of cholera victims in London (Snow, 1855). Snow used descriptive statistics and maps to identify how cholera was transmitted, making recommendations for prevention of future outbreaks. His maps and research continue to attract considerable attention (Koch, 2004; Monmonier,

2005). Barrett (1980) attributes the origins of disease mapping and atlases to Heinrick Berghaus (1845), who produced one of the first physical atlases in which global distributions of cholera, smallpox, and tuberculosis, among others, were shown and correlated with risk factors. The importance of maps to modern health geography is attributed to Jacques May (Pyle, 1979), who advocated a 'disease ecology' approach, in which he placed particular emphasis on the use of maps, since:

> the map of disease represents the sum of the places where requirements of each factor in a complex coincide. By reading a map of disease one can get a clue to all the factors needed for its occurrence, since they must be present in all places where the disease occurs (May, 1958: p. xxiii).

The end of the 1970s also marked the publication of one of the first formal texts on health geography, *Applied Medical Geography* (Pyle, 1979), which focused on "the unity of a small but expanding systematic discipline."

Today, health and wellness researchers use geographic information systems (GIS) and web-based mapping to expand beyond disease mapping to examine a number of scientific hypotheses, such as disease etiology, equitable access to health services, or the social determinants of health (Khan, 2003). For example, mapping of cancer mortality rates in the US between 1950 and 1969 revealed exceptionally high rates of lung cancer along the eastern seaboard (Blot et al., 1978; Devesa et al., 1999). These patterns led to further investigation where several studies found that exposure to asbestos among employees at shipyards accounted for a significant portion of the excessive mortality from lung cancer (Blot et al., 1978, 1980, 1982).

The contemporary GIS is recognized as a powerful information technology to facilitate convergence of disease-specific information and its analysis in relation to population settlements, surrounding social and health services, and the natural environment (WHO, 2007). GIS can help researchers and planners perform analyses of access to services using proximity measures and network functions (Rushton, 2002), or use spatial interaction models for health planning (Bullen, Moon, and Jones, 1996). For example, GIS can be used to examine residential density, the socio-economic characteristics of neighbourhoods, or the access of different neighbourhoods to health services or wellness-related assets such as recreational facilities. Moreover, GIS allow policy makers to easily visualize problems in

relation to existing health and social services and the natural environment, and therefore effectively target resources (WHO, 2007).

The results of GIS analyses can provide valuable information for assessing population wellness measures. Abstract concepts that may affect wellness but that typically are not recorded by administrative data, such as neighbourhood structure, access to recreational facilities, access to grocery stores to obtain nutritious fruits and vegetables, access to public transit which encourages walking, or environmental health determinants, can be calculated using GIS and incorporated with existing data sources to determine wellness indicators. With the development of powerful yet affordable geo-technologies, digital maps and visual displays can be produced (Khan, 2003). GIS are producing important wellness indicators at finer spatial resolutions, which will allow further exploration of the subjective and objective measures of wellness (Sun, 2005). Mapping the spatial distribution of wellness will also help identify concerns of social justice and provide information on the spatial variation of wellness and the extent, intensity, and distribution of wellness variations (Randall, 2003).

Geographical approaches specific to wellness have been very limited to date, however, a significant amount of geographic research has examined quality of life and happiness (Smith, 1973; Townshend, 2001; Cutter, 1985; Rogerson, Findlay, Morris, and Paddison, 1989a, 1989b; Johnston, 1982). These types of studies typically have focused on situations characterized by low quality of life. In the UK, for example, the continuing decline of inner city areas has been revealed by analyses that showed high concentrations of the unemployed, the low-skilled, the aged, and ethnic minorities accompanied by high levels of overcrowding, amenity deficient housing, and out-migration (Pacione, 1999). Similarly, research in the US has focused on the deteriorating physical structure of the city and quality of life implications (Midgley and Livermore, 1998; Waste, 1998). Whether it is low or high levels of quality of life, geographers view the concepts as a measurement of the conditions of place (Randall and Williams, 2002).

A geographical approach by Pacione (2003) examined the usefulness of measuring quality of life or human well-being in terms of outputs of value to social scientists and policy makers. He used a five-dimensional model in two exemplar case studies: 1) the geography of the quality of life in Glasgow with particular attention to the conditions of the disadvantaged end of the population;

2) the landscapes of fear in the city of Glasgow, again especially in locations identified as disadvantaged. This quality of life study proved useful in a number of ways. It provided:

- some baseline measures to examine trends over time;

- knowledge of how satisfaction and dissatisfaction are distributed through society and across space;

- an understanding of the structure and dependence or interrelationship of various life concerns;

- an understanding of how people combine their feelings of individual life concerns into an overall evaluation of quality of life;

- a better understanding of the causes and conditions which lead to individuals' feelings of well-being, and of the effects of such feelings on behaviour;

- identification of problems meriting special attention and possible societal action;

- identification of normative standards against which actual conditions may be judged in order to inform effective policy formulation;

- monitoring of the effect of policies on the ground; and

- promotion of public participation in the policy-making process.

Canadian Health-Related Mapping

Quality of life is a topic of increasing interest in Canada. The Speech from the Throne of the 36th Parliament was titled "Building a Higher Quality of Life for All Canadians" (Governor General of Canada, 1999). Considering the large geographic extent of Canada, and its diverse communities, a geographic approach to addressing the quality of life of Canadians is important. Recognizing this, a number of organizations in Canada have commenced collecting data on quality of life. For example, the Federation of Canadian Municipalities (FCM) has developed the "FCM Quality of Life Reporting System," which generates annual reports providing evaluations for 18 of the largest municipalities in the country (Federation of Canadian Municipalities, 2001). The Canada Mortgage and Housing Corporation (CMHC) also has promoted several pilot case studies from which a set of quality of life indicators are determined (Canada Mortgage and Housing Corporation, 1996). The objective of such data collection mechanisms is to establish standardized reporting systems to analyse the geographic distribution of quality of life across Canada.

Mapping of quality of life indicators and the use of GIS have played an important role in the development and implementation of initiatives to examine quality of life in Canada and elsewhere. According to Helburn (1982), geographers study quality of life because its "utility value as a policy tool is so tied to place and as such it is a goal of which geographers must be cognizant and to which geographers can make important contributions." Geographically localized communities, such as provinces, cities, neighbourhoods, or census divisions, can serve as the basis for examining physical, social, environmental, and political action with respect to issues that affect quality of life or wellness.

The *Atlas of Canada* (2004) recently produced quality of life maps for Canada. To assess quality of life across Canada, indicators were used to represent what are judged to be the most important aspects of a person's life, which include, for example, education, employment, and household finances. The individual indicators were then categorized into three broad groups: the social environment, economic environment, and physical environment. The indicator data were used to generate three quality of life maps for each environment, and then combined to produce an overall quality of life map for Canada. Census subdivisions were used to georeference the data, since they are the geographic areas that best represent different communities or urban areas across Canada (*Atlas of Canada*, 2004). The goal of the *Atlas of Canada* quality of life initiative was to apply a consistent set of indicators and a common methodology to map broad general patterns in quality of life among communities across Canada. Quality of life was not intended to reflect happiness or overall satisfaction with life; rather, the maps show that some locations in Canada present a higher quality of life than other locations, based solely on these indicators (*Atlas of Canada*, 2004)

The *Atlas of Canada* model was developed from the methodology put forth by Randall (2003), who examined the spatial and temporal variations of quality of life within Saskatoon, Saskatchewan from 1991 to 1996. The model incorporated objective and subjective indicators to measure the social and physical environments that contribute to quality of life, and combined Cutter's (1985) geographical model of quality of life and Myers' (1987) concept of community quality of life. Sun (2005) expanded on Randall's research by examining a methodology to produce geographic quality of life measures at a neighbourhood scale. The results of this study suggest that neighbourhood quality of life indicators may be used to measure specific attributes and the overall status of liveability of neighbourhoods; however, some issues, such as how best to characterize the indicators and how to incorporate subjective measures, were recognized to require further attention.

One of the most impressive arrays of health-related atlases comes from the Institute for Clinical Evaluative Sciences (ICES) in Toronto, which has produced approximately 20 separate atlases on different health-related topics between 1994 and 2006 (ICES, 2007). Mapping techniques provide the first step, or the road map, on the path to understanding health variations in populations. These atlases, as with the BC Atlas of Wellness, do not try to explain differences in spatial patterns of disease processes and the resulting health effects. They simply function as a starting point to raise awareness and to frame questions. Answers to these questions, among other explanations, lie in the many risk factors associated with health patterns, including the psychological/social environment, the physical environment, the biological endowment, the economic environment, individual responses, health status and function, and the health care system. The Canadian Institute for Advanced Research (1991), Hayes, Foster, and Foster (1994), and the Canadian Population Health Initiative (Canadian Institute for Health Information, 2004, 2005, 2006a) describe some of these factors, the social gradients in health status, and the resulting impacts on population health. Statistics Canada also has developed a series of reports comparing various quality of life and wellness and health indicators among the key Census Metropolitan Areas based on the 2001 census and other data. More recently, the Canadian Population Health Initiative (CPHI) also has published a major report on place and health (Canadian Institute for Health Information, 2006b). The analysis and understanding of the effects of these factors on population health have been enhanced through the use of mapping techniques and the production of atlases.

Health Mapping in BC

In BC, health mapping has been used in the Provincial Health Officer's Annual Report of 1992 (Millar, 1993) and at the Division of Vital Statistics since 1988 through Annual Reports, Quarterly Digests, and Feature Reports (Danderfer and Foster, 1993; Danderfer and Cronin, 1994, 1995; Foster, Burr, and Mohamed, 1994). Over the past 15 years, health-related atlases and publications have become important in representing data geographically within the province. For example, the first mortality atlas was published in 1992 (Foster and Edgell,

1992), and a health map supplement showing a variety of health-related indicators, including demographics, standardized morbidity rates by gender, maternal and child health rates, immunization, and health care system utilization rates at the Local Health Area level, was published by the Ministry of Health (Nicholls, Ho, and Foster, 1993). Later, this was supplemented by comprehensive health atlases presented by the Centre for Health Services and Policy Research (CHSPR) at the University of British Columbia (McGrail, Schaub, and Black, 2004; McGrail and Schaub, 2002; Watson, Kreuger, Mooney, and Black, 2005; CHSPR, nd). In addition, maps and atlases related to early child development and health have been produced through the Human Early Learning Partnership (HELP) at the University of British Columbia (Hertzman, McLean, Kohen, Dunn, and Evans, 2002; Kershaw et al., 2005; HELP, 2005), and maps have been developed for selected youth health and development indicators (Foster, 2005). An online updated mortality atlas was published in 2006 (www.geog.uvic.ca/mortality), and this has been followed by the BC Atlas of Youth Health and Behaviour (Foster and McKee, 2007). British Columbia Statistics today has an impressive array of indicators that have been mapped and are readily available for downloading. Of particular note is the set of maps that show a series of hardship indicators at several geographical administrative levels (BC Stats, 2007).

Goals of the Atlas: Why Wellness?

The vast majority of the mapping initiatives noted above focus on mapping what is "bad" rather than what is "good," "deficits" rather than "assets," "mortality" rather than "life," and "illness" rather than "wellness." In other words, mapping exercises to date have tended to focus on the negative rather than to accentuate the positive. This is not meant as criticism. Obviously, focusing on problem areas and issues helps get public, political, and management attention so that improvements can be achieved. However, sometimes it may be beneficial to report conditions by placing a focus on the positive.

What we provide in this BC Atlas of Wellness, and to our knowledge this is the first comprehensive atlas of its kind, is a unique focus on the positive rather than the negative. Over 120 indicators are used to build a picture of wellness within BC. We take the optimist's half-full approach rather than the pessimist's half-empty approach, which, as noted above, has been the usual strategy taken in health mapping to date. Instead of mapping illness, we map wellness, or assets that can help determine, maintain, and improve wellness at the population level within the province. Instead of mapping obesity, we map healthy weights; instead of mapping smoking rates, we map smoke-free rates; instead of mapping low birth weight we map healthy birth weight; instead of mapping infant mortality we map infant survival, and many more such indicators.

We noted earlier that researchers have discovered that maps and atlases often are used by readers to compare their own neighbourhood to others (Keller, 1995). In health mapping, the tradition is to compare oneself using maps that communicate degrees of something wrong. This atlas instead facilitates comparison by focusing on what is right, and hopefully what can be learned by others from this.

The conditions we have selected to show are all assets for wellness, just as obesity or smoking or low birth weight are risk factors for illness, poor development, and premature mortality. Focusing on wellness indicators and those areas that achieve high values on particular wellness assets can help provide some understanding of what is achievable for those areas and communities that feel they need to make improvements. The best values can become benchmarks for others to achieve as these values have been attained by a relatively large segment of the population in the province. And the ones who are doing best can strive to do even better, thus raising the wellness bar. One area can learn from another area in terms of what works, and adopt some of the strategies used by the communities who demonstrate high levels of "wellness" (Foster, Burr, and Mohamed, 1992, 1994). Communities can also evaluate which of the indicators that we provide in the Atlas are important ones to them and decide whether to focus on improving them over time.

Some may question the wisdom of this wellness approach as it could lead to the conclusion that all is "well" in the province, thus potentially undermining the need to focus attention on problem issues. This is clearly not our intent. A quick glance at many of the maps and tables will show that there are major "gradients" or differences in wellness between various areas in the province and between different groups within the province. There are certainly areas that need improvement, and can be improved. Studying the areas that appear to be the "best" on a particular wellness indicator may assist others to try to emulate their results by finding out what they are doing "right" to achieve these results. These areas will become clear when using the Atlas.

The following chapter presents a review of the key academic literature that has been written over the past few years on the topic of wellness. How is it defined? What are its dimensions? How can it be measured? This, in turn, is followed by a summary of the key determinants of health and wellness and these two sections provide the basis for the indicators that are mapped and discussed later in this Atlas.

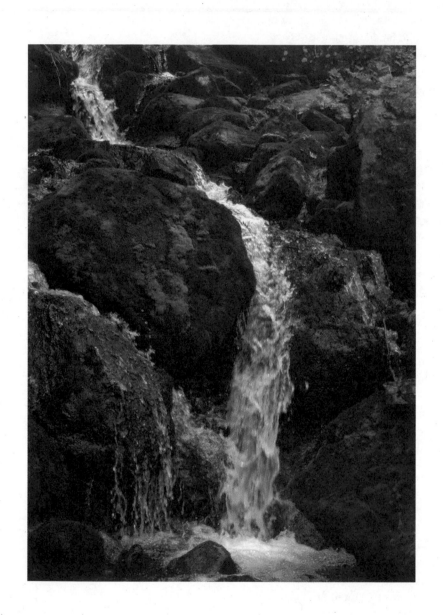

2

Defining Wellness and Its Determinants

Introduction

Wellness is not an easy concept to define. The term
is used in everyday language with an assumption that
everyone knows what it means. Many have made
attempts to define wellness. The first part of this
chapter looks at wellness from a holistic perspective.
It summarizes definitions and conceptualizations of
wellness within the literature of the past 30 years
and looks at the major comprehensive studies to
identify dimensions of wellness. It is based largely
on a discussion paper produced as a background
document for this Atlas. This was based on an extensive
review of the wellness literature, involving online
database keyword searches, screening of abstracts,
and assessing the relevance of articles. Over 200
journal articles, books, and websites were examined
to determine how wellness was defined, and to locate
research and wellness models to support the *BC Atlas
of Wellness* (Miller, 2007). The second section of the
chapter focuses on the importance of the determinants
of population health and wellness. This approach to
considering factors that are important to understanding
health and wellness status has become very prominent
over the past 15 years or so, and is an important way of
considering health and wellness from a perspective that
is more community- or population-based. These two
approaches to assessing the dimensions of health and
wellness provide a basis for understanding the reasons
for the inclusion of many of the mapped indicators that
appear in the later sections of this Atlas.

Wellness from a Holistic Perspective

Holism emerged from the approach used by scientists
to study complex phenomena such as organisms and
ecosystems (Richards and Bergin, 1997), and from a
shift in society toward a worldview that is more holistic
and relational (Larson, 1999). The term wellness
appeared as part of a parallel transformation in the
definition of health toward a more holistic perspective
that is interrelational, positive in nature, and focuses on
the examination of healthy human functioning (Westgate,
1996). Previous definitions held the view that health was
concerned with illness and the body was considered
in terms of isolated physiological systems (McSherry
and Draper, 1998). The holistic perspective completely
transformed this notion of health and the wellness
movement was perhaps the catalyst that began
this transformation.

The wellness movement began after the end of World
War II largely because society's health needs changed.
Advances in medicines and technology meant vaccines
and antibiotics reduced the threat of infectious diseases,
which until that time had been the leading cause
of death (Seaward, 1997, 2002). Instead, chronic
and lifestyle illnesses (e.g., heart disease, diabetes,
cancer), associated with numerous stressors in life and
the workplace, became the primary health concern.
This introduced an expanded concept of health as
encompassing all aspects of the person (mind, body,
spirit) (Donatelle, Snow, and Wilcox, 1999), a concept
that had been lost by western but not by indigenous
societies (Elliott and Foster, 1995).

This expanded view of health allowed the development
of preventive health measures and a focus on optimal
health as practitioners address the whole person,
and consider the causes of lifestyle illnesses rather
than just their symptoms. But the language used to
describe health and, similarly, wellness has become
more complex and confusing. Current literature reveals
additional terms corresponding and interrelating to the
notion of wellness, namely well-being, quality of life, life

satisfaction, happiness, and general satisfaction, the latter being a term similarly understood by many cultures and used in international studies.

Conceptualizing Wellness

Several authors have attempted to define and filter out major concepts around the meaning of wellness (Table 1). It has been argued that wellness is subjective, inherently has a value judgement about what it is and what it is not, and that an accurate definition and measurement of the construct is difficult (Kelly, 2000; Sarason, 2000). Therefore, authors have conceptualized wellness on a continuum and not as an end state (Clark, 1996; Dunn, 1977; Jonas, 2005; Lafferty, 1979; Lorion, 2000; Myers, Sweeney, and Witmer, 2005; Sackney, Noonan, and Miller, 2000; Sarason, 2000).

Larson (1999, p. 123) states that the World Health Organization (WHO) was the first to introduce a holistic definition of health as "a state of complete physical, mental, and social well-being and not merely the absence of disease and infirmity" (1948), and many subsequent conceptualizations of wellness include this central concept. The President's Council on Physical Fitness and Sport for the US has been very involved in defining wellness, and Oliphant (2001) explains that the suggestion by WHO (1967) that health has a positive component led to the now widely used term "wellness."

Dunn (1977) emphasized wellness as a positive state, one that is beyond simply non-sickness, elaborating on the WHO definition by emphasizing the varying degrees of wellness and its interrelated, ever-changing aspects.

He detailed the interconnected nature of wellness of the mind, body, and environment, which exists as a dynamic equilibrium as one tries to balance between each. Dunn (1977) conceptualized the dimensions of wellness fluctuating as people make active choices moving toward or away from their maximum potential.

Egbert (1980) summarized the central areas of wellness as being a combination of having a strong sense of identity, a reality-oriented perspective, a clear purpose in life, the recognition of a unifying force in one's life, the ability to manage one's affairs creatively and maintain a hopeful view, and the capability of inspired, open relationships. WHO (1986, p. 2) further clarified the definition, noting that to reach a state of health "an individual or a group must be able to realize aspirations and satisfy needs, and to change or cope with the environment," while Bouchard and colleagues (1994, p. 23) suggest that "positive health pertains to the capacity to enjoy life and withstand challenges." Lastly, Witmer and Sweeney (1992) defined wellness in terms of life tasks that include self-regulation, work, friendship, spirituality, and love.

Many researchers have explored and defined the various components, or interrelated areas, that comprise wellness. Depken (1994) noted that most college health textbooks describe wellness as encompassing physical, psychological/emotional, social, intellectual, and spiritual dimensions. Lafferty (1979) defined wellness as a balanced amalgamation of these five factors and purposeful direction within the environment. Similarly, Greenberg (1985) defined wellness as the integration of the five dimensions and high-level wellness as the balance among them, but utilized the term mental

Table 1: Dimensions of wellness

	Physical	Emotional Psychological	Social	Intellectual	Spiritual	Occupational	Environmental
Adams et al., 1997	x	x	x	x	x	x	
Anspaugh et al., 2004	x	x	x	x	x	x	x
Crose et al., 1992	x	x	x	x	x	x	
Durlak, 2000	x		x	x			
Hales, 2005	x	x	x	x	x	x	x
Helliwell, 2005	x	x	x		x	x	x
Hettler, 1980	x	x	x	x	x		
Leafgren, 1990	x	x	x	x	x	x	
Renger et al., 2000	x	x	x	x	x		x
Ryan and Deci, 2001	x	x					x
Ryff and Singer, 2006	x	x	x				x

wellness in place of intellectual wellness. Hettler (1980) included an occupational dimension and stressed wellness as the process of becoming aware of wellness and actively making choices towards optimal living.

Towards the end of the last millennium, Adams, Benzer, and Steinhardt (1997) conceptualized wellness from a systems approach, where all subsystems have their own elements and are an essential part of the larger system. The authors described wellness as health-focused, and emphasized the importance of including multiple factors such as cultural, social, and environmental influences from a systems perspective. They included the additional dimension of psychological wellness relating to positive outcomes in response to life's circumstances.

An emphasis on an "integrated and positive spiral of mind-body influences" has been suggested by Ryff and Singer (1998, p. 14). They contend that "zestful engagement in living and loving…remains primarily the purview of philosophy." They indicate that perceptions, beliefs, and cognitions are clearly linked to their physiological responses to the world. They state that well-being obviously includes good mental health, but emotional health does not have to be linked to physiological substrates to be beneficial. The two authors offer a reasonable list of contributing factors gathered from a range of sources, and these health constituents include social support, dispositional optimism, relationship quality, leading a life of purpose, achieving mastery, and possessing positive self regard.

Renger and co-authors (2000) defined wellness as consisting of physical, emotional, social, intellectual, and spiritual dimensions, and added environmental wellness to recognize the important impact of one's surroundings, a concept also discussed by Sackney, Noonan, and Miller (2000). Renger and co-workers stressed the importance of knowledge, attitude, perception, behaviour, and skill in each of several wellness areas, as well as integration and balance.

Adams (2003) has defined four main principles of wellness: 1) wellness is multi-dimensional; 2) wellness research and practice should be oriented toward identifying causes of wellness rather than causes of illness; 3) wellness is about balance; and 4) wellness is relative, subjective, and perceptual. Schuster and colleagues (2004, p. 351) state there is general consensus that definitions of health include multiple domains, among them physical, psychological (mental, intellectual, emotional), social, and spiritual. Wellness is described as "a higher order construct integrating these domains, drawing on individual self-perception."

Myers, Sweeney, and Wittmer (2005, p. 252) define wellness as being "a way of life oriented toward optimal health and well-being in which the body, mind, and spirit are integrated by the individual to live more fully within the human and natural community." The notion that wellness is more a psychological than a physical state has been a focus of several researchers. Anspaugh and co-authors (2004) and Hales (2005) refer to seven dimensions of wellness: physical, emotional, social, intellectual, spiritual, environmental, and occupational.

Jonas (2005, p. 2) elaborates on the difference between health and wellness, saying that health is a state of being, whereas wellness is a process of being. Wellness is defined as:

> a way of life and living in which one is always exploring, searching, finding new questions and discovering new answers, along the three primary dimensions of living: the physical, the mental, and the social; a way of life designed to enable each of us to achieve, in each of the dimensions, our maximum potential that is realistically and rationally feasible for us at any given time in our lives.

Rickhi and Aung (2006) believe creating wellness can mean focusing on practices that benefit one or all of the three dimensions—body, mind, and spirit. Physical wellness includes drinking water, healthy eating, healthful touch such as massage, and physical activity. Mental and spiritual wellness requires mind/body-based stress reduction programs, adapting the body to nature and being aware of the senses.

Recently, Smith and Kelly (2006) have suggested that lack of community may be spurring wellness tourists to seek a sense of community within a holistic centre, a yoga retreat, at a New Age festival, or on a pilgrimage.

Dimensions of Wellness

The above summary of key researchers indicates that there are several main dimensions to defining wellness: physical; psychological/emotional; social; intellectual; spiritual; occupational; and environmental. These are briefly discussed further, below.

Physical Wellness

In general, physical wellness includes physical activity, nutrition, and self-care, and involves preventative and proactive actions that take care of one's physical body. Cooper (1968, 1970, 1975, 1977) studied the relationship of exercise to health and longevity, particularly how exercise reduced the risk of heart disease. His findings revolutionized the fitness industry's understanding of health and wellness and advanced the understanding of the relationship between living habits and health.

Physical wellness encompasses maintenance of cardiovascular fitness, flexibility, and strength. Actions to improve physical wellness include maintaining a healthy diet and becoming in tune with how the body responds to various events, stress, and feelings by monitoring internal and external physical signs. This includes seeking medical care when appropriate, and taking action to prevent and avoid harmful behaviours (e.g., tobacco use and excess alcohol consumption) and detect illnesses (Hettler, 1980; Renger et al., 2000; Leafgren, 1990). Crose and co-workers (1992) included medical history and medications, body awareness, and image. Durlak (2000) and Anspaugh and colleagues (2004) detailed physical wellness to include physical indices (muscle tone, cholesterol level, blood pressure) and behaviours (eating habits, exercise levels). Problems in physical wellness included physical injuries and disabilities, and sexually transmitted diseases.

Helliwell (2005) found optimism about good health resulted in higher wellness scores. He also found that age was of great interest because one might assume happiness decreases with age, whereas in fact 18- to 24-year-olds and 55- to 64-year-olds are equally the happiest of all age groups, with 35- to 44-year-olds being the least happy. Even 65 year olds and above were a lot happier than this 35- to 44-year-old cohort.

Ryff and Singer (2006) found that avoiding negative behaviours such as smoking and inactive living, as well as body type, affects physical wellness, with benefits including better autoimmune functioning. Ryan and Deci (2001) note that physical wellness, however, does not always correlate to one's sense of well-being: a person can be ill and have a positive state of mind, while a physically healthy person can experience a poor sense of well-being.

Psychological/Emotional Wellness

Relatively few discuss psychological wellness, but there is some agreement that it is one's sense of expectation that positive outcomes result from the events and experiences of life. Emotional wellness is conceptualized as awareness and control of feelings, as well as a realistic, positive, and developmental view of the self, conflict, and life circumstances, coping with

stress, and the maintenance of fulfilling relationships with others (Adams, Bezner, and Steinhardt, 1997; Leafgren, 1990). Hettler (1980) considered emotional wellness to be a continual process that included an awareness and management of feelings, and a positive view of self, the world, and relationships.

Renger and co-workers (2000) defined emotional wellness as related to one's level of depression, anxiety, well-being, self-control, and optimism. Emotional wellness includes experiencing satisfaction, curiosity, and enjoyment in life, as well as having a positive anticipation of the future, or optimistic outlook. Ryan and Deci (2001) describe the self-determination theory (SDT) as another perspective that fits within the concept of self-realization as a central definitional aspect of wellness, and that SDT specifies both what it means to actualize the self and how this can be accomplished. This involves the fulfillment of basic psychological needs: autonomy, competence, and relatedness resulting in psychological growth (e.g., intrinsic motivation); integrity (e.g., internalization and assimilation of cultural practices); and well-being (e.g., life satisfaction and psychological health); as well as the experiences of vitality (Ryan and Frederick, 1997) and self-congruence (Sheldon and Elliot, 1999). Ryff and Singer (2006) indicate that quality ties to others are central to optimal living and are connected to psychological factors. Self-actualizers have strong feelings of empathy and affection for all human beings and have a greater capacity for love and deep friendships and more complete self-identification with others than non-actualizers. This, they indicate, develops with maturity.

Personality is one of the strongest indicators of well-being (Diener, Eunkook, Suh, Lucas, and Smith, 1999), with genes accounting for 40% of positive emotionality and 55% of negative emotionality. Features of the environment, one's behaviour, and one's personality may mutually influence each other and affect subjective well-being. According to Harrington and Loffredo (2001), personality aspects of individuals may affect life satisfaction, citing people who are more self-conscious and introverted scoring lower levels of life satisfaction than extroverts. The discussion of extroversion demonstrates varying results, with Diener and colleagues (1999) suggesting that social involvement is required by the demands of society and extroverts are more comfortable in social situations. Pavot and co-authors (1990) found that extroverts were happier in all situations, whether social or in isolation. Diener and co-workers (1999) proposed an intriguing idea that the characteristics of extroverts are actually an outcome of higher levels of positive affect. DeNeve and Cooper (1998) quote Wilson (1967) as stating that a happy individual is one who is extroverted, optimistic, and worry-free.

Longitudinal studies (Sheldon and Kasser, 1998, p. 1322) suggest that, "whereas progress toward intrinsic goals enhances wellness, progress toward extrinsic goals such as money either does not enhance wellness or does so to a lesser extent." Ryan and Deci (2001, p. 154) summarize reviews of the literature on the topic of wealth and happiness by stating that: "The relation of wealth to well-being is at best a low positive one, although it is clear that material supports can enhance access to resources that are important for happiness and self-realization. There appear to be many risks to poverty but few benefits to wealth when it comes to well-being." In addition, studies show that valuing wealth and material goods above intrinsic self-realizational goals adversely affects psychological wellness.

Hales (2005) includes trust, self-esteem, self-acceptance, self-confidence, self-control, and the ability to bounce back from setbacks and failures as important wellness attributes. Maintaining emotional wellness requires monitoring and exploring thoughts or feelings, identifying obstacles to emotional well-being, and finding solutions to emotional problems, if necessary with the help of a therapist.

Social Wellness

Social wellness encompasses the degree and quality of interactions with others, the community, and nature. It includes the extent to which a person works toward supporting the community and environment in everyday actions, such as volunteer work (Hettler, 1980). Included in the definition of social wellness is getting along with others and being comfortable and willing to express one's feelings, needs, and opinions; supportive, fulfilling relationships (including sexual relations), and intimacy; and interaction with the social environment and contribution to one's community (Renger et al., 2000). Leafgren (1990) and Crose and colleagues (1992) confirm the importance of significant relationships and the quality and extent of one's social network. Crose and colleagues (1992) examine the nature of relational styles and patterns, focusing on one's attitude toward relationships and seeking help from others as key to social wellness. Ryff and Singer (2006) cite epidemiological studies stating that mortality is

significantly lower among persons who are more socially integrated. Features of social support consist of the size or density of one's social network and frequency of contact with relatives and friends.

Durlak (2000) includes peer acceptance, attachments/bonds with others, and social skills (communication, assertiveness, conflict resolution) as fundamental to social wellness. Helliwell (2005) found that married people are happier, and separated individuals are the least happy, even less so than those who are divorced. Anspaugh and colleagues (2004) also include the ability to maintain intimacy, to accept others different from yourself, and to cultivate a support network of caring friends and/or family members.

Intellectual Wellness

Intellectual wellness is the degree to which one engages in creative and stimulating activities, as well as the use of resources to expand knowledge and focus on the acquisition, development, application, and articulation of critical thinking. It represents a commitment to life-long learning, an effort to share knowledge with others, and development of skills and abilities to achieve a more satisfying life (Hettler, 1980). The perception of being energized by an optimal amount of intellectually stimulating activity that involves critical reasoning is also important (Adams et al., 1997). Hales (2005) concurs and includes having a sense of humour as important.

Awareness of cultural events is viewed by numerous authors as central to intellectual wellness (Crose, Nicholas, Gobble, and Frank, 1992; Leafgren, 1990; Renger et al., 2000). Renger and co-authors (2000) also defined intellectual wellness as one's orientation and attitude toward personal growth, education, achievement, and creativity. This includes attending cultural events and seeking out opportunities to gain and share knowledge, particularly knowledge of current local and world events.

In addition to attending cultural events, Leafgren (1990) cites that stimulation can come from reading, studying, travelling, and exposure to media. Crose and colleagues (1992) defined intellectual wellness as one's education and learning history, mental status, cognitive style and flexibility, and attitude toward learning. Durlak (2000) includes the development of talents and abilities, learning how to learn, and higher order thinking skills in intellectual wellness. Furthermore, he defined the problem areas as underachievement, test anxiety, and school dropouts.

Spiritual Wellness

Spiritual wellness is possibly the most developed and discussed topic in the wellness literature (Banks, 1980; Hatch, Burg, Naberhaus, and Hellmich, 1998; Ingersoll, 1994; Pargament, 1999). Spirituality is not synonymous with religion (Adams et al., 1997). Rather, religiosity and spirituality are overlapping but distinct concepts (Westgate, 1996). Spirituality can be considered to be the broader concepts of beliefs and values, whereas religiosity can be thought of as behaviours and the means of implementing one's spirituality (Westgate, 1996; Hatch et al., 1998), although Pargament (1999) has challenged this viewpoint and argued that religiosity is the broader concept.

Hettler (1980) and others (Adams et al., 1997; Renger et al., 2000) defined spiritual wellness as the process of seeking meaning and purpose in existence. It includes the appreciation of the depth and expanse of life and the universe, questioning the meaning and purpose in life, as well as recognizing, accepting, and tolerating the complex nature of the world and accepting that the universe cannot be completely understood. Hettler (1980) adds that spiritual wellness is focused on harmony with the self, and with others and the universe, and the search for a universal value system. This value system includes the formation of a worldview that gives unity, purpose, and goals to thoughts and actions.

Applying an adaptation of the Delphi Technique to define spiritual wellness, Banks (1980) cited the following key elements: gives meaning or purpose to life, principles or ethics to live by, sense of selflessness, and feeling for others. Other important elements include: a commitment to God or ultimate being, perception of what it is that makes the universe operate as it does, recognition of powers beyond the natural and rational, a matter of faith in the unknown, involving a survival issue, and finally a pleasure-producing quality of humans.

Ingersoll (1994) initially defined spiritual wellness in terms of seven integrated dimensions that operate synergistically, but later proposed the following 10 dimensions: conception of the absolute or divine; meaning (life meaning, purpose, and sense of peace); connectedness (with people, higher power, community, and environment); mystery (how one deals with ambiguity, the unexplained, and uncertainty); sense of freedom (play, seeing the world as safe, willingness to commit); experience/ritual/practice; forgiveness; hope; knowledge/learning; and present centredness.

Westgate (1996) defined spiritual wellness in terms of holistic dimensions, proposing four spiritual wellness dimensions: meaning in life, intrinsic values, transcendence, and spiritual community. The meaning in life dimension was described as an innate human need where purpose and life satisfaction provide hope. Intrinsic values were defined as the basis of human behaviour and the principles that people live by. Transcendence signifies a relationship with a higher force and the universe, recognition of the sacredness of life, and motivation by truth, beauty, and unity. Lastly, the fourth dimension of spiritual community was defined as giving and sharing with others, shared values, myths and symbols, and the experience of community and mutual support through gathering, singing, praying, and chanting. To some extent, Hales (2005) reflects a similar view of spiritual wellness.

As noted earlier, Helliwell (2005) found age a factor in well-being, with 18- to 24-year-olds and 55 and older equally happiest of all ages. There has been some debate as to whether the higher value in the older age group is related to faith, since those who believe God is important in their lives are happier than those who don't.

Occupational Wellness

Hettler (1980) and Anspaugh and colleagues (2004) defined occupational wellness as the level of satisfaction and enrichment gained by one's work and the extent one's occupation allows for the expression of values. Furthermore, occupational wellness included the contribution of one's unique skills and talents to the community in rewarding, meaningful ways through paid and unpaid work. Lastly, occupational wellness incorporated the balance between occupational and other commitments.

Leafgren (1990) stated that occupational wellness is one's attitude about work and the amount of personal satisfaction and enrichment gained from work, while Crose and co-workers (1992) included work history, patterns and balance between vocational and leisure activities, and vocational goals. Helliwell (2005) found large reductions in well-being from being unemployed.

Environmental Wellness

In their definition of environmental wellness, Renger and co-authors (2000) include the balance between home and work life, as well as the individual's relationship with nature and community resources (i.e., involvement in a recycling or community clean-up effort). Ryan and Deci (2001) found cultural differences when looking at wellness across 61 nations, suggesting that the cultural environment is an important factor. Anspaugh and colleagues (2004) and Hales (2005) further express concerns such as safety of food and water supply, infectious diseases, violence in society, ultraviolet radiation, air and water pollution, and second-hand tobacco smoke.

Ryff and Singer (2006) describe environmental mastery as a dimension of wellness and state that, to make the most of our lives and our world, we need to advance the science of interpersonal flourishing (p. 41).

Studying political and government structures, Helliwell (2005, p. 4) looks at the social capital of environments from a global perspective and proposes that:

> Analysis of well-being (wellness) data provides means for combining income, employment, government effectiveness, family structure and social relations together in ways that permit the external effects of institutions and policies to be assessed.

An international study of about 50 different countries was conducted by Helliwell (2005) utilizing data from three waves of the World Values survey (Annas, 1993). Increased income inequality is associated with lower rates of economic growth (Persson and Tabellini, 1994) and worse health. Individuals attaching high subjective values to financial success have lower values for subjective well-being, even when their financial aspirations are met (Kasser and Ryan, 1993, 1996). Higher levels of subjective well-being occur not in the richest countries, but in those where social and political institutions are effective, mutual trust is high, and corruption is low.

Summary of Wellness Definitions and Dimensions

In summarizing the various conceptualizations of wellness, many of the models and definitions are based upon similar core elements. First, most authors incorporated the idea that wellness is not just absence of illness, as first outlined by the WHO wellness definition. Second, wellness is described in terms of various factors that interact in a complex, integrated, and synergistic fashion, and the dynamic interaction of the dimensions causes the sum of the dimensions to be greater than the whole. Each dimension is integral to the whole and no one dimension operates independently. The

wellness approach is holistic within the person and with the environment. Third, many authors outlined the necessity of balance or dynamic equilibrium among dimensions. Fourth, several models define wellness as the movement toward higher levels of wellness or optimal functioning and assert that wellness is, therefore, partially dependent on self-responsibility and individual motivation. Finally, wellness is viewed on a continuum, not as an end state.

Several key dimensions of wellness have emerged. Physical wellness is the active and continuous effort to maintain the optimum level of physical activity and focus on nutrition, and includes self-care and healthy lifestyle choices (e.g., use of medical services, preventative health measures, abstinence from drugs, tobacco, and excessive alcohol use, safe sex practices).

Emotional wellness includes one's attitudes and beliefs toward self and life. Definitions include a positive and realistic self-concept, identity, and degree of self-esteem, and the awareness and constructive handling of feelings. It might also include the core elements of self-view and awareness of one's actions, feelings, relationships and their management, the realistic assessment of one's limitations, and a developmental focus. It is the ability to act autonomously, cope with stress, as well as to have a positive attitude about life, oneself, and the future.

Social wellness is broad in scope because it includes the interaction of the individual with others, the community, and nature. It includes the interaction (quality and extent) with, and support of, others, the community, and the social and natural environment. Besides the interaction of the individual, society, and nature, social wellness includes the motivation, action, intent, and perception of interactions. Social wellness is comprised of the skills and comfort level one is able to express in the context of interacting with others, the community, and nature. In sum, social wellness is the movement toward balance, and integration of the interaction between the individual, society, and nature.

Intellectual wellness is the perception of, and motivation for, one's optimal level of stimulating intellectual activity by the continual acquisition, use, sharing, and application of knowledge in a creative and critical fashion. This is for both personal growth of the individual and the betterment of society.

The key aspects of spiritual wellness seem to be purpose and meaning in life; the self in relation to others, the community, nature, the universe, and some higher power; shared community and experience; and the creation of personal values and beliefs. In summary, spiritual wellness is the innate and continual process of finding meaning and purpose in life, while accepting and transcending one's place in the complex and interrelated universe. Spiritual wellness is a shared connection or community with others, nature, the universe, and a higher power.

Occupational wellness is the extent to which one can express values and gain personal satisfaction and enrichment from paid and non-paid work; one's attitude toward work and ability to balance several roles; and the ways in which one can use one's skills and abilities to contribute to the community.

Finally, environmental wellness has a broad dimension that considers the nature of an individual's reciprocal interaction with the environment on a global level (e.g., balance, impact, control). The environment includes home, work, community, and nature.

Measuring Wellness

While there is extensive literature on the definition of wellness, there are relatively few empirical explorations of the structure of wellness. Several authors have commented on the difficulty of capturing the dynamic nature of wellness and the inadequacy of the existing measures (Adams et al., 1997; Renger et al., 2000). However, several techniques have been developed to measure wellness at an individual level. These include the Life Assessment Questionnaire (LAQ) (National Wellness Institute, 1983), developed to measure the six wellness dimensions outlined by Hettler (1980), and a modification called TestWell (Owen, 1999); the Perceived Wellness Survey (PWS) (Adams et al., 1997); the Optimal Living Profile (OLP) (Renger et al., 2000); and a Wellness Inventory (WI), developed by Travis (1981), to mention a few.

There are also several scales developed to assess spiritual wellness and well-being. These include: the Spiritual Well-Being Scale (SWBS) by Paloutzian and Ellison (1982); the Spiritual Involvement and Beliefs Scale (SIBS) (Hatch et al., 1998); the Duke Religion Index (DUREL) (Koenig, Parkerson, and Meador, 1997); the Intrinsic Religious Motivation Scale (Hoge, 1972); the Spiritual Well-Being Questionnaire (SWBQ) (Moberg, 1984); and the Expressions of Spirituality Inventory (ESI) (MacDonald, 2000).

Other researchers have conducted large-scale studies using a variety of wellness-related instruments. Mookerjee and Beron (2005) examined the influence of gender and religion on levels of happiness in 60 industrialized and developing nations using two sources of information: 1) The World Database of Happiness (Veerhoven, 2001); and 2) quality of life measuring tools including the Human Development Index, the Gastil Index of Civil Liberty, the Index of Economic Freedom, the Gini Coefficient of Income Inequality, and the Corruption Perception Index.

The urban planning field is evaluated through a set of visions rather than empirically supported theories, since consumers find it difficult to imagine what plans will look like and usually shy away from innovative ideas. Van Kamp and co-authors (2003) describe a review of urban planning visions by Smith and colleagues (1997) in terms of quality and need principles. Important elements include livability, character, connection, mobility, personal freedom, and diversity. On the basis of this physical form, criteria were developed with respect to community quality (i.e., open space areas, outdoor amenities, and 'walkability'). Van Kamp and co-authors (2003) found a need for the development of a conceptual framework that evaluates physical, spatial, and social indicators of well-being in terms of urban environmental quality, livability, sustainability, and quality of life. Both environmental quality and quality of life relate to the person, the environment, and the relationship between the two. Three approaches are used: 1) the economical; 2) the sociological (normative); and 3) the psychological (subjective). Van Kamp found authors whose studies report meaningful relationships between crowding and behaviour, housing quality and functioning of children, and the amount of green in the neighbourhood and coping behaviour (Evans, Saegert, and Harris, 2001; Moser and Corroyer, 2001; Kuo, 2001).

Ardell and Jonas (2005) have developed the Wellness Process for Healthy Living (WPHL), which is a tool for implementing the wellness concept. The five steps of the WPHL are: 1) assessment—both self-assessment and assessment by health practitioners; 2) defining success; 3) goal setting; 4) establishing priorities; and 5) mobilizing motivation. These steps provide a single common mental pathway for preparing to successfully make health-promoting behaviour change. It is necessary to be at a point of wanting to make a change before change can be made. A variety of tools can be used to measure Quality of Life (QOL), subjective well-being, and wellness. Skevington and co-workers (2004) analysed the WHOQOL-BREF, a 26-item version of the WHOQOL-100 assessment, as a valid assessment tool. This tool came from 10 years of development research on QOL and was tested in 24 countries and available in most of the world's major languages. Sick and well respondents were sampled and the self-assessment completed, as well as socio-demographic and health status questions.

Of interest within Canada, Ekos Research Associates (2006) are devising the Canadian Index of Well-being (CIW), which will be used to account for changes in Canadian human, social, economic, and natural wealth by capturing the full range of factors that affect Canadians' well-being. The CIW encompasses seven domains that are at different stages of development, including: Living Standards, Healthy Populations, Time Allocation, Educated Populace, Ecosystem Health, Community Vitality, and Good Governance (Civic Engagement). The Atkinson Charitable Foundation, with the support of the United Way of Canada and their local agencies, as well as CIW project partners at local and national levels, consulted to find out if these seven domains capture what really matters to Canadians. The participants described the CIW as "an excellent and timely idea and a needed alternative to traditional economically based ways of measuring progress" (Ekos Research Associates 2006, p. 3).

Determinants of Health and Wellness

The influence of social factors on health outcomes has been observed since vital statistics were routinely collected in Britain more than 150 years ago. At that time, average age at death was demonstrated to be systematically associated both with occupation (unskilled labourers had a much lower average age at death than skilled labourers, whose average, in turn, was lower than the administrative occupations) and region (with counties in the north of England having a lower average age at death than those in the south) in a socially graded fashion. Interestingly, these patterns persist in England today, although occupational classifications have changed dramatically since then (Gregory, Dorling, and Southall, 2001).

In 1977, the government of the United Kingdom appointed an expert group, chaired by Sir Douglas Black, to examine the distribution of health outcomes in the UK after nearly 40 years of the National Health Service (NHS). The Black Report (Townsend and Davidson, 1982) analysed health outcomes by occupational classification for males and females across the full spectrum of age groups of 5 and 10 year intervals across the life span. Mortality (death), morbidity (chronic and short-term illnesses), and activity limitation (physical

consequences of poor health) were measured for general and disease-specific causes. The report found that relative differences in health outcomes by occupation had actually increased over the nearly 40 years of public health care, and reflected a social gradient. The Report offered four possible explanations for the observed patterns: reverse causality (people who are sicker or more likely to die are less able to acquire the skills needed for higher occupational status jobs); artifact (the size of occupational groups have changed, leaving behind the most difficult cases); lifestyle (lower occupational groups make poorer health choices); and social structural and material factors (groups are systematically exposed to greater hazards in the environment—higher risk, fewer choices, and fewer resources—and the cumulative effect of these combined factors causes premature 'weathering' or wearing-out of the body). The Report gave greatest weight to the last explanation, but acknowledged that lifestyle or personal health practices were also involved. It found little evidence to support reverse causality or artifact explanations. Though all groups had experienced improvements in health outcomes, rates of improvement experienced by the higher status occupational groups (those associated with higher incomes and greater prestige) were faster than those experienced by lower status groups, so relative differences increased.

The Black Report stimulated several questions about the role of social circumstance in shaping health and wellness outcomes that galvanized international research and policy interest. Since the release of the Report, health and wellness outcomes have been observed to follow a social gradient practically everywhere the distribution of outcomes from a population health perspective has been studied. Several explanations have been offered to account for observed gradients, including materialist, psycho-social, and eco-social perspectives. While there are subtle differences between these explanations, they all have a great deal in common. Most pronounced is the shared view that our bodies respond to environmental influences, especially those emanating from our social relationships, although obviously exposure to non-social environmental factors such as UV radiation, particulate matter, noxious gases, or toxic substances also affect us. The combined influences of our material (i.e., money and the things money buys) and non-material (our abilities to problem solve, communicate our needs, and negotiate with others, often associated with education) resources appear to profoundly influence our health and wellness outcomes through various direct and indirect pathways.

The interplay of our social selves (how we imagine ourselves and our place in the world—our identity) and our biological selves (genetic factors and how our bodies function as biological systems) condition how we feel, how our bodies operate, and, ultimately, shape our health and wellness experiences. We use various markers of this complex interaction, such as income, education, or occupation, to group people into categories of social similarity and observe the aggregated impact of these processes at the population level.

Several so-called 'determinants of health' have been identified. The Public Health Agency of Canada (PHAC) identifies 11 health determinants: income and social status, social support networks, education, employment and working conditions, social environments, geography, physical environments, healthy child development, health services, gender, and culture (Public Health Agency of Canada, 2006). Participants in a Canadian conference entitled *Social Determinants of Health Across the Life-span*, held at York University in 2002, identified a similar list of social determinants of health, including income and its distribution, early life, Aboriginal status, education, employment and working conditions, food security, health care services, housing, the social safety net, social exclusion, and unemployment and employment security (Raphael, 2004). Note the subtle but important differences between the two lists. Housing, food security, distribution of income, the social safety net, social exclusion, and Aboriginal status are issues not explicitly identified (though may be implied) in the PHAC list, while gender, culture, and geography (including social and physical environments) are not explicitly identified in the list developed through the York conference. In part, the differences between the lists reflect the subtle differences embodied by the different theoretical perspectives identified above. They also reflect differences in the way language is used and concepts are treated by government-based agencies and academic/advocacy communities.

Health, Wellness, and Place

Empirical and theoretical understanding of how the interplay between daily life circumstances and human biology influences health and wellness outcomes at the population level is a central concern for makers, implementers, and researchers of social policy. This concern has, in turn, stimulated an interest in the relationship between health and wellness and place. Several researchers have examined how the socio-spatial structure of cities (or land use, property ownership, density, proximity to services, etc.) is bound up in the empirical distribution of health and wellness outcomes across socio-economic groups and reflected in small area differences in health status (see Berkman and Kawachi, 2000; Kawachi and Berkman, 2003; Dunn and Hayes, 2000; Ross et al., 2004; Oliver and Hayes, 2007). Others have attempted to assess the quality of social relationships through surveys examining feelings of safety and security, the degree of social cohesion among neighbours, participation in community organizations and civil life, and the opportunity structures available within specific locations (e.g., to purchase food, access to cultural and recreational activities, public transportation modes, etc.) (Macintyre, Ellaway, and Cummins, 2002; Oliver and Hayes, 2005).

Research focusing on the relationship between health and place has frequently (but not always) demonstrated an effect of place on health over and above the effects arising from strictly individual factors (Diez-Roux, 1998; Pickett and Pearl, 2001). That is, research indicates that the quality of the environments of everyday life does influence health outcomes, such that persons of the same income or educational attainment or occupational status may experience health and wellness outcomes that are better or worse than expected, based on the attributes of their surrounding environment. Of course, this result is hardly surprising given that all living things must constantly adapt to their environments. Yet, focusing on the specific qualities of the places we live, and understanding how these qualities influence human health outcomes draws attention to the often-overlooked issues associated with community design, or where poverty and disadvantage are concentrated. It takes our understanding of these issues and spatializes them— puts them into the landscape and into everyday life rather than leaving them in highly abstract and placeless domains of tables or figures in research reports.

Another consequence of focusing attention on how health and wellness outcomes are distributed across space (and within specific places) is that it reinforces the fact that our ability to maintain our well-being is shaped by influences of everyday life, and to understand these requires a life-course perspective. When the real world distribution of health and wellness outcomes is considered, it draws attention to issues of housing, nutritious food availability and security, recreational opportunities, and the quality of interpersonal relationships. These issues get far less attention in discussions about health, wellness, and well-being than they should according to research evidence.

The public seems obsessed with issues of health care—or so it would appear if news coverage is anything to go by. Analysis of coverage of health-related stories in both English- and French-language newspapers found that two-thirds of all stories focus on issues of health care and that only about 5% concern all topics associated with the social determinants (Hayes et al., 2007). A survey conducted by the Canadian Institute for Health Information (CIHI) discovered that two of every three Canadian adults do not immediately understand or identify social determinants of health (Canadian Institute for Health Information, 2005a). Astonishingly, these findings come about 30 years after the release of the federal government white paper entitled *A New Perspective on the Health of Canadians* (Lalonde, 1974). That report, which received world-wide acclaim, gave rise to health promotion in Canada. It argued that health (and wellness) does not equal health care, and that a focus on other factors outside the health sector was required. About 40% of our public resources are invested in health care. If support for health-enhancing policies relating to the provision of child care, housing, employment, recreation and culture, and community design is to be obtained by politicians and policymakers from the general public, a greater appreciation of the research literature illustrating why these factors are important to health is required. CIHI's new report, *Improving the Health of Canadians: An Introduction to Health in Urban Places* (Canadian Institute for Health Information, 2006b), is one example of an attempt to make information about the relationship between health and place more accessible to the public.

Summary

Describing wellness has an extensive literature and it has been shown to have several key dimensions that include physical, emotional and psychological, social, intellectual, spiritual, occupational, and environmental attributes. Most of all, wellness is generally viewed from a holistic perspective; it represents a perceived positive state of being and embraces a body-mind-spirit concept. Many factors contribute to wellness in a series of complex and interacting ways, but wellness, like health, is more than the absence of disease; it involves important subjective concepts by individuals about themselves.

Measuring wellness has received much less treatment by researchers and tends to focus on assessments of individuals mainly through the use of questionnaires. Currently, there are several initiatives under way to try to measure wellness concepts at a population or national level. While not discussed in this chapter, it is worth noting that there have also been several approaches to measuring health and wellness at the community level (Hancock, Labonte, and Edwards, 1999; Canadian Institute for Health Information, 2005b).

By contrast, there are numerous studies that measure the determinants of health and wellness at a population level, and much of the research has helped to inform policies related to health promotion. There are well over a dozen so-called determinants, which include income, its distribution and social status, social support networks, education, security of employment and actual working conditions, social environments, physical environments, healthy child development, health services, gender, and culture. Other factors include Aboriginal status; food security; housing quality, affordability, and security; and last, but not least, geography.

Increasingly, researchers and policy makers today are recognizing the importance of place in determining health and wellness. Place involves where individuals live, work, play, and study. How factors vary across space is very much the focus of the *BC Atlas of Wellness*. The maps provided throughout this Atlas ought to be interpreted not discretely, but as simultaneously occurring and dynamic influences operating day-in and day-out. The information upon which the Atlas is based originates from static, cross-sectional data collected at discrete intervals. It is crude, to be sure; but it does give food for thought to imagine the more dynamic aspects of everyday life that so profoundly shape the health and wellness experiences of populations. The focus on wellness draws attention to the fact that health is a resource for everyday living; emphasizing factors that enhance our abilities to thrive (and not simply survive) creates a positive frame of reference for discussion of how public policies can be developed to better nurture the human condition and spirit.

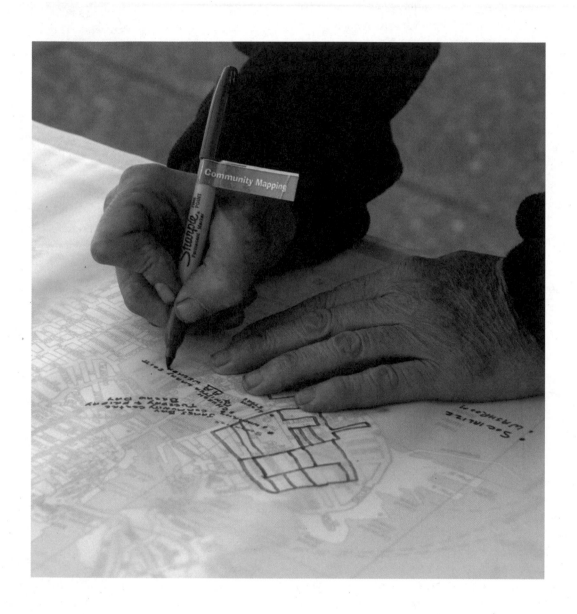

3

Data, Information, and Map Reading

Introduction

In producing the maps contained in this Atlas, several key data sets and information sources were used. Key criteria for including data are as follows:

- Data are readily available. No new data have been collected specifically for the analysis included in the Atlas. Rather, existing data are brought together from a variety of different sources in order to develop the maps.

- Data are collected on an ongoing or periodic basis. This allows an opportunity to measure changes and trends over time.

- Data can be analysed on a geographical basis, primarily for the 16 Heath Service Delivery Areas (HSDAs) of the province. This ensures that geographical differences can be measured, and patterns detected. For some maps, depending on the data source, School Districts (59), Economic Development Regions (8), or BC Games Zones (8) are used (see following pages). In others, "custom" maps are presented, based on a single, novel indicator.

- Data have not been mapped and published elsewhere. In large part, the maps included in the Atlas are unique and have been constructed specifically for the purposes of this Atlas. In a couple of instances this is not the case, as key maps and data are necessary to provide context for the maps that follow.

The following are the key data sources that were used for mapping purposes.

Canadian Community Health Survey (CCHS-3.1)

The Canadian Community Health Survey (CCHS) is undertaken by Statistics Canada, in partnership with Health Canada, on a regular basis across the country. There is a standard set of questions asked of all participants, whose ages range from 12 years and up. Provinces can buy extra modules of questions dealing with a variety of different health- and wellness-related factors (*www.statcan.ca/english/concepts/health/ cycle3_1/overview.htm*). BC, for example, purchased additional modules related to such areas of interest as social supports in the latest survey, which was undertaken throughout 2005 and for which results are now readily available (Ibid.). More than 14,000 BC residents participated in the survey.

As noted above, respondents are limited to those 12 years of age and older and, as the title suggests, the survey collects information from respondents living in the general community. Therefore, data are limited, in that individuals living in institutions (e.g., care or health institutions, jails) or living on Indian reserves or Crown lands, full-time members of the Canadian Armed Forces, and residents of very remote regions are not included. Some of these groups, particularly Aboriginal peoples, are known to have, on average, generally poorer health and wellness status than the remainder of the population (see, for example, Kendall, 2002, 2007; Foster, Macdonald, Tuk, Uh, and Talbot, 1996). As a consequence, the data presented from the survey may be biased toward more positive values of wellness, although approximately 98% of the Canadian population aged 12 and older are covered. Given the relatively large numbers of remote communities, particularly Indian reserves, in the province, it is likely that the coverage may be less than the national average of 98% for BC. As with any survey data, although best attempts are made to ensure clarity of questions, honesty of responses, and randomness in the selection of respondents, these criteria may not always be fully met, and caution should always be practiced when studying the data and making conclusions based on the resulting analyses.

For BC, survey data are available at the HSDA level, and numerous indicators based on the survey are mapped in this Atlas. In most cases, for each indicator, five separate maps are provided consisting of results for the total population, for males and females separately, and for two separate age cohorts—12 to 19 year olds, and those aged 65 years or older. The values of the indicators are given as percentages (%) of respondents answering a question in a certain way. In some cases, the value for the Canadian population as a whole is provided, usually when there is a statistically significant difference (as determined through confidence intervals—see below) between provincial results and Canadian results. Occasionally, specific values are provided just for selected variables for Aboriginal respondents, but only at the provincial level. The sample size for the Aboriginal population is too small to undertake geographical mapping. The Aboriginal identifier used was whether the respondent reported being an Aboriginal person or having Aboriginal origins.

Confidence intervals have been calculated so that statistical significance can be determined at the 95% confidence level. This enables statements to be made on the significance of variations in values by geography (HSDA), gender, and age groups. Confidence intervals are used when values are calculated based on a survey sample of the population. They estimate the margin of error and give a range within which the true value lies. The ranges used for determining significance for these mapped indicators are at the 95% level. This means that, if the survey were repeated, the same results would occur within this range 95 times out of 100. Thanks is given to Statistics Canada for the use of these data.

2001 Canadian Census Data

Every 5 years, the Government of Canada undertakes a general census of the total population and its characteristics. Although the 2006 census has been completed, detailed data are not available to the public as of yet. Consequently, 2001 census data are used in this Atlas. Key determinants of wellness and health are available from this data source, and several are mapped to provide a sense of the "assets" or "positives" available at the population level to support wellness. The data for our purposes, although owned by Statistics Canada, have been provided by BC Statistics and by the Ministry of Health Data Warehouse. Once gain, the provision for use of these data is gratefully acknowledged. One caution with respect to census data is that several of the population characteristics depend on self-identification, such as "Aboriginal heritage." This may be underestimated as a result.

School District Data

There is a variety of data related to wellness indicators available from school districts. For several years, the BC Ministry of Education has undertaken annual satisfaction surveys of students in selected grades, canvassing various issues, such as physical activity, bullying, and school safety, to name a few. These data are readily available at the school district level (*www. bced.gov.bc.ca/apps/imcl/imclWeb/Home*). A number of indicators have been mapped at this geographic level, including physical activity/nutrition and school safety. Although a survey instrument was used for Grades 3/4, 7, 10, and 12, all students were surveyed, eliminating the need for developing confidence intervals, as was necessary for the CCHS data. Given the young age of some of the respondents, caution should be exercised when interpreting results. Educational outcome data are also available. Key indicators include high school graduation. Data are available at the Ministry of Education website, and other maps are available in Foster and McKee (2007).

The Human Early Learning Partnership (HELP) at the University of British Columbia continues to collect "readiness to learn" data on entry level kindergarten students throughout the province of BC using the Early Development Instrument (EDI). Only a limited number of maps are included in the *BC Atlas of Wellness*, as many are available elsewhere (*www.earlylearning.ubc.ca/*). In 2005, the first edition of the *British Columbia Atlas of Child Development* was produced for the province as a whole (Kershaw et al., 2005), and contains numerous maps for the interested reader.

McCreary Centre Society Adolescent Health Survey

Over the past decade or so, the McCreary Centre Society, a non-profit agency in Burnaby focused on youth health and behaviour, has undertaken three major surveys of students in Grades 7 to 12 in BC. The last survey, which included over 30,000 respondents, was undertaken in 2003, while the next is scheduled for 2008. There are well over 100 questions in the survey instrument, which is administered in randomly selected classes throughout most school districts. While this is a very rich and robust data set, not all school districts in the province elected to be included in the survey, leaving several areas of the province without data, particularly in the northeast and the Fraser Valley. Data, while collected at the school level, are sampled and weighted based on the characteristics of the school population in each HSDA. For 2003, data gaps occur for the Fraser South, Fraser East, and Northeast HSDAs. More information about the McCreary survey, along with numerous reports based on their surveys, can be found on their website (*www.mcs.bc.ca*). Additional maps are available in Foster and McKee (2007).

BC Vital Statistics Data

The BC Vital Statistics Agency collects a variety of data on births, deaths, and marriages, as well as data related to congenital anomalies and handicapping conditions contained within its Health Status Registry (*www.vs.gov. bc.ca*). Important wellness data on maternal conditions, perinatal conditions, and outcomes for newborns and infants (first year of life) are collected through the Physician's Notice of Birth (PNOB). A healthy beginning for a child is related to healthy development through to adulthood. Important data used in this Atlas include, among others, age of mother giving birth, birth weight, and length of pregnancy before delivery—all key wellness factors for newborns (Kierans, Collison, Foster, and Uh, 1993; Kierans et al., 2004; Kierans, Kendall, Foster, Liston, and Tuk, 2006; Kierans, Kendall, et al., 2007a; Kierans, Verhulst, Mohamed, and Foster, 2007). Some caution is required with the use of the PNOB data as they rely on individual physicians to complete all of the required components of the form, and data are not always complete. Also, the data presented in the Atlas only cover events that occurred in the province. Events occurring to BC residents elsewhere are not included, and this is particularly problematic for the northeast and southeast of the province where difficult or risky births may occur in the neighbouring province of Alberta (Burr, McKee, Foster, and Nualt, 1995). Again, caution is required when analysing the maps.

Women's and Children's Hospital Perinatal Data Base

An important database related to new mothers and babies has been developed by Women's and Children's Hospital in Vancouver. It records information on each birth in the province, including characteristics of the mother and the baby. Key data used in this Atlas include non-smoking behaviour in pregnancy, and breastfeeding of newborns on discharge from the hospital, both of which are key assets for the wellness of newborns and their healthy development into adulthood. In all, data are available on approximately 150,000 babies who were discharged from BC's hospitals between April 2000 and March 2004.

BC Recreation and Parks Association (BCRPA)

Over the past 3 years, the BCRPA has sponsored three key surveys of assets related to wellness. These include selected public recreation facilities (BCRPA, 2004), selected sports and recreation outdoor assets (BCRPA, 2006a), and selected community-based activity centres (BCRPA, 2006b). While the first survey of local government had a response rate of 100%, the later two both had response rates of 88% of the 185 entities surveyed, and so some caution is required in interpreting results. These data are mapped at the HSDA level. In addition, BCRPA is responsible for promoting increased physical activity at the community level through its promotion of Active Communities. The population living in registered active communities within HSDAs are mapped using data provided by BCRPA. Thanks to this organization for access to its data.

Sports BC Membership Data

Sports BC is a non-profit agency that represents more than 80 sport organizations, including over 60 designated provincial sports organizations. Membership registration is collected for numerous sports and games activities by Sports BC. Key rates of participation, as measured by registration in different sports activities, have been used in the Atlas based on the data provided by Sports BC for 2005. These data do not include sports activities undertaken through schools and, as such, participation rates are likely an underestimate of actual sports participation in the province. Thanks is given to Sports BC for allowing access to its data.

Other Data Sources

There is a variety of other data sources used to map different indicators. These include, among others, public transit, public library use, combined child and senior dependency ratios, heart and stroke walking clubs, municipal and school district no smoking bylaws, as well as several climatic change and physical feature maps.

Interpreting the Maps and Tables

In total, there are more than 270 maps and supporting tables provided in the BC Atlas of Wellness to show specific patterns and values of wellness-related indicators, based on the previously mentioned data sources. There are several major map forms included in the Atlas. To the extent possible, data are mapped at the Health Service Delivery Area (HSDA) administration level, of which there are 16 in the province. As noted earlier, this is the most detailed unit for which much of the data are available and thus it represents the base mapping unit for the Atlas. Using a common mapping unit enables an examination of the values of different indicators for any HSDA, thus allowing the ability to build an overall wellness picture of that HSDA based on numerous indicators related to wellness determinants/ assets, smoke-free environments, nutrition and food security, activity, healthy weights, and healthy pregnancy and birth. These are the key components of the ActNow BC initiative. In addition, indicators based on wellness outcomes are included.

The second geographical area used in the Atlas is the school district administrative unit, of which there are 59 for mapping purposes (an additional school district, Ecole Scolaire Francophone, is not geographically based, but is generally included in the total values for the provincial school population). Several key indicators are available at this level for kindergarten to Grade 12 students, for total students and for male and female students separately, and for school districts themselves.

Thirdly, a series of maps uses the larger BC Games Zone administrative area, consisting of eight zones,

and the eight Economic Development Regions are used for several maps. Finally, there is a series of individual maps that provide information on novel indicators and may not conform to administrative boundary maps: they are what we refer to as "custom" maps. These cover a variety of information sources, and provide information as point sources (e.g., Farmers Markets) or as isolines (e.g., hours of bright sunshine).

Where possible, data are divided into quintiles for mapping purposes. A quintile represents one-fifth or 20% of the administrative units being mapped for any particular indicator. Different colours differentiate between the quintile groupings. Most range from GREEN for those geographical units with indicator wellness values in the highest or best quintile (or top 20%) through colour gradations to RED for the lowest quintile (or bottom 20%) value areas. The following section provides an example of the most frequent map page form, along with a supporting table. The CCHS map model is used, but the majority of other maps are of a similar nature for presentation and analysis purposes.

Cautions and Caveats

When using maps to view information and data the user should be aware of a couple of major cautions, especially for many of the maps presented in this Atlas. While we are able to show variations in indicator values between different HSDAs, or school districts, we do not show variations within HSDAs. In many instances, such as Vancouver, which has large variations in many socio-economic characteristics among the smaller areas within the HSDA, the variations in the indicator values may be greater than those between Vancouver and all other HSDAs. Secondly, the population in BC is very much concentrated in the extreme southwest of the province and southern part of Vancouver Island. Much of the interior, north, and southeast of the province is very sparsely populated, but covers large tracts of land. Users must be cautioned against coming to a conclusion that much of the province has high or low values related to a certain indicator. While technically that may be correct from the perspective of land mass covered, it would not be correct to say those values occur to most of the population in the province.

The following pages provide base maps for HSDAs, School Districts, BC Games Zones, and Economic Development Regions, along with a brief guide on how to interpret and analyse the maps and tables used in this Atlas.

Health Service Delivery Areas

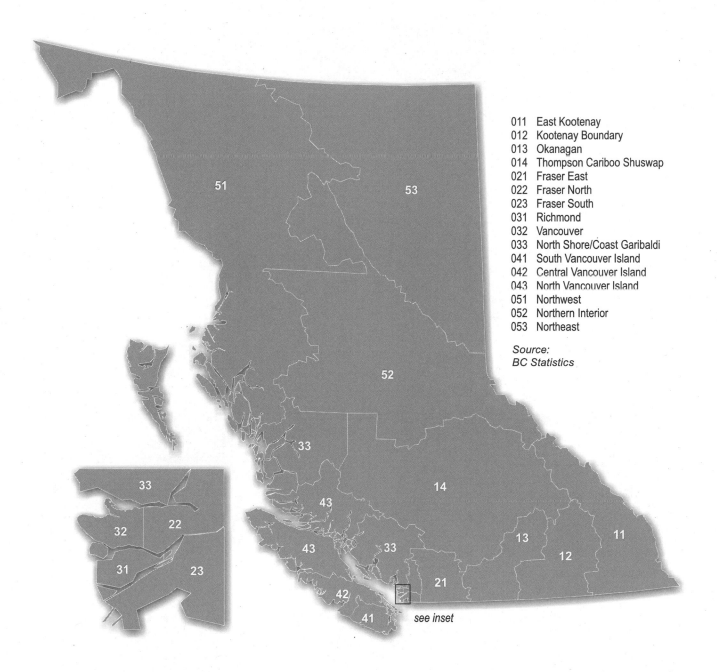

011	East Kootenay
012	Kootenay Boundary
013	Okanagan
014	Thompson Cariboo Shuswap
021	Fraser East
022	Fraser North
023	Fraser South
031	Richmond
032	Vancouver
033	North Shore/Coast Garibaldi
041	South Vancouver Island
042	Central Vancouver Island
043	North Vancouver Island
051	Northwest
052	Northern Interior
053	Northeast

Source:
BC Statistics

see inset

School Districts

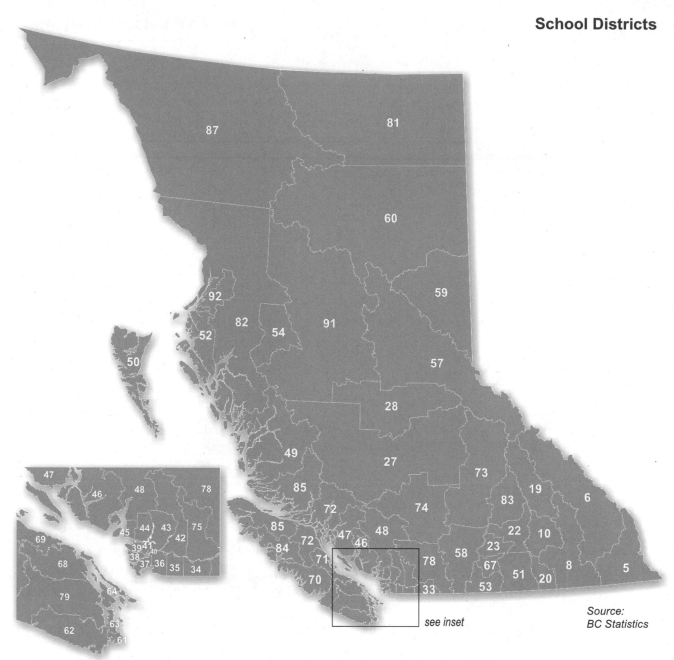

005	Southeast Kootenay	
006	Rocky Mountain	
008	Kootenay Lake	
010	Arrow Lakes	
019	Revelstoke	
020	Kootenay-Columbia	
022	Vernon	
023	Central Okanagan	
027	Cariboo-Chilcotin	
028	Quesnel	
033	Chilliwack	
034	Abbotsford	
035	Langley	
036	Surrey	
037	Delta	
038	Richmond	
039	Vancouver	
040	New Westminster	
041	Burnaby	
042	Maple Ridge-Pitt Meadows	
043	Coquitlam	
044	North Vancouver	
045	West Vancouver	
046	Sunshine Coast	
047	Powell River	
048	Howe Sound	
049	Central Coast	
050	Haida Gwaii/Queen Charlotte	
051	Boundary	
052	Prince Rupert	
053	Okanagan Similkameen	
054	Bulkley Valley	
057	Prince George	
058	Nicola-Similkameen	
059	Peace River South	
060	Peace River North	
061	Greater Victoria	
062	Sooke	
063	Saanich	
064	Gulf Islands	
067	Okanagan Skaha	
068	Nanaimo-Ladysmith	
069	Qualicum	
070	Alberni	
071	Comox Valley	
072	Campbell River	
073	Kamloops/Thompson	
074	Gold Trail	
075	Mission	
078	Fraser-Cascade	
079	Cowichan Valley	
081	Fort Nelson	
082	Coast Mountains	
083	North Okanagan-Shuswap	
084	Vancouver Island West	
085	Vancouver Island North	
087	Stikine	
091	Nechako Lakes	
092	Nisga'a	

Source:
BC Statistics

BC Games Zones

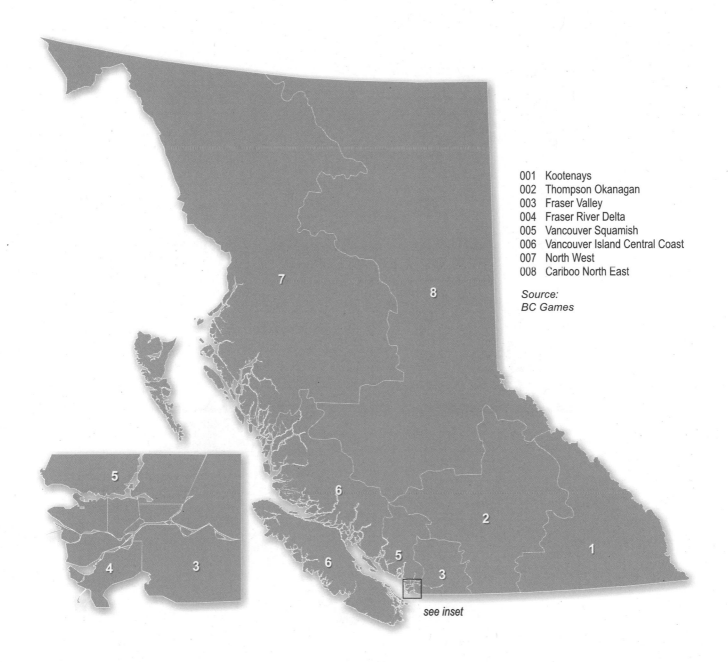

001   Kootenays
002   Thompson Okanagan
003   Fraser Valley
004   Fraser River Delta
005   Vancouver Squamish
006   Vancouver Island Central Coast
007   North West
008   Cariboo North East

Source:
BC Games

see inset

Economic Development Regions

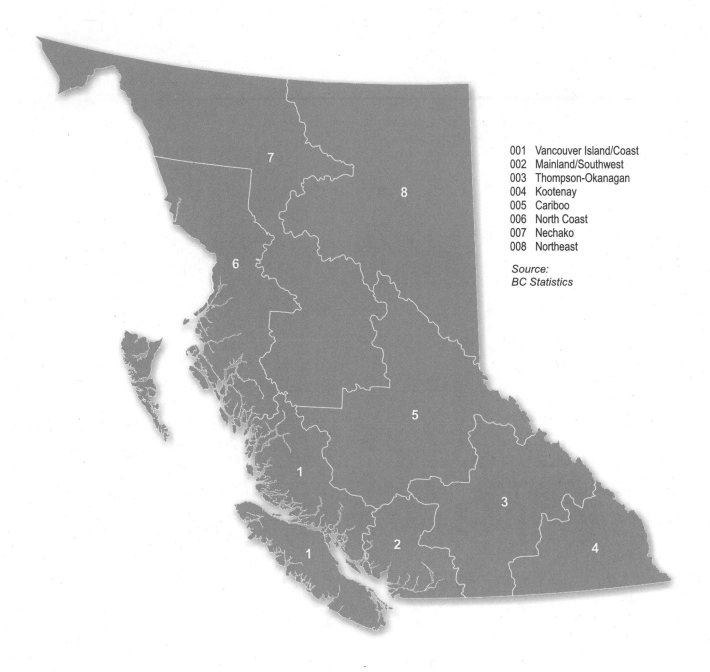

001   Vancouver Island/Coast
002   Mainland/Southwest
003   Thompson-Okanagan
004   Kootenay
005   Cariboo
006   North Coast
007   Nechako
008   Northeast

Source:
BC Statistics

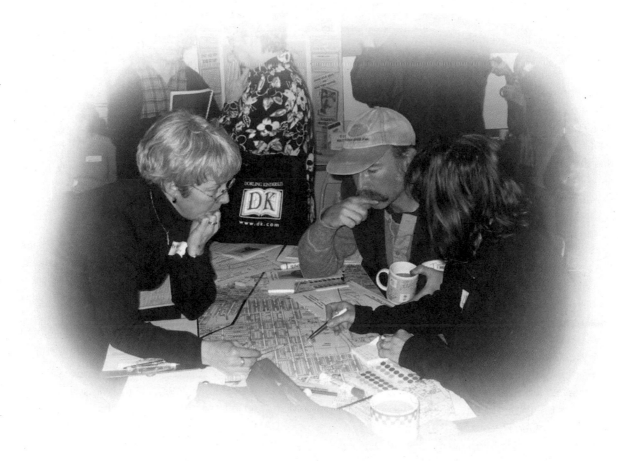

Canadian Community Health Survey—sample data

The five maps plot, by quintile, the values in percent (%) for the total respondents who answered the CCHS question in a positive way from a wellness asset perspective. The colour index at the side of the maps provides the range of the values of the five quintiles used for mapping. For example, the **DARK GREEN** or highest wellness quintile has a range of 38.17–52.44% for the larger top map and includes the three HSDAs (East Kootenay #11, Central Vancouver Island #42, South Vancouver Island #41) with the highest values; the next highest quintile, in **LIGHT GREEN**, has a range of 25.57–32.63% and includes the three HSDAs with the next highest values; the middle quintile (which has four HSDAs because the 16 HSDAs cannot be divided into five equal groupings) contains the four HSDAs with the middle values which are coloured **BEIGE**; the next three HSDAs are coloured **ORANGE** and have lower values than the middle group; and finally the three HSDAs with the lowest values are **RED** and have a range of 18.94–19.14% (Fraser East #21, North Vancouver Island #43, Richmond #31). When HSDAs are **GREY** it indicates that data are not available for mapping, usually because the sample size is too small (less than 30) to report for that HSDA (see map at bottom left opposite). This follows the convention developed by Statistics Canada for these survey data.

CROSSHATCHED HSDAs have values that are significantly different statistically from the overall provincial value (see Fraser East, North Vancouver Island, and Richmond, which are all significantly lower than the provincial average). An inset for the lower mainland HSDAs is provided; although these have a small land mass, this is where the majority of the province's population resides.

Four smaller maps below the larger map focus on characteristics of the CCHS respondents. The first two look at the patterns for males and females individually, and also note by CROSSHATCHING any HSDAs that have significantly higher or lower values statistically than

Health Service Delivery Area	All respondents (%)	Males (%)	Females (%)	Ages 12-19 (%)	Ages 20-64 (%)	Ages 65+ (%)
011 East Kootenay	52.44	52.49	52.39	55.33	51.79	52.99
042 Central Vancouver Island	38.49	41.79	35.33	32.92	42.92	27.09‡
041 South Vancouver Island	38.17	33.65†	42.25†	34.06	40.24	32.67
012 Kootenay Boundary	32.63	32.08	33.18	F	34.18	30.25
014 Thompson Cariboo Shuswap	29.93	32.35	27.52	F	32.79	21.28E
022 Fraser North	25.57	22.97	28.12	31.97	26.47	14.43E‡
053 Northeast	25.51	19.55E	31.91	F	26.41	F
033 North Shore/Coast Garibaldi	25.01	25.67	24.38	F	26.61	21.12
051 Northwest	24.56	29.43	19.30	F	27.82	F
052 Northern Interior	23.73	24.17	23.26	F	26.15	F
013 Okanagan	20.83	18.47	23.06	21.93	22.44	15.09E
023 Fraser South	20.59	19.40	21.75	22.80	21.25	14.64
032 Vancouver	19.20	18.75	19.64	F	21.51	12.20E‡
021 Fraser East	19.14	17.02	21.20	F	19.50	19.47
043 North Vancouver Island	19.01	16.93E	21.07E	F	19.92E	F
031 Richmond	18.94	20.87	17.13	F	18.16	F
999 Province	**25.30**	**24.40**	**26.18**	**23.77**	**26.70**	**19.79‡**

‡ Age group differs significantly from 20-64 group.
E Interpret data with caution (16.77< coefficient of variation <33.3).
F Data suppressed due to Statistics Canada sampling rules.
† Males differ significantly from females.

the provincial average by gender (see East Kootenay #11 in both cases). The second two maps focus on the age "book ends" of the data. One looks at the youngest or youth/teen age group of 12- to 19-year-olds, while the other looks at the 65 and over seniors age group. A key focus of ActNow BC is to work on healthy developments for children and youth and healthier living for seniors.

The table above supports the maps opposite. Using the same colour scheme and hatching symbols as the maps, the left hand column shows the values of the HSDAs from highest to lowest. The other columns keep the HSDA order of the left hand column and provide the actual data for each HSDA by gender and for three separate age cohorts. The † symbol indicates that there is a significant difference (statistically) between males and females within a particular HSDA; ‡ indicates there is a significant difference between the 12 to 19 age group and the 20 to 64 age group, or between the 65 and over age group and the 20 to 64 age group within the HSDA. (Note that no separate map is provided for the population aged 20-64 years because of space constraints. In most cases, the pattern is very similar to that for "All respondents.") The symbol **F** denotes that the sample size is too small or has a very large coefficient of variation, and the symbol **E** denotes caution in interpretation because of unstable values (large coefficient of variation). This allows the user to get a more complete picture of any of the wellness-related indicators mapped and provides a tabular mosaic of the values of the indicator by HSDA.

Canadian Community Health Survey—sample map

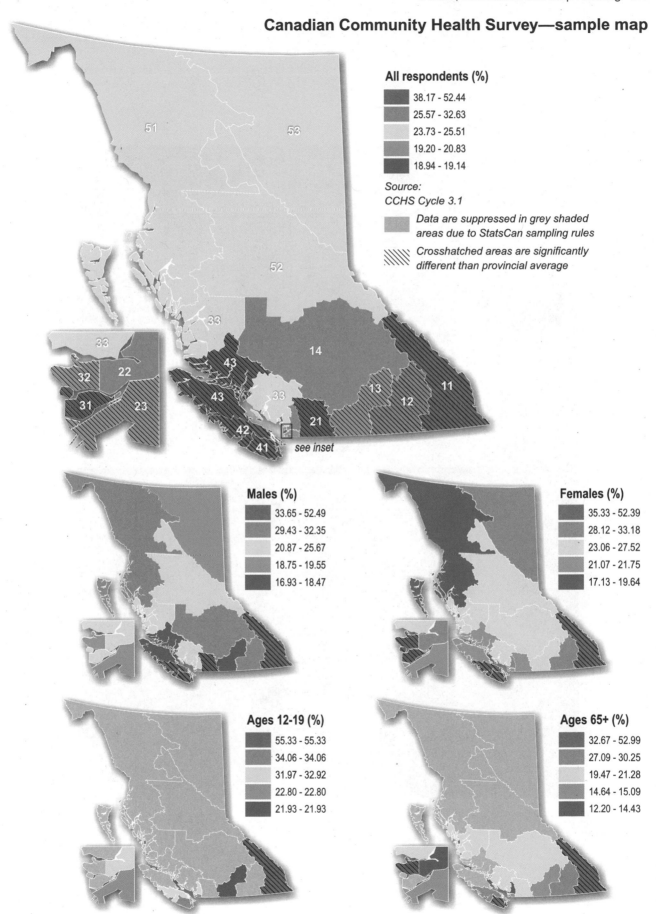

All respondents (%)

- 38.17 - 52.44
- 25.57 - 32.63
- 23.73 - 25.51
- 19.20 - 20.83
- 18.94 - 19.14

Source:
CCHS Cycle 3.1

Data are suppressed in grey shaded areas due to StatsCan sampling rules

Crosshatched areas are significantly different than provincial average

Males (%)

- 33.65 - 52.49
- 29.43 - 32.35
- 20.87 - 25.67
- 18.75 - 19.55
- 16.93 - 18.47

Females (%)

- 35.33 - 52.39
- 28.12 - 33.18
- 23.06 - 27.52
- 21.07 - 21.75
- 17.13 - 19.64

Ages 12-19 (%)

- 55.33 - 55.33
- 34.06 - 34.06
- 31.97 - 32.92
- 22.80 - 22.80
- 21.93 - 21.93

Ages 65+ (%)

- 32.67 - 52.99
- 27.09 - 30.25
- 19.47 - 21.28
- 14.64 - 15.09
- 12.20 - 14.43

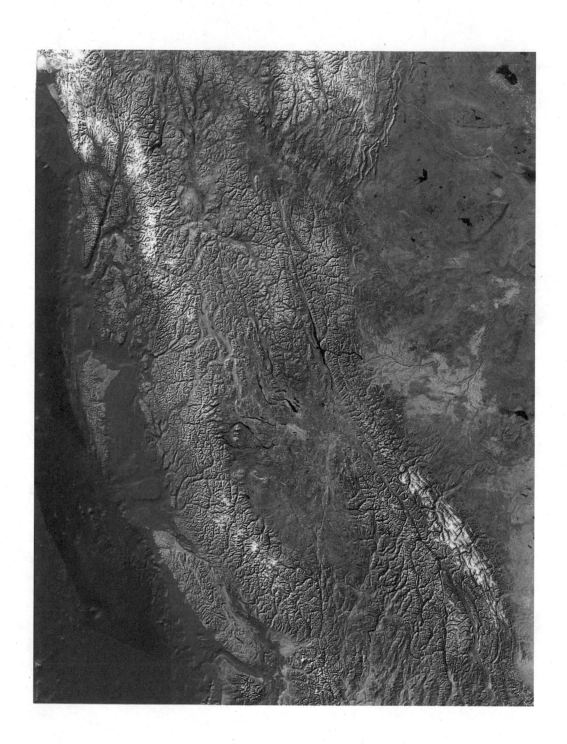

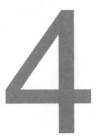

The British Columbia Context

Introduction

This chapter of the Atlas provides some background material on the Province of BC from both a physical geography perspective and a demographic perspective. The first section presents a brief overview of some of the major characteristics of BC's physical environment, including several key climate indicators, followed by provincial population indicators. These indicators and maps all provide a context for the rest of the Atlas. Some of the key indicators can be viewed as wellness assets themselves, as they influence the patterns that appear in the maps in later sections of the Atlas.

The first section presents nine maps showing physical and important climatic indicators that can influence wellness. The first three maps provide information on the major physiographic regions of the province, with supporting maps showing days of bright sunlight and precipitation-free days. These two climate-related indicators have been chosen because of their relationship to health and wellness. Sunlight is a wellness asset in many ways. It is an important source of Vitamin D and also important in countering the debilitating effects of Seasonal Affective Disorder Syndrome (SADS). Of course, too much sun can be damaging to the skin. The precipitation-free days indicator was chosen because research has shown that individuals are more likely to engage in outdoor physical exercise on precipitation-free days and in the summer (Canadian Institute for Health Information, 2006a).

A report by the Ministry of Water, Land and Air Protection (2002) provides numerous maps and data related to the "wellness" of the province's environment and ecosystems. Information is provided on human health and environment, toxic contaminants, climatic change, stewardship, and biodiversity. For interested readers, an updated report by the Ministry of Environment is anticipated in the future.

Given its importance to health and wellness in BC (Ministry of Water Land and Air Protection, 2004), the next set of six maps present key information related to climatic change. These include four maps providing information on changing precipitation patterns over the past 50 years or so, and two maps on temperature changes within the province.

In the second section, there are 10 maps in all that provide key indicators on the population and demographic make-up of the province. The first two maps show population density and where the population lives by HSDA. The second two maps provide similar information on the province's Aboriginal population. While the Aboriginal population is relatively small as a percentage of the BC population, it is an important group in that both the health and wellness status of Aboriginal peoples are substantially less than for the population as a whole (Stephenson, Elliott, Foster, and Harris, 1996; Kendall, 2001, 2002, 2007). Included in various sections of the Atlas are specific data related to Aboriginal peoples, but in many cases, as noted previously, the data can not be mapped geographically because relatively small numbers do not allow their reporting.

These maps are followed by three maps showing information on how the age make-up of the province varies regionally by HSDA. The final three maps show information related to language and recent immigrant data, again at the HSDA level. Over the past two decades, BC's cultural make-up has changed substantially as a result of major immigration from south and east Asia, and these maps show some of the patterns within the province associated with these trends.

Physiography of BC

Geographically, BC is the western-most province of Canada, although parts of the Yukon Territory lie further west. It has a land area of nearly 95 million hectares and has a diverse group of physiographic characteristics, as shown.

As noted in the 1992 Mortality Atlas (Foster and Edgell, 1992), its key physical features run in a general northwest to southeast direction. The western-most part of the province consists of Haida Gwaii (Queen Charlotte Islands) in the north and Vancouver Island in the south. Both these islands are the Outer Mountain region. To its east is the Coast Trough region, which is paralleled to the east by the Coast Mountain region. These three features make up what is referred to as the Western System of BC.

The Fraser River plain in the southwestern-most part of the mainland, along with the southeast tip of Vancouver Island and the eastern part of the Island, is where the majority of people live (Strohmaier and Burr, 1992).

The Interior System, to the east, consists of three major physiographic groupings. The Northern and Southern Plateaus and Mountain areas, the Central Plateau and Mountain area, and to the east the very dominant Rocky Mountain Trench. East of the Trench lies the Rocky Mountains which go north to the Mackenzie Mountain area, while the northeast part of the province is part of the Alberta Plateau.

The province is characterized by large river drainage systems, particularly the Fraser and Thompson systems and Columbia system which flow to the south. The Peace system drains eastward while the Liard system flows north. In the northwest, the Stikine, Nass, and Skeena systems flow west to the Pacific Ocean. In addition to these large systems there are numerous lakes and smaller rivers.

WESTERN SYSTEM

Coast Mountain Area

Coast Trough

Outer Mountain Area

INTERIOR SYSTEM

Northern and Southern Plateaus and Mountain Areas

Central Plateau and Mountain Area

Rocky Mountain Trench

EASTERN SYSTEM

Rocky Mountain Area

Mackenzie Mountain Area

Alberta Plateau

Precipitation in the province exhibits major variations based on its mountainous relief and the generally westerly atmospheric flow of weather patterns. Parts of the interior of the province get 25 centimetres of precipitation annually—rain and snow combined— while over 500 centimetres is not uncommon on the coastal mountains. Precipitation falls mainly in winter, but as Foster (1987) noted, overall climate, like the province's physiography, is very diverse: "Variations in latitude, elevation, land and sea distribution, and relief combine to create a complex climatic mosaic in BC. Climates range from marine temperate on the coast to continental steppe and subarctic in the interior and north of the province, respectively" (p. 45).

Precipitation-free days

Similar to the previous map, the trend in terms of precipitation-free days shows a northwest to southeast gradient, but the pattern is somewhat more complex than the previous maps. The range varies from a high of over 285 to a low of less than 125 precipitation-free days.

The areas with most precipitation-free days are in the central interior part of the province and the areas with the least occur on the coast. The extreme west of Haida Gwaii has the lowest number of precipitation-free days (darkest blue). There is also a region in the eastern central part of the province (darker blue) with fewer precipitation-free days.

There are very steep gradients, or changes, in the number of precipitation-free days over a short distance, particularly along the coastal mountains and western flanks of the Rocky Mountains.

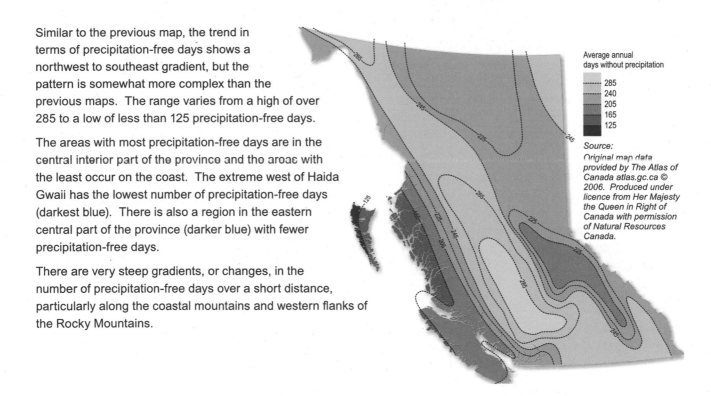

Average annual
days without precipitation

285
240
205
165
125

Source:

Original map data provided by The Atlas of Canada atlas.gc.ca © 2006. Produced under licence from Her Majesty the Queen in Right of Canada with permission of Natural Resources Canada.

Hours of bright sunshine

As with the previous two maps, there is a similar northwest to southeast trend with hours of bright sunlight. There is a range from over 2,000 hours per year to less than 1,000 hours per year and, generally, bright sunshine hours increase from the west to the east of the province.

In the southwest tip of the province, and around the Strait of Georgia between the lower half of Vancouver Island and the mainland where much of the population resides, there is an area with higher levels of bright sunshine than areas immediately to the east. The southern central part of the interior also is an "island" of bright sunshine.

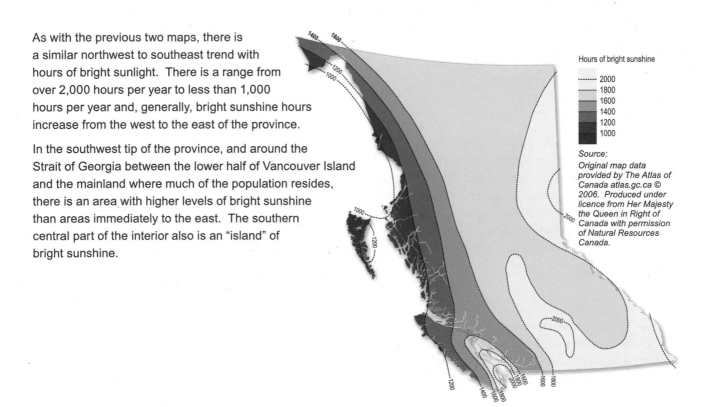

Hours of bright sunshine

2000
1800
1600
1400
1200
1000

Source:

Original map data provided by The Atlas of Canada atlas.gc.ca © 2006. Produced under licence from Her Majesty the Queen in Right of Canada with permission of Natural Resources Canada.

Seasonal trends in precipitation

Precipitation, while it can discourage outdoor activities, is important from many other perspectives: a source of water supply; a source for continuing the life of rivers and lakes and the associated aquatic flora and fauna; an important resource for recreation when it falls as snow; an important resource for agriculture; and a source of water for hydroelectric power, to name but a few.

The four maps opposite provide information related to the trends in seasonal precipitation throughout the province between 1961 and 1990. Changes in precipitation patterns can have major effects, both positive and negative, on individuals, communities, and the environment.

Winter

The winter season trends, seen at top left on the opposite page, show a general north to south orientation. The lightest colour area depicts little change in the amount of precipitation. Generally, winter precipitation has decreased over time as one moves west to east. An increase in winter precipitation has occurred in the Dease Lake area in the north and offshore around Haida Gwaii. Areas west of a line from Dease Lake in the north to Quatsino on Vancouver Island have experienced increases (up to 25%), while areas east of that line have seen decreases, some as much as a 45% reduction (east of Summerland in the Okanagan and around Golden in the east of the province).

Spring

Most areas of the province have received increased precipitation during this season as noted on the map at the top right opposite. Only the areas between Ft. Nelson and Ft. St. John in the northeast and the area just east of Prince George show reductions (in the order of 5% to 15%). The southern interior region around Kamloops and the Okanagan shows an increase of 35% and more.

Summer

The map at the bottom left of the page opposite shows that, for the summer period, much of the province has witnessed modest increases in precipitation, except in the northeast of the province, as far south as Prince George. The southern part of Vancouver Island is also an area that has not seen an increase during this season. Larger increases in precipitation are found in the interior around Kamloops and south, and in the Golden area in the east (both over 35%).

Autumn

For the autumn or fall season, while there are trends throughout the province, they are not as dramatic nor as consistent as in some of the other seasons. Much of the province has witnessed small changes. The areas around Kamloops in the interior (25% plus) and to a lesser extent in the northeast and northwest (15% plus) show increases, while decreases are evident (15% plus) in the area west of Golden in the east of the province.

Summary

The four maps opposite indicate that the climate cannot necessarily be expected to remain stable. Although some of these changes may be due to random fluctuation, evidence is clearly mounting that major changes in climate are occurring globally and that BC is far from immune to such changes and their effects. Most of BC experienced wetter springs and summers and drier winters throughout the second half of the last millennium (Ministry of Environment, 2006).

Seasonal trends in precipitation

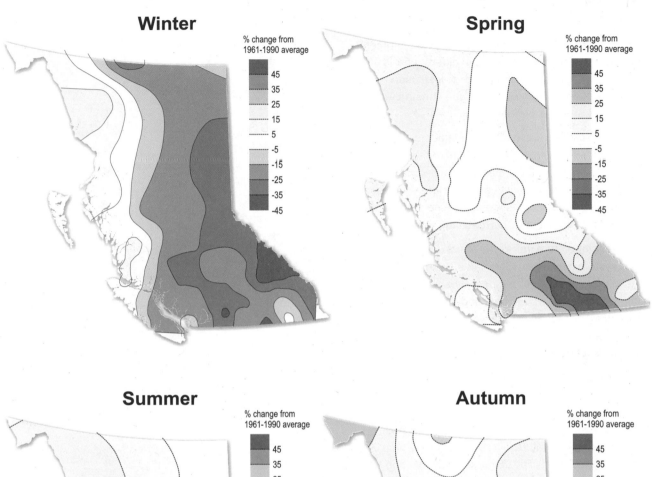

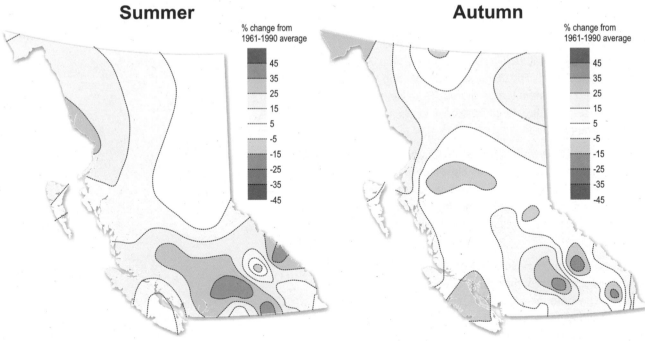

Source: Environment Canada, Adjusted Historical Canadian Climate Data, 2004.

Recent changes in temperatures

The maps opposite provide an indication of the recent changes in average temperature in different parts of the province. Over time, people, their institutions, their architecture, and other key factors are constructed, in part, based on the experience of climate.

Changes in climate can have major impacts, not only on individuals but on whole societies. Increasingly, there is major concern about the impact of climate change and global warming on all societies. Few places appear to be immune from these changes given the global nature of ocean and atmospheric currents and systems.

Average temperature increases affect other components of the system of climate. This can include warmer coastal and inland water temperatures, affecting fish habitats, precipitation regimes, and changes in snow pack. Also, increased severe weather events, such as major storms, heat waves, and dry spells, which favour forest fire conditions, or warmer winters, which allow pests to survive, are part of the overall variability in weather beyond what has normally been expected (Ministry of Water, Land and Air Protection, 2002; 2004) .

Over the past half-century, all of the province has experienced temperature increases (Ministry of Environment, 2006). The increases have been in both minimum and maximum temperatures. Both winter and spring temperatures appear to be rising faster than summer temperatures.

As the Ministry of Environment (2006) has noted, overnight minimum temperatures have increased faster than daytime maximum temperatures, thus creating a narrower daily temperature range, and a longer growing season. It also results in lower winter heating requirements.

Geographically, as the maps indicate, the rises in temperature are lowest (around 0.5 degrees Celsius) in coastal BC, where the majority of the population lives, and increase as one moves northward and eastward from the coastal area for rises in both maximum and minimum temperatures. The greatest increases occur in the northeast (in excess of 2.5 degrees Celsius), although large increases also occur in minimum temperatures in the interior around Kamloops.

Over time, these changes will create the need for adjustments by individuals and the biosphere.

Recent changes in temperatures

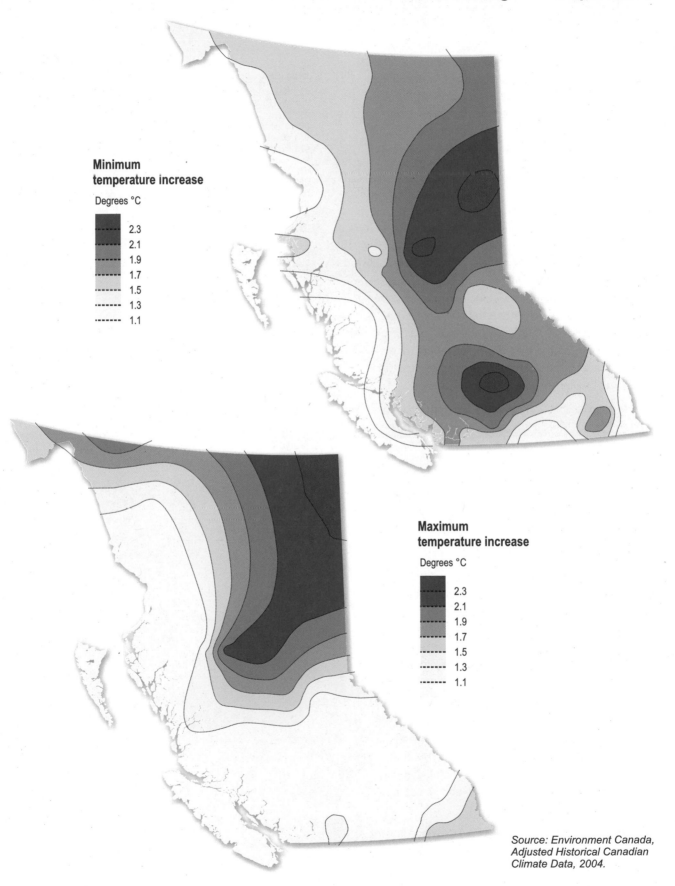

**Minimum
temperature increase**

Degrees °C

2.3
2.1
1.9
1.7
1.5
1.3
1.1

**Maximum
temperature increase**

Degrees °C

2.3
2.1
1.9
1.7
1.5
1.3
1.1

*Source: Environment Canada,
Adjusted Historical Canadian
Climate Data, 2004.*

Population distribution within the province

The two maps opposite provide key indicators related to the province's population in terms of its distribution geographically, and the population density by HSDA, and provide an important context for the maps on wellness that follow. They are based on the P.E.O.P.L.E. 30 population projections developed by BC Statistics for 2005.

Percent of total population

Most of the province's population is concentrated in three regions. Nearly 40% of the population resides in three HSDAs in the extreme southwest part of the province. Fraser South (15.08%), Vancouver (13.93%), and Fraser North (13.13%) dominate the population distribution within the province. Neighbouring HSDAs such as North Shore/Coast Garibaldi, Richmond, and, to a lesser extent, Fraser East, are also considered part of the lower mainland area. Together these HSDAs contain nearly half of the province's population.

The second region of importance is South Vancouver Island. This HSDA contains 8.25% of the province's population. The third main region is the Okanagan in the southern interior of the province with 7.78% of the province's total. The northern half and southeastern parts of the province, which cover the largest land mass, contain relatively few people.

Population density per square kilometre

The population density of the Vancouver HSDA dominates the density distribution map and table. At over 4,500 people per square kilometre, it had more than three times the population density of the next highest HSDA (Richmond with 1,420 people/sq. km.). Fraser South, at 760 people per square kilometre, was also prominent, as was Fraser North with 244 people per square kilometre. These are all in the urbanized part of the lower mainland in the southwest.

South Vancouver Island also has a relatively high population density and, as with other HSDAs, the population within it tends to be concentrated in only a small part of the region as a whole, and so some caution is required in analysing these data.

The whole of the northern half of the province is very sparsely populated, with small settlements scattered throughout the region. Again, some caution is required

Health Service Delivery Area	Percent of total pop.	Pop. density per sq. km
023 Fraser South	15.08	759.56
032 Vancouver	13.93	4,523.44
022 Fraser North	13.13	244.10
041 South Vancouver Island	8.25	149.09
013 Okanagan	7.78	15.49
033 North Shore/Coast Garibaldi	6.45	5.07
021 Fraser East	6.22	21.14
042 Central Vancouver Island	5.94	20.49
014 Thompson Cariboo Shuswap	5.22	1.85
031 Richmond	4.13	1,420.91
052 Northern Interior	3.62	0.92
043 North Vancouver Island	2.79	2.95
051 Northwest	1.98	0.34
011 East Kootenay	1.94	1.84
012 Kootenay Boundary	1.89	2.79
053 Northeast	1.63	0.37
999 Province	**100.0**	**4.50**

given that there are several major towns in which much of the population may be concentrated. Prince George in the Northern Interior, with a population in excess of 77,000, is one such community which dominates the population of the HSDA. The same can be said of other regions: Nanaimo (population of nearly 80,000) for Central Vancouver Island; Kelowna (population of 110,000) in Okanagan; and Kamloops (nearly 83,000) in Thompson Cariboo Shuswap.

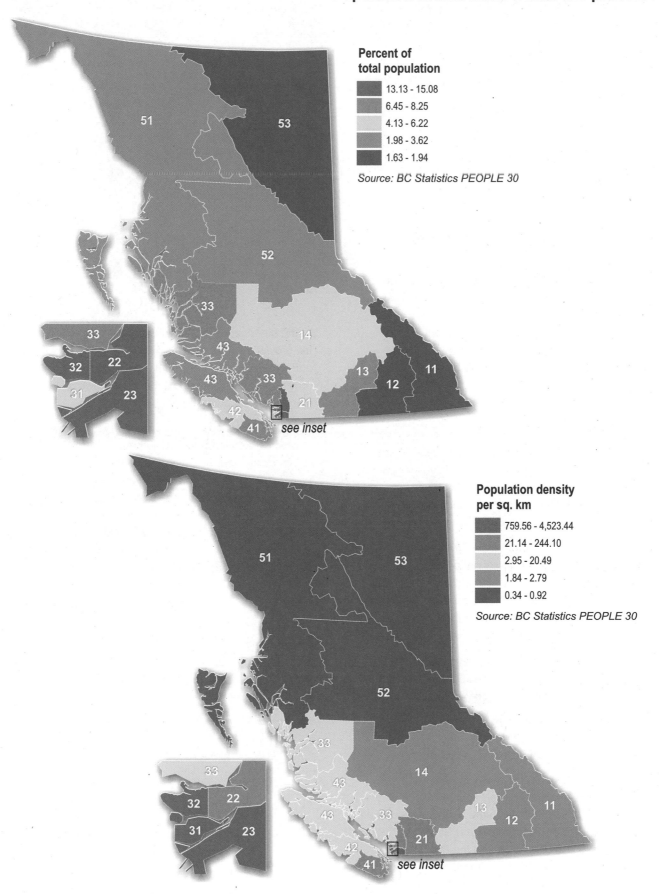

Population distribution within the province

Percent of total population

- 13.13 - 15.08
- 6.45 - 8.25
- 4.13 - 6.22
- 1.98 - 3.62
- 1.63 - 1.94

Source: BC Statistics PEOPLE 30

see inset

Population density per sq. km

- 759.56 - 4,523.44
- 21.14 - 244.10
- 2.95 - 20.49
- 1.84 - 2.79
- 0.34 - 0.92

Source: BC Statistics PEOPLE 30

see inset

Aboriginal population distribution

According to the 2001 census, the Aboriginal population in the province constituted 4.4% of the provincial total, based on self-identification. This may be a slight underestimate, as a few Indian reserves refused to participate in the census exercise, although estimates were made in those instances. Of those identifying themselves as Aboriginal, 70% were North American Indian, and 26% were Metis. If the results of the census are based on Aboriginal ancestry, rather than Aboriginal identity, then the percentage of the BC population with Aboriginal origin (or identity) is higher, at 5.6% (BC Statistics, 2004a)

The Aboriginal population tends to be much younger than the general population (approximately 30% are under 15 years old, almost twice the percentage for the non-Aboriginal population), and the population is reasonably mobile in that many reside on Indian reserves but frequently move between reserve and urban areas.

Percent Aboriginal population

As a percentage of total population by HSDA, there was a major geographic difference in values for percent of Aboriginal populations from more than one-quarter (25.05%) in the Northwest, to less than one percent (0.71%) in Richmond in the lower mainland.

Geographically, the northern half of the province had a greater representation of Aboriginal peoples, with each northern HSDA having more than 10% of its population self-identified as Aboriginal. Northern Vancouver Island and Thompson Cariboo Shuswap, in the interior of the province, also had populations that were approximately 10% Aboriginal.

By contrast, much of the lower mainland urban HSDAs had 2% or less of their population that self-identified as Aboriginal.

Distribution of total Aboriginal population

Based on the 2001 Canada census, the Aboriginal population was distributed geographically all around the province. The HSDAs with the largest Aboriginal populations were Thompson Cariboo Shuswap (20,290), Northwest (20,080), and Northern Interior (16,095). Each had approximately 10% or more.

Health Service Delivery Area	Percent Aboriginal	Distribution of Aboriginal population
051 Northwest	25.05	11.81
053 Northeast	13.27	4.70
052 Northern Interior	11.24	9.47
043 North Vancouver Island	10.75	3.40
014 Thompson Cariboo Shuswap	9.95	11.93
042 Central Vancouver Island	6.06	8.08
011 East Kootenay	5.10	2.25
021 Fraser East	4.90	6.74
033 North Shore/Coast Garibaldi	4.17	6.19
041 South Vancouver Island	3.67	8.14
013 Okanagan	3.51	6.07
012 Kootenay Boundary	3.08	1.37
023 Fraser South	2.04	6.86
032 Vancouver	2.02	6.53
022 Fraser North	1.93	5.78
031 Richmond	0.71	0.69
999 Province	**4.39**	**100.00**

At the other extreme, Richmond has a mere 0.69% of the province's Aboriginal population and East Kootenay and Kootenay Boundary, with 2.25% and 1.37% of the provincial Aboriginal population respectively, also have small numbers of Aboriginal peoples.

Many Aboriginal peoples live on reserve lands, some of which are quite remote (Elliott and Foster, 1995). In 2001, only one-third of those living on reserve did so in large urban areas. In total, 104,000 of the province's 170,000 Aboriginal people are registered under the Indian Act of Canada and belong to a Band, but only 27% live on reserve. Of those who are registered, over 40% live on reserve. Those living on reserve tend to be older (BC Statistics, 2004b).

Aboriginal population distribution

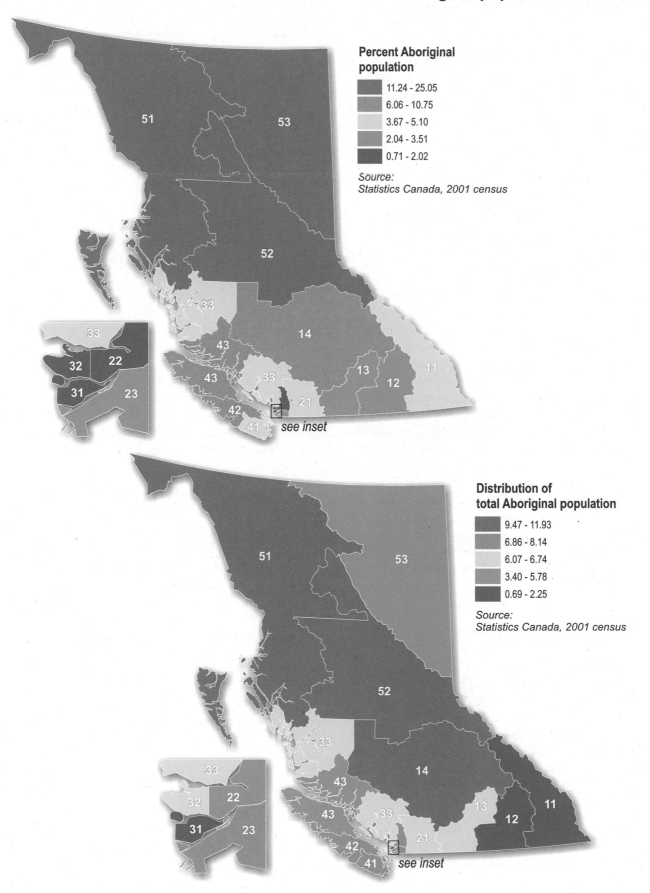

Percent Aboriginal population

- 11.24 - 25.05
- 6.06 - 10.75
- 3.67 - 5.10
- 2.04 - 3.51
- 0.71 - 2.02

Source:
Statistics Canada, 2001 census

Distribution of total Aboriginal population

- 9.47 - 11.93
- 6.86 - 8.14
- 6.07 - 6.74
- 3.40 - 5.78
- 0.69 - 2.25

Source:
Statistics Canada, 2001 census

Population age patterns

The three maps opposite provide a brief summary of the age breakdown of the population in 2005, based on P.E.O.P.L.E. 30 from BC Statistics. The data are provided at the HSDA, or regional, level and show the percentage of each HSDA population in 2005 by three different age categories. The top map looks at the 20 to 64 age cohort in the province and the bottom two maps show the distribution of the population below age 20 and the population in the seniors (age 65 and over) cohort. There are major differences throughout the province in proportions of the population in the three age groups.

Population 20 to 64 years old

This is by far the largest portion of the population, making up nearly two-thirds of the total for the province (63.31%). It consists of the post-war "baby boom" cohort, which is dominant not only in BC but throughout Canada. This group of the population is generally involved in the work environment and raising families. There was a 10 percentage point range between the HSDA with the highest (Vancouver at 68.86%) and lowest (Okanagan at 58.56%) percentage in this age group. Generally speaking, the lower mainland HSDAs in the southwest of the province (Vancouver, Fraser North, and Richmond) had the highest percentage (more than 65%) in the middle age, or 20 to 64 age cohort. Central Vancouver Island, Fraser East, and Okanagan in the interior (all with less than 60%) had the lowest proportion of their population in the 20 to 64 age group. All other HSDAs were between 61% and 64%.

Population below age 20

The percent of total provincial population in this age cohort in 2005 was 22.92%. The range between the highest and lowest HSDAs with population in this age cohort was over 12 percentage points. The northern, more rural HSDAs (Northwest, Northern Interior, and Northeast) all had more than one-quarter of their population in this young age group (more than 27.5%), while Vancouver and Richmond in the lower mainland, and South Vancouver Island, all urban areas, had about one-fifth or less of their population in this category.

Population 65 years or over

This map is almost the opposite of the previous map. The HSDAs with the highest percentage of their

Health Service Delivery Area	Ages <20 (%)	Ages 20-64 (%)	Ages 65+ (%)
032 Vancouver	18.10	68.86	13.04
031 Richmond	20.26	66.52	13.21
022 Fraser North	22.69	65.72	11.59
033 North Shore/Coast Garibaldi	21.77	63.93	14.30
052 Northern Interior	27.67	63.28	9.05
041 South Vancouver Island	20.00	62.73	17.27
023 Fraser South	25.68	62.67	11.66
011 East Kootenay	23.58	62.34	14.08
053 Northeast	30.58	61.94	7.48
051 Northwest	29.77	61.90	8.33
014 Thompson Cariboo Shuswap	23.91	61.79	14.30
043 North Vancouver Island	24.82	61.48	13.70
012 Kootenay Boundary	22.10	61.26	16.61
042 Central Vancouver Island	22.63	59.29	18.08
021 Fraser East	27.25	59.01	13.74
013 Okanagan	21.89	58.56	19.55
999 Province	**22.92**	**63.31**	**13.77**

populations in the seniors group were in the southern part of Vancouver Island and the Okanagan, which have all become favourable places to which people retire, not only from within BC, but also from elsewhere in Canada. By contrast, less than 10% of the northern part of the province were seniors. In total, only 13.77% of the population were seniors in 2005, but it is the fastest growing age group of the three.

Summary

Within the province, there were major variations in the age make-up of the population. The north had a substantial part of its population in the younger age groups, and a relatively small proportion who were seniors. The lower mainland dominated in the 20 to 64 age category, and the southern half of Vancouver Island and the Okanagan had a higher proportion of the seniors population.

Population age patterns

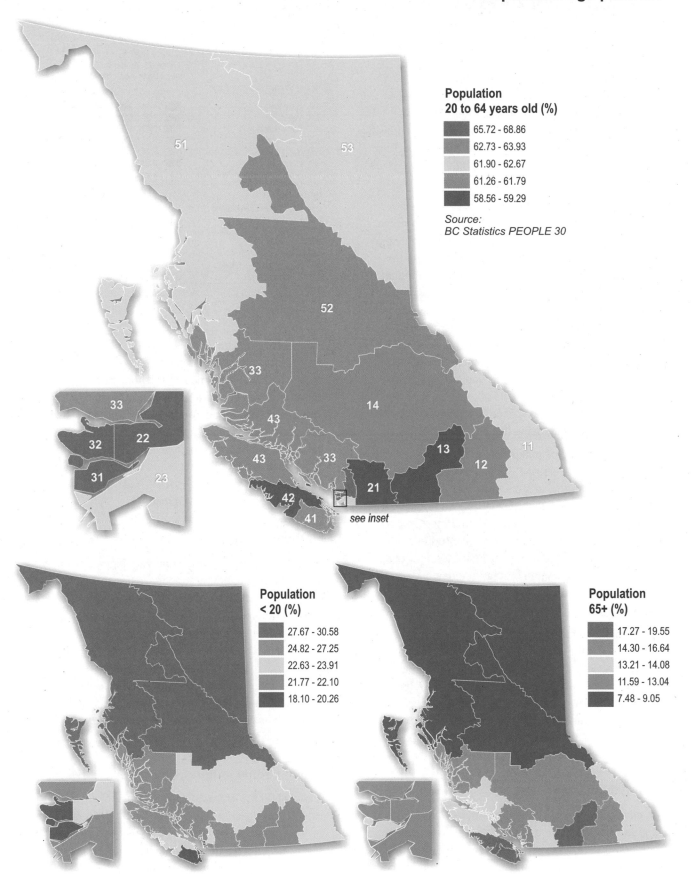

**Population
20 to 64 years old (%)**

- 65.72 - 68.86
- 62.73 - 63.93
- 61.90 - 62.67
- 61.26 - 61.79
- 58.56 - 59.29

*Source:
BC Statistics PEOPLE 30*

see inset

**Population
< 20 (%)**

- 27.67 - 30.58
- 24.82 - 27.25
- 22.63 - 23.91
- 21.77 - 22.10
- 18.10 - 20.26

**Population
65+ (%)**

- 17.27 - 19.55
- 14.30 - 16.64
- 13.21 - 14.08
- 11.59 - 13.04
- 7.48 - 9.05

Recent immigrants and language

Over the past couple of decades, BC has had a major influx of new foreign-born individuals. In 2001, there were over one million such immigrants living in BC, accounting for more than a quarter of the total population. The immigrant population has been growing much faster than the Canadian-born population. This trend will have a major effect on the health and wellness attributes of the BC population.

The majority of immigrants in the province have lived in Canada for more than 20 years. A higher percentage of the early immigrants came from Europe (mainly the United Kingdom or Germany) and the United States, and European immigrants make up more than a third of the province's immigrant population, and more than three-quarters of the immigrants that arrived in Canada prior to 1980. Asian immigrants (mainly from Mainland China, Hong Kong, and India), on the other hand, account for over one-half of the immigrant population and more than three-quarters arrived in Canada after 1980. Approximately two-thirds of these later immigrants were between the ages of 25 and 64 years, with females slightly outnumbering males (BC Statistics, 2003).

Approximately 10% of immigrants in 2001 were unable to speak, write, or understand English or French. This puts many new immigrants at a disadvantage in contributing to those parts of the economy that rely on English as the language of communication. Furthermore, it may also disadvantage, at least initially, the progress of younger children in the school system (Kershaw et al., 2005). The most common mother tongues used by non-English speaking immigrants were Cantonese, Mandarin, Punjabi, Tagalog, Korean, and Farsi.

New immigrants tend to be healthier than native-born Canadians. This "healthy immigrant effect" is related to the fact that potential immigrants are screened on health and medical criteria before being admitted to Canada. In addition, there is some degree of self-selection in the originating countries, which also can affect the wellness of new immigrants entering BC (Ng, Wilkins, Gendron, and Berthelot, 2005).

Recent immigrants

The distribution of new immigrants (those entering Canada between 1996 and 2001) is based on data from the 2001 Canada census. Overall, nearly 1 in every 20 people in the province were new immigrants in

Health Service Delivery Area	Recent immigrant (%)	Mother tongue non-official (%)	Foreign language (%)
031 Richmond	14.58	52.72	24.96
032 Vancouver	9.97	47.87	21.68
022 Fraser North	9.43	34.29	13.18
023 Fraser South	5.37	28.01	10.59
033 North Shore/Coast Garibaldi	5.24	19.70	5.25
021 Fraser East	2.58	19.01	5.78
041 South Vancouver Island	1.41	10.57	2.11
013 Okanagan	1.04	12.19	1.71
053 Northeast	1.01	8.49	1.78
042 Central Vancouver Island	0.81	8.30	1.12
011 East Kootenay	0.75	7.59	0.60
014 Thompson Cariboo Shuswap	0.72	9.61	1.41
051 Northwest	0.67	13.01	1.80
012 Kootenay Boundary	0.63	11.66	0.90
043 North Vancouver Island	0.59	8.01	1.25
052 Northern Interior	0.50	9.61	1.61
999 Province	**4.95**	**24.29**	**8.77**

2001. Geographically, there was a major cluster of new immigrants in the lower mainland area in the southwest of the province. In particular, the population of Richmond was comprised of nearly 15%, while Vancouver and Fraser North both had nearly 10% of their population comprised of new immigrants. Other HSDAs in the lower mainland had relatively high levels of new immigrants when compared to the rest of the province. Outside of the lower mainland, most HSDAs had 1% or less of their population who were new immigrants.

Mother tongue

Some parts of the province had very high numbers of residents whose mother tongue was neither English nor French. The lower mainland HSDAs all had populations of approximately 20% or more whose mother tongue was not one of the official two languages. Richmond with 52.72% and Vancouver at 47.87% had by far the largest numbers of residents with a foreign mother tongue. At the other extreme, East Kootenay in the southeast, North and Central Vancouver Island, Northeast, Thompson Cariboo Shuswap, and Northern Interior all had populations less than 10% with a foreign mother tongue.

Foreign home language

A total of 8.77% of the BC population spoke a language other than English or French at home. The pattern was very similar to the previous two maps described, with the lower mainland HSDAs having the highest percentage of foreign language use in the home.

Recent immigrants and language

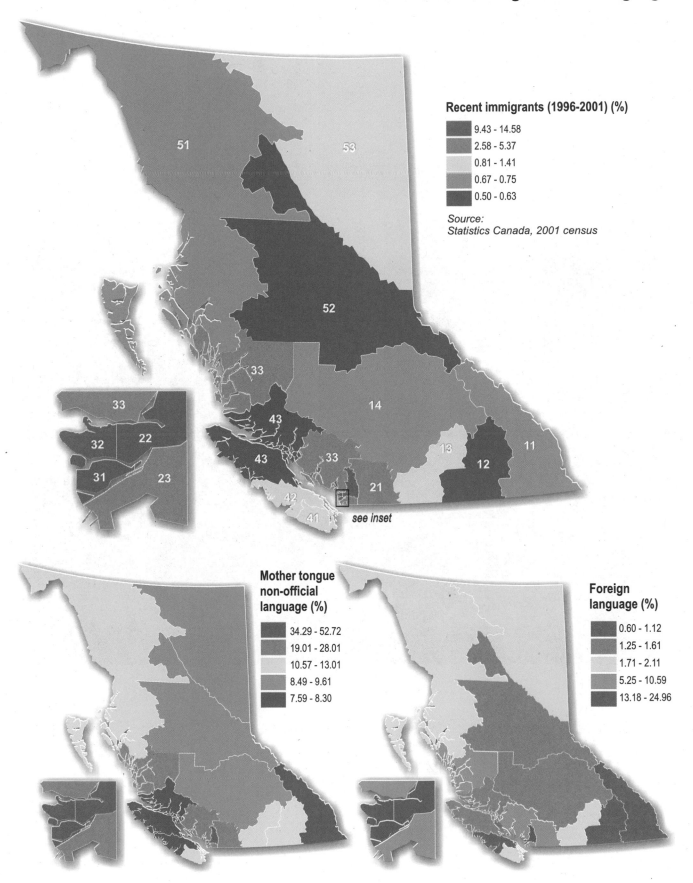

Recent immigrants (1996-2001) (%)

- 9.43 - 14.58
- 2.58 - 5.37
- 0.81 - 1.41
- 0.67 - 0.75
- 0.50 - 0.63

Source:
Statistics Canada, 2001 census

see inset

Mother tongue non-official language (%)

- 34.29 - 52.72
- 19.01 - 28.01
- 10.57 - 13.01
- 8.49 - 9.61
- 7.59 - 8.30

Foreign language (%)

- 0.60 - 1.12
- 1.25 - 1.61
- 1.71 - 2.11
- 5.25 - 10.59
- 13.18 - 24.96

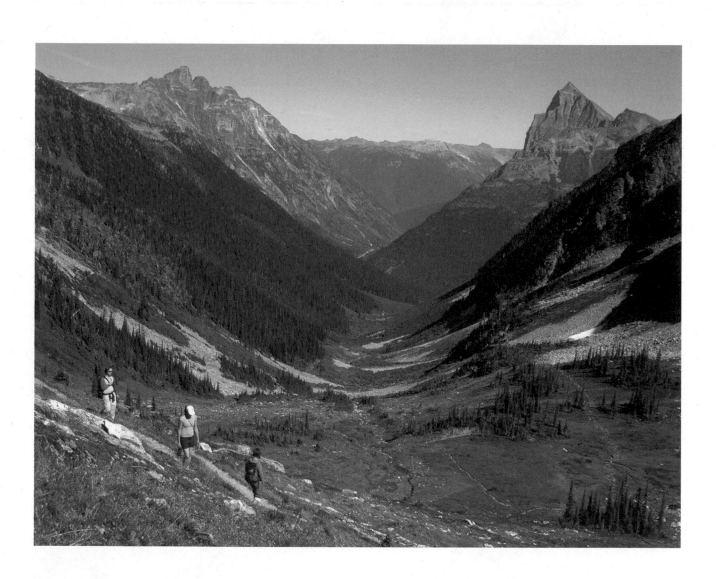

5

The Geography of Wellness in British Columbia

British Columbia, as discussed previously, is a very diverse province geographically. This includes its physical and demographic environments. It is also a province whose environments continue to evolve and change. This chapter presents the main focus of the Atlas, which is the geographical presentation of wellness throughout the province. At the outset, it must be recognized that this is a static snapshot of wellness in BC. Like other aspects of its environment, wellness and its assets and indicators will continue to evolve over time as the population shifts increasingly to a multicultural one, to one that is older, and to one that becomes more concentrated in urban areas, particularly in the southwest part of the province in the lower mainland, southern and eastern parts of Vancouver Island, and in the Okanagan region of the southern interior.

There are seven main sections to this chapter. The first (5.1) presents a variety of mapped indicators that portray a series of assets or determinants of wellness and health. In total, there are more than 60 maps providing data and geographic patterns for approximately 30 wellness indicators. They cover the key areas of family structure and economic characteristics, social assets for and determinants of wellness, educational indicators for several age groups, safety indicators, and finally, civic engagement. Many of these maps provide data at the Health Service Delivery Area (HSDA) level, but some, specifically those related to education, provide data at the school district level.

The second section (5.2) provides information on one of the key ActNow BC pillars—the reduction of smoking throughout the province. More than 30 maps show the geography of smoke-free environments in BC. Maps provide information on school smoking prevention policies and the distribution of population

covered by municipal no smoking bylaws. Most of the maps, however, are based on results from the Canadian Community Health Survey (CCHS) undertaken in 2005. Maps cover smoke-free environments such as public places, workplaces, vehicles, and homes, and also look at variations in non-smoking behaviours throughout the province. Each of these maps provides geographic information at the HSDA level for the total respondents of the survey, and for sub-components based on age cohorts (12 to 19 years, and 65 years and over) and gender. Those HSDAs that are significantly different from the provincial averages are identified.

The third section (5.3) provides a variety of indicators related to a second pillar of ActNow BC—nutrition and food security. Approximately 25 maps provide information on breastfeeding, healthy eating, healthy food education, nutrition policies in schools and school districts, and food availability in the form of farmers' markets.

The fourth section (5.4) provides nearly 50 maps focused on a third pillar of ActNow BC—physical activity. Information is given on available assets that enable individuals to undertake different kinds of activities. These include specific types of recreation facilities such as ice rinks and swimming pools, activity centres such as seniors centres and community halls, as well as outdoor opportunities provided through the availability of sports fields such as soccer pitches and baseball diamonds. Some of these data, which are based on surveys, are incomplete and so caution in analysing the geographic patterns is required. However, it is useful to know that these data on recreation and activity assets exist for those interested in understanding, and planning for, activity levels throughout the province. Information is also provided on the distribution of walking clubs and public transit use and coverage within the province. Membership data in specific sports clubs are also included, along with the location of national and provincial parks.

The fifth section (5.5), which is short, looks at issues related to healthy weights. Healthy weights are closely related to aspects of nutrition and physical activity levels of individuals. Data are provided at the HSDA level based on responses to a couple of questions on the CCHS. In all, 10 maps are presented.

The sixth section (5.6) provides a series of indicators related to healthy pregnancies and childbirth. ActNow BC is concerned with healthy choices in pregnancy related to alcohol consumption and concerns about Fetal Alcohol Syndrome Disorder (FASD), but there are few data available related to this condition for mapping purposes. While one FASD-related indicator is included, we have chosen to provide healthy pregnancy indicators based primarily on data from the Vital Statistics Agency covering the 5 year period 2001 to 2005 inclusive. Indicators show the degree of complications-free perinatal and maternal conditions during pregnancy and childbirth. In addition, maps provide information on the healthiest age for mothers to conceive, and the geography of healthy birth weights, full term deliveries, infants born free of congenital anomalies, and infant survival rates. These are all important factors for the future wellness of individuals. The data are all shown at the HSDA level. Smoking-free behaviour rates in pregnancy are also mapped. Finally, the availability of Pregnancy Outreach Programs is provided.

The final section (5.7) of this chapter provides 50 maps and 10 indicators on self-assessed wellness features based on response data from the CCHS. Topics covered include general health, mental health, both chronic- and injury-free conditions, and the degree of satisfaction with life. All CCHS question indicators are provided at the HSDA level by gender and by age group. A final indicator looks at life expectancy at birth for the total population and for each gender individually by HSDA.

5.1 Assets and Determinants

Research has shown that numerous factors are assets and determinants of health and wellness (see Chapter 2). This section provides a variety of maps that focus on some of these key factors. Individuals and communities that possess these wellness-related factors are more likely to possess better health and wellness status than those without them. Many of the data presented in this section are drawn from the 2001 Canada census. Although several years old, these data are still generally the most current for the purposes of geographic comparisons. Other data, which focus on school children, use information from school districts and the Ministry of Education (2004 to 2006), and also from the latest McCreary Adolescent Health Survey (2003). Other indicators are based on a variety of different sources, including the Ministry of Children and Family Development, the public libraries system, the court system, and the Electoral Office of BC.

The first nine maps look at indicators related to family structure and economics. Children living at home do far better than those living alone or in state care (Kendall, 2001; Foster and Wright, 2002; Kendall and Morley, 2006). Children living with two adults have a greater likelihood of thriving than those in lone parent families. Single parenthood is generally tougher on both parent and child than living in a two adult family, thus potentially compromising wellness. Adults living together are better able to provide many kinds of different supports for each other throughout life, thus increasing wellness for both individuals.

Gender is also important. Women have a longer life expectancy than men, but usually report being less healthy. For some, their final years may be spent alone in relative poverty with chronic disabilities, all of which affect their sense of wellness. In 2000/2001 Canada-wide, more than 4 million women compared with less than 3 million men reported having two or more chronic conditions, and over half a million more women than men reported having disabilities based on an assessment of their functional health (Canadian Institute for Health Information, 2004). A recent study on chronic conditions in BC showed women were much more likely than men to have confirmed chronic conditions and have co-morbidity of such conditions (Broemeling, Watson, and Black, 2005). The percentage

of young and old who are (theoretically) supported by the working age group is also a useful community wellness indicator, as is the diversity of income sources within a community. High levels of income diversity result in more stable communities. Three indicators of family economics complete this cluster of family/community-related wellness factors. The first looks at the employment rate. The second provides median household income, which is that income level that has 50% of the province's households both above and below it. At the population level, health and wellness status increases as income increases. The third indicator, known as the Low Income Cut-off (LICO), is an income threshold, calculated by examining family expenditure data, below which families spend more of their household income on food, clothing, and shelter than would an average family. It is a measure, although not the only one, of relative poverty. This indicator is not without controversy (Statistics Canada, 2006), but one in general use.

The second group of indicators deals with a variety of social issues. A total of 24 maps provide data on issues related to home ownership and housing affordability, as well as attachment to school and family for students, and community attachment for the broader population. Housing is a key asset for wellness. It provides shelter, a place for families to form and bond, and a place where friends and neighbours can gather to socialize and share time, experiences, and support when needed. Shelter is one of the key basic needs of individuals. Housing provides not only protection, but also security and stability. However, not all housing is perfect, and poor housing conditions can lead to health and wellness reduction. The cost of housing can make it very difficult for low income families to find adequate accommodation.

A key indicator that has been shown to be important for positive youth development and wellness is that of family connectedness: youth with high levels of family connectedness have a reduced likelihood of engaging in a variety of risky behaviours, such as early sexual activity, smoking cigarettes or marijuana, other drug use, getting into fights, or experiencing emotional distress or considering suicide (McCreary Centre Society, 2004; Tonkin, 2005).

A student's connectedness to school has been shown to be important for health and wellness and for positive youth development. Based on data from the National Longitudinal Survey of Children and Youth, the Canadian Institute for Health Information has shown that a high level of school engagement for 12- to 15-year-olds was significantly related, statistically, to a variety of factors such as high self-worth, excellent or very good health, low level of anxiety, and a lower likelihood of alcohol, tobacco, and marijuana use and of associating with peers who commit crimes (Canadian Institute for Health Information, 2005). Similar results have been found using the McCreary Adolescent Health Survey data for Grade 7 to Grade 12 students (Tonkin, 2005).

Where people live is important from a wellness perspective. In a speech on determinants of people's health, Roy Romanow made this recommendation: "Be sure to live in a community where you trust your neighbours and feel that you belong: a civil and trusting community promotes health and long life" (as quoted in Canadian Institute for Health Information, 2004, p. 12). The next several maps show data, by gender and age group, indicating the level of social and emotional supports individuals feel they have available to them.

The next cluster of maps (22) indicate education and learning characteristics and opportunities within BC. Health and wellness generally increase with level of education. Getting a good start in life is a key determinant of health and wellness. Prenatal and early childhood events and experiences have been shown to have major impacts on later health and wellness (Canadian Institute for Health Information, 2004). In BC, an Early Development Instrument (EDI), which is a population-based tool, assesses the state of child development for kindergarten students throughout the province. It is generally acknowledged that, because our abilities and choices differ, complete equality in outcomes for individuals across a population is likely unattainable. Rather, it is equality of opportunity that is generally accepted as a desirable, attainable goal. Education is not only a key determinant of wellness, but is important for health, labour market participation, and social inclusion (Canadian Institute for Health Information, 2004). It is one of society's most effective means of providing children from various backgrounds with similar opportunities to attain positive outcomes. For society, universal quality education is the foundation of an egalitarian, socially coherent, and progressive society and essential for future self-fulfilment, economic productivity gains, and poverty reduction.

Not all children at school are in a grade normally associated with their age. Variations between groups of children from different backgrounds or gender can be symptomatic of opportunity inequality. For instance, Aboriginal children, students from socio-economically deprived backgrounds, and children in the care of the state are less likely than other children to be in a grade appropriate for their age (Kendall and Turpel-Lafond, 2007). This measure may also be a useful barometer of general wellness and social well-being and a leading indicator of future graduation rates within a geographic area, in this case, a school district. Four maps are presented based on this indicator.

Graduation from high school is an important event in life's developmental trajectory. It is a major step toward initiating post-secondary education and the lifelong benefits that come from that pursuit: improved employment opportunities, critical thinking, participation in society and social structures, to name but a few. Four maps related to graduation are included.

In a knowledge-based economy, lifelong learning is important for most individuals. It is a process that involves the development of skills, knowledge, and values from early childhood through to adulthood. Several maps are presented on lifelong learning.

Libraries are important institutions for assisting with lifelong learning. While they provide a traditional service of lending out print and other media to the public at no direct charge, they are also important locations for socialization and other activities, including educational opportunities. In particular, most libraries run literacy and reading programs, especially for the young, and literacy, in and of itself, is an important wellness asset. A recent report has suggested that as much as 55% of Canada's adult population may be jeopardizing their health because of an inability to understand prescription information, nutrition labels, or safety instructions (Canadian Council on Learning, 2007). Furthermore, all public libraries in BC provide free access to the internet so that individuals can gain a broader knowledge on a variety of topics, including issues related to health literacy and wellness.

The next six maps provide information on community safety. Students spend a large part of their daily lives in a school setting. There is "a recognition that a strong relationship exists between feelings of safety and belonging and a student's ability to learn" (Ministry of Education, 2004, p. 3). Furthermore, the feeling of safety at school enhances a student's mental health. Crime rates are a measure of community cohesion, safety, and wellness. While crime is a "negative" indicator of community wellness, it is an important consideration when looking at key community indicators.

The final map in this section provides a measure of civic engagement. Community activities of individuals is a useful measure of their commitment to their community. These commitments not only benefit the individual, but usually make the community stronger, more cohesive, and healthier. Civic engagement results in interactions with others through, for example, social clubs, voluntary organizations, school groups for both students and parents, and faith groups. Community wellness and social capital is enhanced by increased civic engagement. While there are many variables, too numerous to mention, that can be used to measure civic engagement, we have focused on one: the rate of voting by registered voters in the last (2005) provincial election.

Family structure

Children living at home

The proportion of children living with their family, rather than being in the care of the province or living independently through a Youth Agreement with the province, is a useful indicator of community and family social and economic well-being. It also measures the effectiveness of community supports for families in need. While socio-economic deprivation is associated with depression, very low self-esteem, substance abuse, and other issues that affect parents' ability to care for their children, factors such as community resources, cohesiveness, and social capital are significant mediators. This is true of all population groups, but it must be acknowledged that Aboriginal children are less likely to be living at home than other British Columbian children (Foster and Wright, 2002; Foster and Wharf, 2007).

In BC throughout 2005, 98.52% of children (individuals aged 0 to 18 years) were living at home for the whole year. This ranged from 99.38% in Richmond to 97.86% in Thompson Cariboo Shuswap. Rates were higher in lower mainland HSDAs and Kootenay Boundary in the southeast interior of the province. A range of approximately 1.5% may seem very small, but children not living at home are but a small proportion of the neediest of all children. From small differences in the rate of children living at home, large differences in the social wellness of communities can be inferred.

Children living in two parent families

Single parents generally experience greater challenges in child rearing. They tend to be poorer economically and have a greater challenge balancing life's requirements around work and family. They are more socially isolated, in general, than two parent families. In short, children with two adults in their life generally do better. Throughout BC in 2001, nearly four out of every five children were being raised in a two parent family. The range within the province went from 85.93% (Richmond) to 75.14% (Central Vancouver Island). The lower mainland (with the exception of Vancouver) and Northeast were above the provincial average on this indicator. The lowest values were in the northern two-thirds of Vancouver Island and Thompson Cariboo Shuswap in the interior.

Health Service Delivery Area	Children living at home (%)	Children in two parent families (%)	Couples living together (%)
031 Richmond	99.38	85.93	59.69
012 Kootenay Boundary	99.22	76.98	61.00
033 North Shore/Coast Garibaldi	99.21	82.93	59.99
022 Fraser North	99.15	81.70	58.12
032 Vancouver	99.08	79.37	49.19
023 Fraser South	98.96	82.90	62.28
053 Northeast	98.81	82.57	62.65
011 East Kootenay	98.63	78.94	63.24
041 South Vancouver Island	98.55	77.03	57.61
043 North Vancouver Island	98.50	75.30	61.87
013 Okanagan	98.47	77.14	62.36
052 Northern Interior	98.32	76.84	60.25
042 Central Vancouver Island	98.28	75.14	61.69
021 Fraser East	98.21	80.25	62.05
051 Northwest	98.00	77.30	60.82
014 Thompson Cariboo Shuswap	97.86	76.55	61.67
999 Province	**98.52**	**79.80**	**58.86**

Couples living together

Adults living together, whether legally married or in a common-law relationship, are able to share many aspects of living, such as income, household duties, and child rearing, to name but a few. Mutual emotional and social supports are provided and, in times of ill health, caring is immediately at hand. For males, those who are married tend to live longer. In BC, nearly 6 out of every 10 adults live in a relationship with another adult. The highest rates were in East Kootenay, Northeast, Okanagan, and Fraser East (all greater than 62%). Most other regions were about average or above, except for Vancouver, where more than half of the adults were not living in a shared relationship.

Family structure

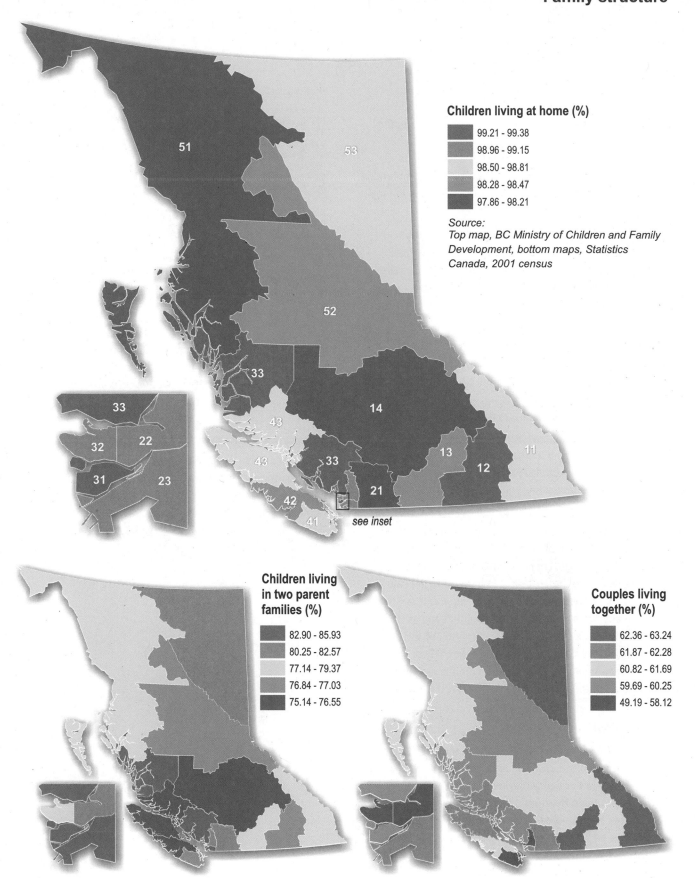

Children living at home (%)

- 99.21 - 99.38
- 98.96 - 99.15
- 98.50 - 98.81
- 98.28 - 98.47
- 97.86 - 98.21

Source:
Top map, BC Ministry of Children and Family Development, bottom maps, Statistics Canada, 2001 census

see inset

Children living in two parent families (%)

- 82.90 - 85.93
- 80.25 - 82.57
- 77.14 - 79.37
- 76.84 - 77.03
- 75.14 - 76.55

Couples living together (%)

- 62.36 - 63.24
- 61.87 - 62.28
- 60.82 - 61.69
- 59.69 - 60.25
- 49.19 - 58.12

Gender, dependency, and income diversity

Gender: Female population

In 2005, 50.78% of the province's population were women. Geographically, however, there were important regional trends in the distribution of women among the HSDAs. Higher than average percentages of women than men were evident in parts of the lower mainland, particularly Richmond and North Shore/Coast Garibaldi, in South Vancouver Island, and in the Okanagan in the interior of the province.

By contrast, several northern and interior HSDAs had more males than females. These included the three northern HSDAs (Northwest, Northeast, and Northern Interior), North Vancouver Island, and East Kootenay in the southeast.

Health Service Delivery Area	Female population (%)	Dependency rate (%)	Economic diversity index
041 South Vancouver Island	52.04	53.30	59
013 Okanagan	51.62	63.10	72
031 Richmond	51.61	44.94	71
033 North Shore/Coast Garibaldi	51.11	50.27	75
042 Central Vancouver Island	51.04	61.08	69
032 Vancouver	50.77	40.97	71
022 Fraser North	50.74	46.51	71
023 Fraser South	50.73	52.75	72
021 Fraser East	50.55	61.20	72
014 Thompson Cariboo Shuswap	50.16	54.29	72
012 Kootenay Boundary	50.15	55.73	72
011 East Kootenay	49.80	52.96	76
052 Northern Interior	49.20	50.48	61
043 North Vancouver Island	49.13	54.82	70
053 Northeast	48.61	53.45	74
051 Northwest	48.60	53.21	68
999 Province	**50.78**	**51.53**	**N/A**

Dependency rate

This looks at the combined number of children (aged 0 to 17 years) and seniors (aged 65 and over) as a percentage of the population in the 18 to 64 age group. This indicator gives a sense of the ability of the "working age population" to support the young and the old, both economically and as their caregivers. The lower the rate, the greater the likelihood that the resident population can support the young and old dependents.

For the province as a whole, the overall dependency rate is 51.53, which means that there are about twice as many people available than those requiring "looking after" or supporting. There are, however, variations in this rate among the HSDAs. The range in the rate is more than 22 points. The HSDAs with the lowest dependency rates occur in the lower mainland HSDAs, particularly Vancouver (40.97), Richmond (44.94), and Fraser North (46.51). By contrast, three HSDAs have rates in excess of 60: Okanagan in the interior, Fraser East in the south, and Central Vancouver Island.

Economic diversity index

This is a measure of the degree of income source diversity within a region. The less dependent a region is on one dominant industry, the more likely it is to be able to weather volatile economic times. The index includes several key economic sectors (Forestry, Mining, Fishing, Agriculture and Food, Tourism, High Technology, Public Sector, Construction, Other, Government Transfers [e.g., pensions], and Non-employment Income). The most

diversified region economically would have its income sources divided equally among the economic sectors and its value would be 100. If its value were zero (0), it would only have one income source (Horne, 2004).

For BC, the diversity index ranges from a high of 76 for East Kootenay, to a low of 59 for South Vancouver Island, which is heavily dependent upon the public sector for its economy. Northern Interior and Northwest, both dominated by the public sector and forestry, also have relatively low indices, while Northeast and North Shore/Coast Garibaldi have more diversified economies.

Gender, dependency, and income diversity

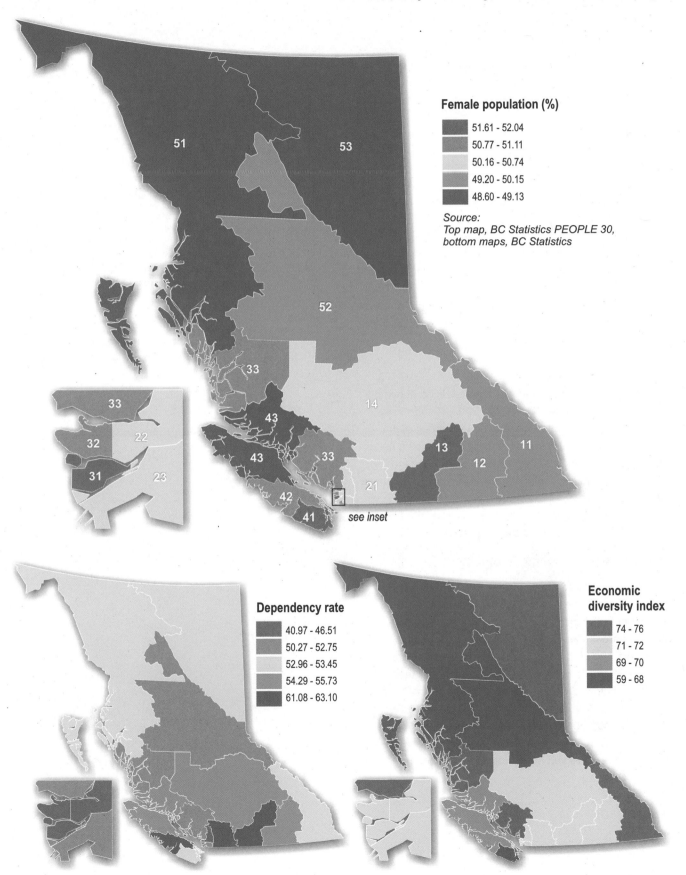

Female population (%)

51.61 - 52.04
50.77 - 51.11
50.16 - 50.74
49.20 - 50.15
48.60 - 49.13

*Source:
Top map, BC Statistics PEOPLE 30,
bottom maps, BC Statistics*

Dependency rate

40.97 - 46.51
50.27 - 52.75
52.96 - 53.45
54.29 - 55.73
61.08 - 63.10

Economic diversity index

74 - 76
71 - 72
69 - 70
59 - 68

Family economics

Income and economic stability are important not only to individuals and families, but also to the communities in which they live. Having a good, enjoyable, and well-paying job is important for health and wellness.

Employment rate

In 2001, the employment rate in BC was nearly 60%, although the range among HSDAs was quite large at 15 percentage points. HSDAs with higher rates of employment were in the north, parts of the lower mainland, and North Vancouver Island (all greater than 60%). At 67.3%, Northeast had the highest employment rate, followed by Fraser South and North Shore/Coast Garibaldi in the southwest, and Northern Interior. The areas with the lowest employment rates occurred in the southern interior and Central Vancouver Island (all about 55% or lower).

Low income cut-off

More than four out of every five families lived above the low income cut-off (LICO) level in 2001. There were major regional variations, however, with much of the northern half and southeast parts of the province being well above the average, while several HSDAs in the lower mainland had relatively fewer families living above the LICO level set for that year. Vancouver, Richmond, and Fraser North were relatively low, all with less than 79% of households above the LICO level.

Median annual family income

For BC as a whole, the median annual family income in 2001 was $46,802, but there was quite a range throughout the province. The higher median family income areas were in the lower mainland and the northern half of the province. Fraser South, with a median family income of nearly $56,000, was the highest, followed by its neighbour North Shore/Coast Garibaldi at over $54,000. The northern HSDAs were all above $50,000, as was Richmond in the southwest. Kootenay Boundary, Okanagan, and Central Vancouver Island all had median household incomes below $41,000.

Health Service Delivery Area	Employment rate (%)	Above LICO (%)	Median income ($ Can)
053 Northeast	67.30	88.52	53225
023 Fraser South	63.20	84.46	55945
033 North Shore/Coast Garibaldi	62.60	86.28	54128
052 Northern Interior	62.20	85.71	50134
022 Fraser North	61.70	78.62	49877
043 North Vancouver Island	60.00	84.83	46055
051 Northwest	59.80	86.49	51754
032 Vancouver	59.60	72.95	42090
021 Fraser East	59.40	85.42	45207
041 South Vancouver Island	59.20	85.66	45733
011 East Kootenay	59.10	86.93	43948
031 Richmond	58.80	76.14	50060
014 Thompson Cariboo Shuswap	57.20	85.00	42879
012 Kootenay Boundary	55.40	85.92	39673
013 Okanagan	53.60	85.49	40002
042 Central Vancouver Island	52.60	83.84	40973
999 Province	**59.60**	**82.25**	**46802**

Family economics

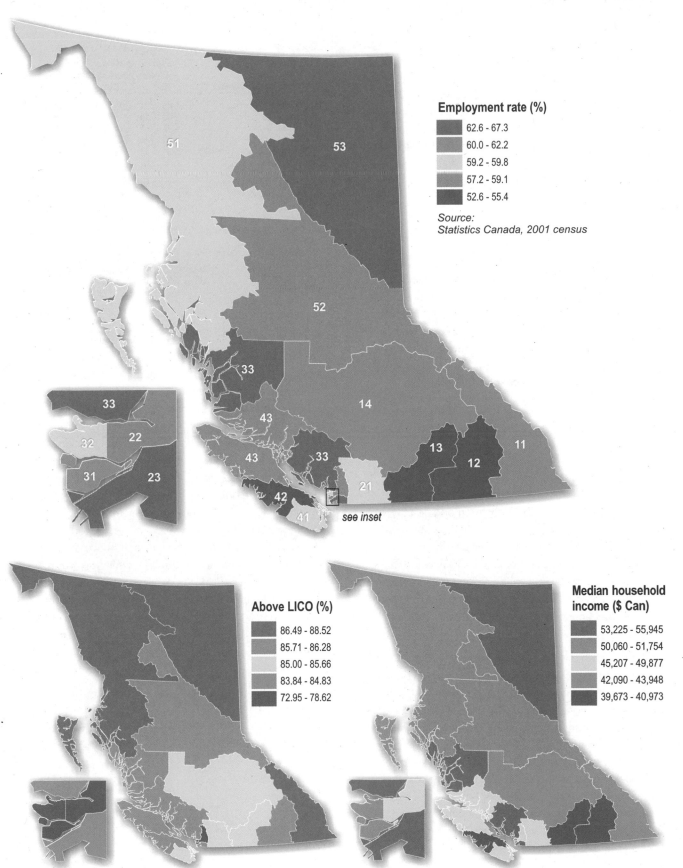

Employment rate (%)

- 62.6 - 67.3
- 60.0 - 62.2
- 59.2 - 59.8
- 57.2 - 59.1
- 52.6 - 55.4

Source:
Statistics Canada, 2001 census

see inset

Above LICO (%)

- 86.49 - 88.52
- 85.71 - 86.28
- 85.00 - 85.66
- 83.84 - 84.83
- 72.95 - 78.62

Median household income ($ Can)

- 53,225 - 55,945
- 50,060 - 51,754
- 45,207 - 49,877
- 42,090 - 43,948
- 39,673 - 40,973

Selected housing characteristics

Three indicators related to housing provide information that shows the percentage of the population exhibiting certain housing characteristics based on the 2001 census. The three indicators, which are mapped opposite, are as follows: a measure of those who moved in the 12 month period immediately prior to the census, owner occupied housing, and households spending more than 30% of their income on accommodation.

Moved in the past year

Stability of residence is significant in terms of developing social capital and cohesive neighbourhoods and communities. It is also important for learning outcomes for children (Kershaw et al., 2005). In the 12 months prior to the census, 16.39% of households moved. The most stable HSDAs were in the southwest (Richmond and Fraser South) and southeast (Kootenay Boundary) parts of the province. Households in Northeast, Vancouver, and South Vancouver Island were the most likely to have moved.

Owner occupied dwelling

Home ownership is an important desire of most individuals and families. It provides security and stability. Stability helps to build strong and healthy neighbourhoods as well as healthy communities, one of the objectives of ActNow BC initiatives. In 2001 in BC, nearly two-thirds of households (66.31%) owned their own accommodation, indicating a reasonable amount of stability and security for the population. It also indicated an important financial investment that families make for the future.

Home ownership varied dramatically by HSDA throughout the province, as shown on the map opposite. Home ownership was greatest in the southeast part of the province (more than three-quarters of households in Kootenay Boundary and East Kootenay owned their own accommodation) and there were ownership rates above the provincial average throughout most of the province. Rates for the southwest lower mainland, particularly Vancouver and Fraser North, were below the provincial rate, as was South Vancouver Island. These HSDAs are also where much of the province's population resides.

Health Service Delivery Area	Moved in past year (%)	Owner occ. dwelling (%)	Less than 30% on housing (%)
012 Kootenay Boundary	13.91	76.97	77.10
031 Richmond	14.18	70.90	68.97
023 Fraser South	14.61	73.71	71.28
011 East Kootenay	15.17	76.59	79.34
033 North Shore/Coast Garibaldi	15.37	69.24	72.75
051 Northwest	15.63	71.17	79.10
014 Thompson Cariboo Shuswap	15.90	73.58	75.64
042 Central Vancouver Island	15.96	73.82	74.28
022 Fraser North	15.96	63.71	69.97
021 Fraser East	16.10	71.51	70.98
052 Northern Interior	16.19	73.00	77.82
043 North Vancouver Island	16.61	71.54	77.64
013 Okanagan	16.64	73.17	72.99
041 South Vancouver Island	17.34	65.63	72.08
032 Vancouver	19.73	43.79	64.55
053 Northeast	20.16	70.30	80.29
999 Province	**16.39**	**66.31**	**71.52**

Spending less than 30% on housing

Spending less than 30% of the household income on housing is viewed as a desirable goal. More than this amount and households have to reduce expenditures on other necessities, such as food. Within BC in 2001, more than 7 out of every 10 households (71.52%) spent less than the 30% "limit" on their accommodation. Most of the province, geographically, was above the provincial average, and much of the northern and interior parts of the province had rates in excess of 75% spending less than 30% of household income on housing. The urban southwest of the province, however, had rates below 70%, and in Vancouver, less than two-thirds of households were within the 30% limit. It is worth noting that, since 2001, the average residential price in BC has jumped from almost $221,000 to more than $390,000 in 2006, and costs are especially high in the lower mainland, lower Vancouver Island, and Okanagan. These costs continue to climb.

Selected housing characteristics

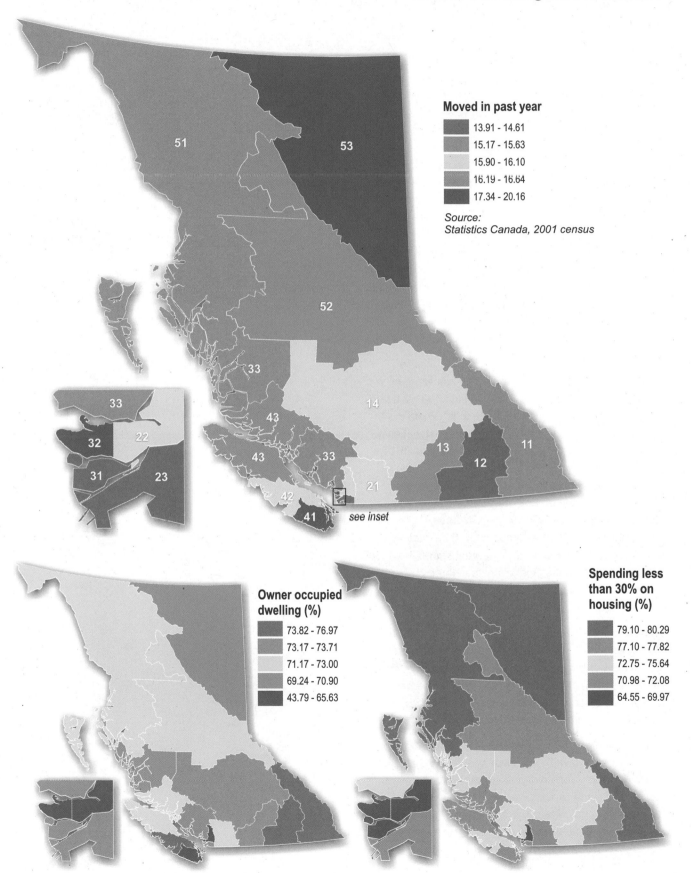

Moved in past year

- 13.91 - 14.61
- 15.17 - 15.63
- 15.90 - 16.10
- 16.19 - 16.64
- 17.34 - 20.16

Source:
Statistics Canada, 2001 census

see inset

Owner occupied dwelling (%)

- 73.82 - 76.97
- 73.17 - 73.71
- 71.17 - 73.00
- 69.24 - 70.90
- 43.79 - 65.63

Spending less than 30% on housing (%)

- 79.10 - 80.29
- 77.10 - 77.82
- 72.75 - 75.64
- 70.98 - 72.08
- 64.55 - 69.97

Family connectedness for youth

The family connectedness scale used here includes 11 items from the McCreary Adolescent Health Survey. The questions ask about the extent to which students feel their family understands them, pays attention to them, and has fun together. It includes separate items about their relationships with mothers and fathers, such as how close they feel and how much they feel cared about by their mother or their father, how much their mothers or fathers are warm and loving towards them, how satisfied they are with their relationships with their mother or father, and so on. Students who have only one parent or who live with other relatives can still receive a score if they have responded to a minimum of three questions in the scale. The Family Connectedness score is created by averaging the responses of the questions answered, standardized on a scale of 0 to 1, with 1 being the highest connectedness and 0 being the lowest (Saewyc, 2007). The scores here have been multiplied by 100.

Overall, youth in BC had a connectedness score of 78.02 (out of a possible score of 100) in 2003. While the range went from a high of 79.65 to a low of 76.34, several HSDAs were significantly different statistically from the provincial score. The lower mainland HSDAs of North Shore/Coast Garibaldi and Fraser North, along with South Vancouver Island, all had scores of 79 or higher. At the other extreme, Vancouver had a statistically significantly lower than average score, as did Northern Interior. Geographically, there was no clear macro regional pattern observable throughout the province. (Note that school districts in three HSDAs are not represented as they did not participate in this survey, and so the middle "quintile" has only one HSDA.)

There were significant differences between genders. Males (with a score of 79.30) had statistically significantly stronger family connectedness than females (score of 76.76). Not only was this difference observed for the province as a whole, but eight of the HSDAs had statistically significant differences between the genders.

Geographically, North Shore/Coast Garibaldi and South Vancouver Island were statistically significantly higher for males, and Vancouver and Northern Interior were statistically significantly lower. For females, North Shore/Coast Garibaldi and Fraser North were statistically significantly higher than the provincial average for female students, while East Kootenay, Northern Interior, and Vancouver were statistically significantly lower.

Health Service Delivery Area	Family connectedness index	Males	Females
033 North Shore/Coast Garibaldi	79.65	80.98†	78.19†
041 South Vancouver Island	79.39	80.92†	77.87†
022 Fraser North	79.00	79.89	78.04
051 Northwest	78.34	79.62	77.10
042 Central Vancouver Island	78.20	79.74†	76.76†
012 Kootenay Boundary	78.15	80.03†	76.37†
013 Okanagan	78.11	80.02†	76.41†
043 North Vancouver Island	78.07	79.47	76.59
014 Thompson Cariboo Shuswap	77.85	80.23†	75.69†
031 Richmond	77.82	78.68	76.89
011 East Kootenay	77.37	79.60†	74.90†
052 Northern Interior	76.70	78.11†	75.44†
032 Vancouver	76.34	77.28	75.41
021 Fraser East	F	F	F
023 Fraser South	F	F	F
053 Northeast	F	F	F
999 Province	**78.02**	**79.30†**	**76.76†**

† Males differ significantly from females.
F Data not available.

Family connectedness for youth

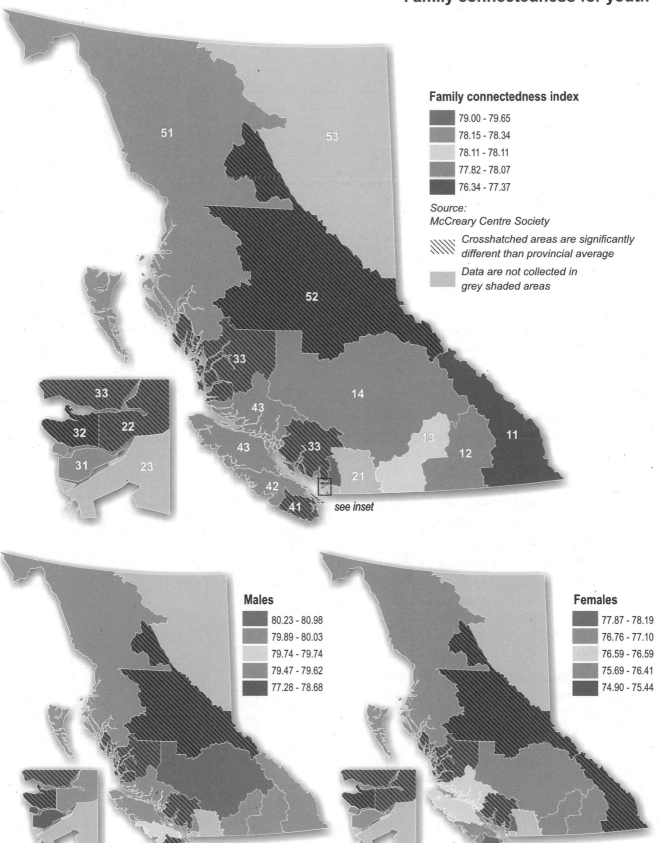

Family connectedness index

- 79.00 - 79.65
- 78.15 - 78.34
- 78.11 - 78.11
- 77.82 - 78.07
- 76.34 - 77.37

Source:
McCreary Centre Society

Crosshatched areas are significantly different than provincial average

Data are not collected in grey shaded areas

see inset

Males

- 80.23 - 80.98
- 79.89 - 80.03
- 79.74 - 79.74
- 79.47 - 79.62
- 77.28 - 78.68

Females

- 77.87 - 78.19
- 76.76 - 77.10
- 76.59 - 76.59
- 75.69 - 76.41
- 74.90 - 75.44

School connectedness for youth

A school connectedness indicator has been developed based on the McCreary Adolescent Health Survey. It is comprised of seven items that assess the extent to which students feel teachers care about them, they feel like they are part of their school, they feel happy to be at school, they feel safe at school, they get along with teachers and students, and they feel that teachers treat them fairly. Students received a school connectedness score if they answered 75% of the questions in the scale. The score is created by averaging the responses to the number of questions answered, standardized on a scale of 0 to 1, with a higher score denoting greater connectedness (Saewyc, 2007). The score has been multiplied by 100 for analysis purposes.

For Grade 7 to 12 students in BC, the level of school connectedness falls from Grade 7 through to Grade 10 and then rises again (McCreary Centre Society, 2004). Overall, for these grades, the average school connectedness score was 66.72 (out of a possible 100) in 2003. There were clear geographical variations between the 13 HSDAs included in the survey. Lower mainland HSDAs had statistically significantly higher than average scores (Richmond, Fraser North, and North Shore/Coast Garibaldi), while East Kootenay and Thompson Cariboo Shuswap in the interior, Northern Interior in the north, and North Vancouver Island all had statistically significantly lower than provincial average values.

Females (provincial score of 68.29) had a statistically significantly higher score than males (score of 65.11). This is a reversal from family connectedness, discussed previously. Not only was this the case provincially, but 10 of the 13 HSDAs were significantly higher, statistically, for females than for males.

Among males, Richmond, Fraser North, and North Shore/Coast Garibaldi had statistically significantly higher school connectedness scores, while Central and North Vancouver Island, Kootenay Boundary and East Kootenay in the southeast, Thompson Cariboo Shuswap in the interior, and Northern Interior in the north all had significantly lower scores, statistically, than the province.

Among females, only Richmond had a significantly higher score than the provincial average for females, while Thompson Cariboo Shuswap, North Vancouver Island, Northern Interior, and East Kootenay all had significantly lower values than the provincial score.

Health Service Delivery Area	School connectedness index	Males	Females
031 Richmond	68.88	67.16†	70.70†
022 Fraser North	67.84	66.55†	69.24†
033 North Shore/Coast Garibaldi	67.49	66.11†	68.98†
041 South Vancouver Island	67.28	65.62†	68.91†
013 Okanagan	67.20	65.53†	68.69†
032 Vancouver	66.45	64.71†	68.16†
042 Central Vancouver Island	66.40	64.21†	68.40†
051 Northwest	66.14	65.02	67.21
012 Kootenay Boundary	65.66	63.09†	68.03†
014 Thompson Cariboo Shuswap	65.59	63.90†	67.10†
043 North Vancouver Island	64.29	63.04	65.60
052 Northern Interior	63.43	62.01†	64.68†
011 East Kootenay	63.37	62.17	64.67
021 Fraser East	F	F	F
023 Fraser South	F	F	F
053 Northeast	F	F	F
999 Province	**66.72**	**65.11†**	**68.29†**

† Males differ significantly from females.
F Data not available.

School connectedness for youth

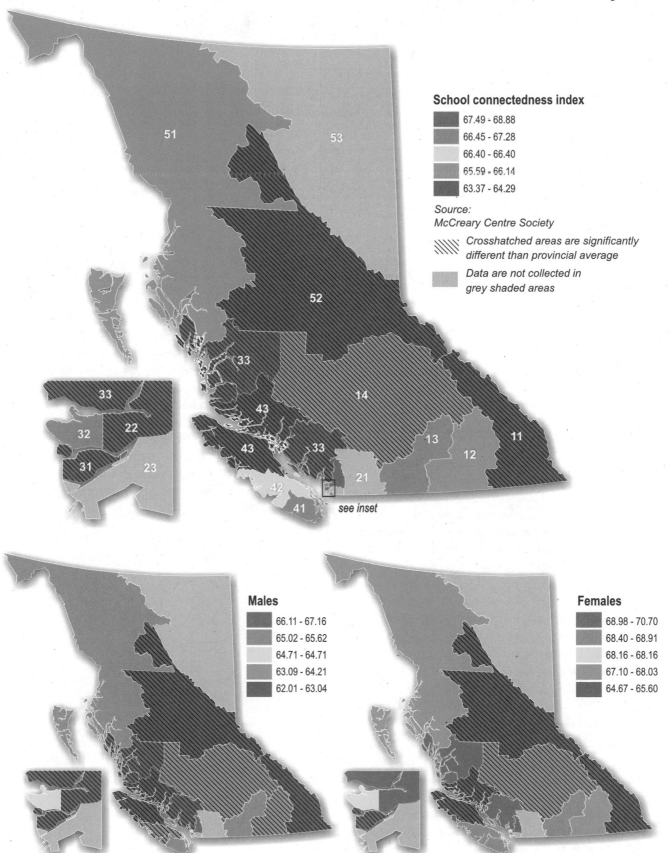

School connectedness index

- 67.49 - 68.88
- 66.45 - 67.28
- 66.40 - 66.40
- 65.59 - 66.14
- 63.37 - 64.29

Source:
McCreary Centre Society

Crosshatched areas are significantly different than provincial average

Data are not collected in grey shaded areas

Males

- 66.11 - 67.16
- 65.02 - 65.62
- 64.71 - 64.71
- 63.09 - 64.21
- 62.01 - 63.04

Females

- 68.98 - 70.70
- 68.40 - 68.91
- 68.16 - 68.16
- 67.10 - 68.03
- 64.67 - 65.60

Sense of belonging to local community

Sense of belonging to one's local community is a measure of the degree of connection that individuals have built up within their neighbourhood or community. This may be achieved through membership in local organizations or through helping others out when needed and vice versa.

The CCHS asked respondents: *"How would you describe your sense of belonging to your local community? Would you say it is very strong, somewhat strong, somewhat weak, or very weak?"* More than two-thirds (67.32%) of BC respondents indicated that they felt a very strong or somewhat strong connection to their local community. This was significantly higher statistically than the response for Canadians overall (62.36%). The BC Aboriginal response was lower than for BC residents as a whole, but not statistically significantly so (64.64%).

For all respondents combined, there was a 16 percentage point spread in responses between the lowest and highest HSDAs, depicting important geographic variations across the province. The Northwest, Kootenay Boundary, and Thompson Cariboo Shuswap regions were all statistically significantly greater than the BC provincial average. Each had more than 74% of respondents indicating a strong attachment to their local community. (The use of the word significantly throughout the description of all CCHS data refers to statistically significant, which means there is a real difference between the HSDA/region and the average value for the indicator provincially.) While not statistically significantly different, the lower mainland HSDAs showed lower attachments than their interior counterparts.

There was no significant difference between genders, although for males, Northwest (81.51%) was significantly higher than for males as a whole. Among females, several HSDAs had significant differences from the female average. Thompson Cariboo Shuswap females were significantly higher (75.27%), and East Kootenay (60.72%) and Fraser North (62.53%) were significantly lower than the female provincial average.

Health Service Delivery Area	All respondents (%)	Male (%)	Female (%)	Ages 12-19 (%)	Ages 20-64 (%)	Ages 65+ (%)
051 Northwest	79.04	81.51	76.36	81.06	78.68	78.54
012 Kootenay Boundary	74.89	71.29	78.52	79.33	72.37	81.65
014 Thompson Cariboo Shuswap	74.29	73.32	75.27	78.64	74.53	69.84
043 North Vancouver Island	70.23	62.82	77.57	61.58	71.47	72.17
041 South Vancouver Island	70.04	65.85	73.83	76.88	68.02	73.82
033 North Shore/Coast Garibaldi	69.32	70.10	68.58	77.23	67.45	72.25
013 Okanagan	68.93	69.88	68.04	69.93	68.81	68.74
042 Central Vancouver Island	68.58	66.66	70.42	70.31	67.69	70.51
021 Fraser East	66.71	63.71	69.63	82.35‡	63.01	68.85
023 Fraser South	66.69	64.32	69.01	67.51	66.26	68.29
011 East Kootenay	66.33	71.80	60.72	69.48	65.65	66.80
053 Northeast	66.09	63.09	69.30	68.64	65.01	70.73
052 Northern Interior	65.36	62.31	68.57	68.33	64.62	66.48
022 Fraser North	64.50	66.52	62.53	64.66	63.65	69.49
031 Richmond	64.19	62.80	65.48	66.60	64.29	61.94
032 Vancouver	63.21	61.00	65.37	71.49	61.83	68.43
999 Province	**67.32**	**66.02**	**68.59**	**71.34‡**	**66.14**	**69.84‡**

‡ Age group differs significantly from 20-64 group.

A stronger sense of belonging was evident among teens or youth (12- to 19-year-olds) and seniors (65 and over) when compared to the middle age cohort (20 to 64 years). This difference was significant statistically. Fraser East teens had a higher sense of belonging to their community than other teens around the province, and this sense of belonging was also statistically significantly higher than the 20 to 64 age group in their region. Kootenay Boundary seniors had a significantly greater sense of belonging to their community than other seniors in the province.

Sense of belonging to local community

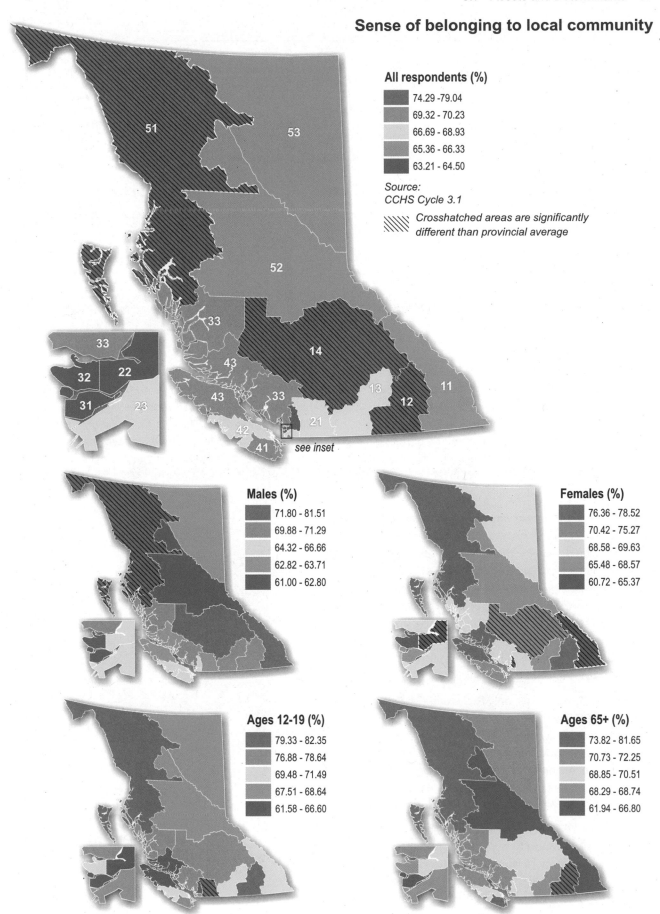

All respondents (%)

- 74.29 - 79.04
- 69.32 - 70.23
- 66.69 - 68.93
- 65.36 - 66.33
- 63.21 - 64.50

Source:
CCHS Cycle 3.1

Crosshatched areas are significantly different than provincial average

Males (%)

- 71.80 - 81.51
- 69.88 - 71.29
- 64.32 - 66.66
- 62.82 - 63.71
- 61.00 - 62.80

Females (%)

- 76.36 - 78.52
- 70.42 - 75.27
- 68.58 - 69.63
- 65.48 - 68.57
- 60.72 - 65.37

Ages 12-19 (%)

- 79.33 - 82.35
- 76.88 - 78.64
- 69.48 - 71.49
- 67.51 - 68.64
- 61.58 - 66.60

Ages 65+ (%)

- 73.82 - 81.65
- 70.73 - 72.25
- 68.85 - 70.51
- 68.29 - 68.74
- 61.94 - 66.80

Social support index

The CCHS developed an index based on the response to four questions: "Do you have someone to: have a good time with; get together with for relaxation; do things to get mind off things; and, do something enjoyable with?" The index measures the degree of social support that an individual has available to them. It has a scale from 0 to 16, with higher scores denoting greater social supports. We have focused our work on mapping those whose overall score was 15 to 16. Altogether, 48.76% of BC respondents scored in this range. The score for Canada as a whole is a little higher at 50.53%, and this is significant statistically. Not all provinces and territories participated in these questions, and so extreme caution is required in interpreting this difference. In BC, 43.71% of Aboriginal respondents scored in the 15 to 16 range, but this value was not significantly different from the provincial average for all respondents.

The range in index scores was nearly 18 percentage points, indicating major geographical differences throughout the province. The lowest scores were in the urban areas of the southwest. Both Vancouver and Richmond were significantly lower statistically than the provincial average. The regions with the highest percentage scoring 15 to 16 on the social support index tended to be in the interior regions, which are more rural in nature. Okanagan (55.25%) was significantly higher than the provincial average.

Geographically, for males, only Richmond (34.72%) and Vancouver (38.70%) were significantly different (lower) from the average for males. For females, Northern Interior (58.56%) was higher and, as was the case for males, Vancouver and Richmond were lower than the average for females overall. These differences were significant statistically.

Youth and the 20- to 64-year-olds had relatively similar values overall, provincially, but there were differences for some HSDAs. Northern Interior youth had significantly lower social supports than the 20- to 64-year-olds in their HSDA. The middle age group had a similar pattern

Health Service Delivery Area	All respondents (%)	Males (%)	Females (%)	Ages 12-19(%)	Ages 20-64(%)	Ages 65+(%)
013 Okanagan	55.25	55.42	55.09	52.97	56.94	51.20
053 Northeast	54.81	56.21	53.31	55.46	56.06	43.00
052 Northern Interior	54.28	50.22	58.56	39.38‡	58.35	46.16
014 Thompson Cariboo Shuswap	53.21	55.64	50.80	56.34	55.29	41.75‡
011 East Kootenay	53.17	53.12	53.21	61.19	53.58	44.51
023 Fraser South	52.56	53.32	51.82	53.68	52.50	51.78
042 Central Vancouver Island	52.39	49.76	54.92	45.95	53.50	52.61
012 Kootenay Boundary	52.15	50.61	53.71	50.94	54.71	43.04
021 Fraser East	51.13	53.48	48.84	47.97	53.73	42.41
033 North Shore/Coast Garibaldi	49.51	50.81	48.27	50.15	49.54	48.87
041 South Vancouver Island	49.43	45.87	52.64	51.16	50.19	45.53
043 North Vancouver Island	49.43	46.17	52.66	56.54	47.20	53.25
022 Fraser North	46.00	48.06	44.00	54.42	46.49	35.50‡
051 Northwest	45.93	44.65	47.32	50.96	44.83	46.36
032 Vancouver	39.58	38.70	40.44	44.62	41.49	26.02‡
031 Richmond	37.43	34.72	39.97	41.19	36.08	41.77
999 Province	**48.76**	**48.57**	**48.94**	**50.74**	**49.52**	**43.60‡**

‡ Age group differs significantly from 20-64 group.

to that for all respondents combined, although Northern Interior was significantly high. Seniors, provincially, had significantly lower percentages on this index than 20- to 64-year-olds. Three HSDAs, Thompson Cariboo Shuswap, Fraser North, and Vancouver, had significantly lower values statistically than their younger counterparts. Among seniors, Vancouver had significantly lower social supports (26.02%) than other HSDAs.

Social support index

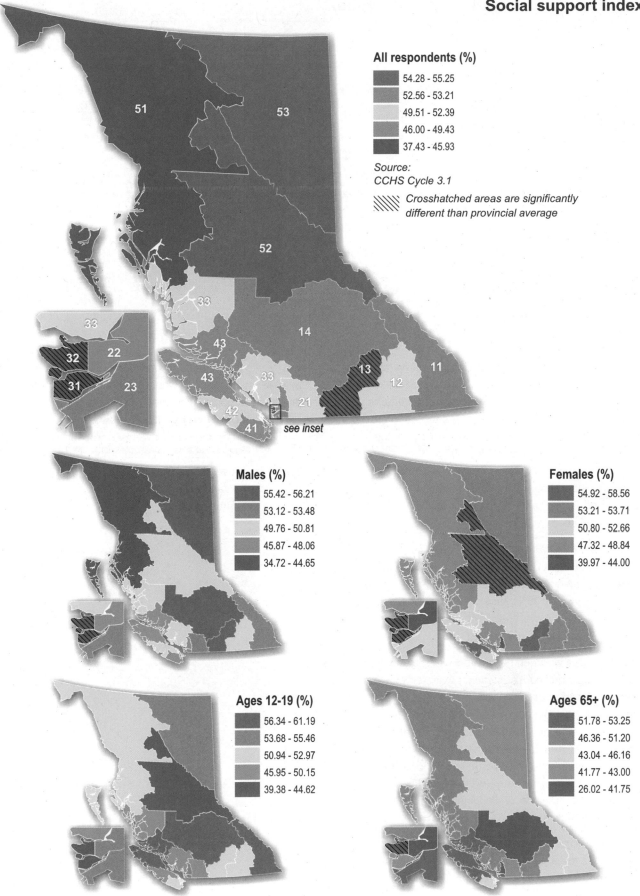

All respondents (%)

- 54.28 - 55.25
- 52.56 - 53.21
- 49.51 - 52.39
- 46.00 - 49.43
- 37.43 - 45.93

Source:
CCHS Cycle 3.1

Crosshatched areas are significantly different than provincial average

Males (%)

- 55.42 - 56.21
- 53.12 - 53.48
- 49.76 - 50.81
- 45.87 - 48.06
- 34.72 - 44.65

Females (%)

- 54.92 - 58.56
- 53.21 - 53.71
- 50.80 - 52.66
- 47.32 - 48.84
- 39.97 - 44.00

Ages 12-19 (%)

- 56.34 - 61.19
- 53.68 - 55.46
- 50.94 - 52.97
- 45.95 - 50.15
- 39.38 - 44.62

Ages 65+ (%)

- 51.78 - 53.25
- 46.36 - 51.20
- 43.04 - 46.16
- 41.77 - 43.00
- 26.02 - 41.75

Emotional or informational support index

A second index developed from a variety of CCHS questions measures emotional and informational support available to individuals. As the earlier reviews on wellness and determinants in the Atlas suggest, this is an important wellness asset and determinant. The index is made up of the results from eight individual questions as follows: *"Do you have someone to: listen; receive advice about a crisis; help understand a problem; confide in; give advice; share most private worries and fears; turn to for suggestions for personal problems; and, who understands problems."*

Health Service Delivery Area	All respondents (%)	Males (%)	Females (%)	Ages 12-19 (%)	Ages 20-64 (%)	Ages 65+ (%)
014 Thompson Cariboo Shuswap	53.39	53.58	53.20	54.54	56.48	39.10‡
052 Northern Interior	52.77	46.51	59.36	41.98	56.35	42.26
013 Okanagan	52.66	50.44	54.74	51.96	54.92	45.87
021 Fraser East	52.04	51.09	52.96	50.40	55.28	39.07‡
042 Central Vancouver Island	51.81	48.10	55.39	41.74	54.96	47.45
012 Kootenay Boundary	51.25	45.38	57.14	52.59	52.61	44.99
023 Fraser South	51.13	48.10	54.11	52.63	51.10	49.81
053 Northeast	50.87	48.43	53.48	48.71	53.31	33.82‡
033 North Shore/Coast Garibaldi	50.39	49.40	51.33	38.98	52.94	46.85
041 South Vancouver Island	49.11	43.86	53.86	46.21	50.69	44.81
011 East Kootenay	48.61	49.46	47.74	F	50.48	43.45
043 North Vancouver Island	47.43	40.54	54.25	F	46.82	53.64
022 Fraser North	45.33	45.92	44.75	46.92	46.29	38.10
051 Northwest	44.40	43.65	45.20	41.94E	44.72	45.81
032 Vancouver	41.05	39.55	42.52	43.53	43.25	27.40‡
031 Richmond	37.65	37.13	38.13	44.39	35.66	43.14
999 Province	**48.23**	**46.13†**	**50.28†**	**47.30**	**49.52**	**42.19‡**

‡ Age group differs significantly from 20-64 group.
† Males differ significantly from females.
E Interpret data with caution (16.77< coefficient of variation <33.3).
F Data suppressed due to Statistics Canada sampling rules.

The results of these eight questions were amalgamated to create the index, which has a score from 0 to 32, with the higher score depicting greater emotional or informational support. The data used for the maps and table here are based on the percentage of the respondents who scored between 29 and 32. For BC, 48.23% of respondents fell into this category. For Aboriginal respondents in the province, 39.87% scored between 29 and 32. While lower, this difference was not statistically significant.

For all respondents combined, the range between the highest and lowest regions (HSDAs) was nearly 16 percentage points. Two HSDAS, Richmond (37.65%) and Vancouver (41.05%), had significantly lower values than the provincial average. Higher value areas tended to be concentrated in interior HSDAs.

The difference between the average for males and females was significant statistically, with females having greater support. For males, the pattern was quite similar to that for the population as a whole, and only Vancouver was significantly different. The range for females, at 21 percentage points, was higher than that for males. Females in the Northern Interior (59.36%) had significantly greater support than the average for females in the province, while Richmond and Vancouver were significantly lower.

There was no significant difference between teens or youth (12 to 19 years) and the middle (20 to 64 years) cohort. Two HSDAs had too few data to report the results for the teen group. Seniors (age 65 and over) in the province, however, had significantly fewer emotional supports than the middle age cohort. Four regions (HSDAs) had significantly lower support than the younger groups. These were Thompson Cariboo Shuswap, Fraser East, Northeast, and Vancouver. North Vancouver Island had significantly higher support, and Vancouver significantly lower support than seniors provincially.

Emotional or informational support index

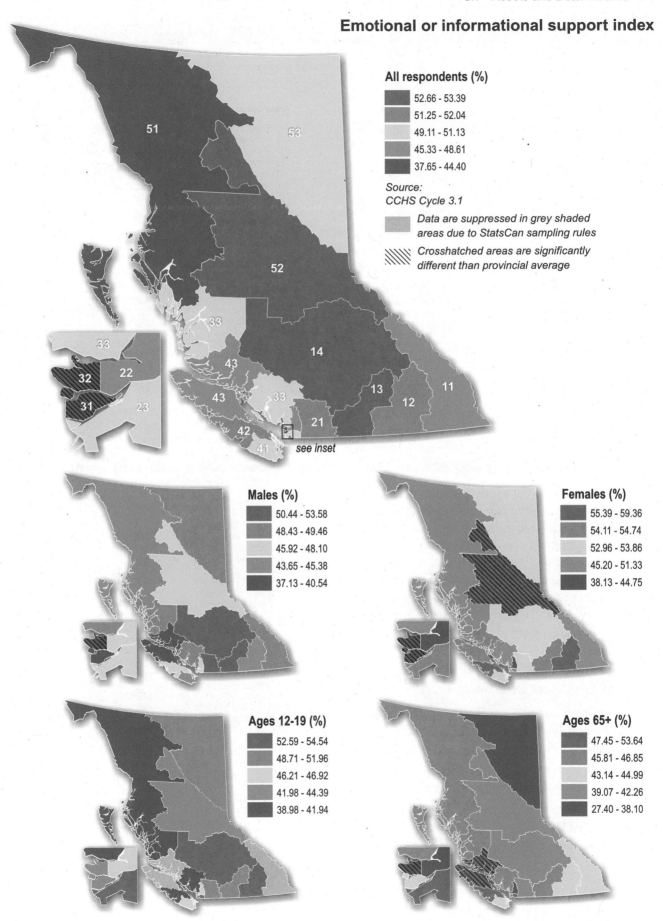

All respondents (%)

- 52.66 - 53.39
- 51.25 - 52.04
- 49.11 - 51.13
- 45.33 - 48.61
- 37.65 - 44.40

Source:
CCHS Cycle 3.1

Data are suppressed in grey shaded areas due to StatsCan sampling rules

Crosshatched areas are significantly different than provincial average

Males (%)

- 50.44 - 53.58
- 48.43 - 49.46
- 45.92 - 48.10
- 43.65 - 45.38
- 37.13 - 40.54

Females (%)

- 55.39 - 59.36
- 54.11 - 54.74
- 52.96 - 53.86
- 45.20 - 51.33
- 38.13 - 44.75

Ages 12-19 (%)

- 52.59 - 54.54
- 48.71 - 51.96
- 46.21 - 46.92
- 41.98 - 44.39
- 38.98 - 41.94

Ages 65+ (%)

- 47.45 - 53.64
- 45.81 - 46.85
- 43.14 - 44.99
- 39.07 - 42.26
- 27.40 - 38.10

Readiness to learn

Getting a good start in life is a key determinant of health and wellness. Prenatal and early childhood events and experiences have been shown to have major impacts on later health and wellness (Canadian Institute for Health Information, 2004). In BC, an Early Development Instrument (EDI), which is a population-based tool, assesses the state of child development for kindergarten students throughout the province. This checklist covers five domains: physical health and well-being; social competence; emotional maturity; language and cognitive development; and communication skills and general knowledge. On average, 10% of students perform below developmental expectations and are considered to be vulnerable in each domain (Kershaw et al., 2005).

The approach taken here is to map the results by school district for kindergarten students based on the percentage who are not vulnerable. These maps differ from those developed elsewhere, which have been based on the percentage of kindergarten students who are vulnerable in specific domains (Hertzman et al., 2002; Kershaw et al., 2005; more information and maps are available at www.earlylearning.ubc.ca/).

Readiness to learn

On average, only three out of every four students (73.67%) were developing in a satisfactory manner in all of the five domains. The students in the highest performing school districts were found in the southeast of the province and in the lower mainland and Vancouver Island. At the other end of the spectrum, several school districts had less than 60% of their students with no vulnerabilities. They tended to be coastal communities. The range in values was from 86.86% to 42.86%, indicating major geographical variations throughout the province.

Physical health and well-being

The pattern for this domain was quite similar to that for the first map. The range was from 95.51% for Revelstoke to 73.21% for Prince Rupert.

Emotional maturity

The range in values for this domain went from a high of 95.51% (West Vancouver) to a low of 77.19% (Stikine). The geographical pattern was again similar to the other two maps.

School District	Readiness to learn (%)	Physical health & well-being (%)	Emotional maturity (%)
045 West Vancouver	86.86	94.23	95.51
020 Kootenay-Columbia	84.76	95.17	92.57
006 Rocky Mountain	83.44	93.36	94.69
072 Campbell River	81.75	92.94	93.78
019 Revelstoke	80.90	95.51	94.38
022 Vernon	80.82	91.96	95.00
035 Langley	80.56	90.35	92.10
051 Boundary	80.54	95.11	91.89
008 Kootenay Lake	80.35	91.57	92.51
044 North Vancouver	79.79	93.35	90.89
043 Coquitlam	79.23	91.59	92.77
005 Southeast Kootenay	78.67	90.74	90.48
083 North Okanagan-Shuswap	78.62	89.88	92.14
037 Delta	77.66	92.17	92.21
062 Sooke	76.66	89.57	89.93
060 Peace River North	76.34	89.02	92.20
079 Cowichan Valley	76.33	86.29	91.82
064 Gulf Islands	76.00	90.00	87.94
091 Nechako Lakes	76.00	86.91	91.67
042 Maple Ridge-Pitt Meadows	75.70	88.14	87.64
061 Greater Victoria	75.59	89.32	91.23
053 Okanagan Similkameen	75.59	90.29	90.81
073 Kamloops/Thompson	75.57	89.07	90.27
071 Comox Valley	75.38	90.72	88.26
054 Bulkley Valley	75.32	88.54	84.81
057 Prince George	75.13	87.03	90.25
010 Arrow Lakes	75.00	82.50	82.50
070 Alberni	74.69	90.05	92.38
063 Saanich	74.57	91.40	86.80
046 Sunshine Coast	74.57	90.04	89.61
036 Surrey	74.26	91.86	91.15
033 Chilliwack	74.05	90.13	87.71
028 Quesnel	73.82	85.09	95.26
023 Central Okanagan	73.39	88.42	89.64
034 Abbotsford	73.35	90.49	89.29
027 Cariboo-Chilcotin	72.86	88.21	91.44
069 Qualicum	72.66	85.51	90.65
067 Okanagan Skaha	72.53	86.49	87.70
074 Gold Trail	72.03	85.59	84.62
038 Richmond	70.42	91.30	87.18
078 Fraser-Cascade	69.63	89.20	87.26
068 Nanaimo-Ladysmith	69.45	86.95	87.06
059 Peace River	69.09	87.34	88.61
082 Coast Mountains	69.06	84.46	87.34
050 Haida Gwaii/Queen Charlotte	68.85	81.97	85.25
058 Nicola-Similkameen	68.75	84.38	91.25
047 Powell River	68.08	87.30	86.32
048 Howe Sound	67.92	87.06	89.40
040 New Westminster	67.87	88.43	86.60
041 Burnaby	67.31	90.15	87.43
075 Mission	67.23	86.96	86.51
081 Fort Nelson	67.12	89.04	89.04
085 Vancouver Island North	65.68	82.63	82.98
087 Stikine	63.16	85.96	77.19
052 Prince Rupert	59.82	73.21	84.30
084 Vancouver Island West	59.38	78.13	84.38
039 Vancouver	59.06	81.47	85.64
049 Central Coast	47.06	76.47	88.24
092 Nisga'a	42.86	82.14	88.29
999 Province	**73.67**	**89.23**	**89.89**

Readiness to learn

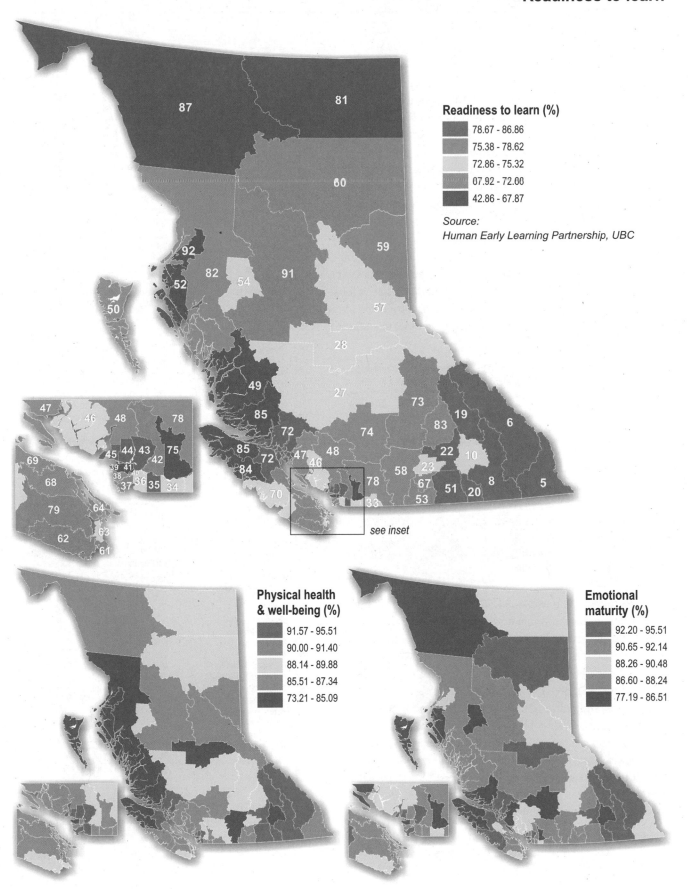

Readiness to learn (%)

- 78.67 - 86.86
- 75.38 - 78.62
- 72.86 - 75.32
- 07.92 - 72.00
- 42.86 - 67.87

Source:
Human Early Learning Partnership, UBC

see inset

Physical health & well-being (%)

- 91.57 - 95.51
- 90.00 - 91.40
- 88.14 - 89.88
- 85.51 - 87.34
- 73.21 - 85.09

Emotional maturity (%)

- 92.20 - 95.51
- 90.65 - 92.14
- 88.26 - 90.48
- 86.60 - 88.24
- 77.19 - 86.51

Age-appropriate grade

If a child is of the age normally associated with a particular grade no earlier than September 1st of the year before they start that grade, they are considered to be age-appropriate. For example, a student entering Grade 1 in 2005 could have been born as early as September 1, 1998. Birthdates and maximum ages for age-related grade levels are given below. Accelerated children, or children who are considered young for their grade level, are still considered to be in an age-appropriate grade. All students and grades are combined for each school district to provide the percentage of students who are in an age-appropriate grade. Generally, students in lower grades are more likely to be age-appropriate than students in the higher grades. There is a rapid drop off in age-appropriate grade beyond Grade 7, especially for relatively disadvantaged students, such as those from income assistance families, children in the care of the state, and Aboriginal students, and after Grade 9 for other students (Danderfer, Wright, and Foster, 2006).

Grade	Earliest birthdate to be considered age-appropriate	Maximum grade-related age on September 1, 2005
1	9/1/1998	7
2	9/1/1997	8
3	9/1/1996	9
4	9/1/1995	10
5	9/1/1994	11
6	9/1/1993	12
7	9/1/1992	13
8	9/1/1991	14
9	9/1/1990	15
10	9/1/1989	16
11	9/1/1988	17
12	9/1/1987	18

For the province as a whole, 94.56% of public school students were at the age-appropriate grade in 2005/6, but there was a range of over 30 percentage points between the school districts with the highest and lowest values. Overall, Conseil Scolaire Francophone, which is not a geographically based school district, had the highest value, with 97.85% of students at the age-appropriate grade. Coquitlam, Delta, West Vancouver, Surrey, Burnaby, and Maple Ridge-Pitt Meadows in the lower mainland also rated highly, as did Revelstoke in the southeast, Okanagan Skaha in the southern interior, and Greater Victoria, Campbell River, and Nanaimo-Ladysmith on Vancouver Island. Many of the interior and northern districts were in the lower two quintiles for age-appropriate grades.

There is a difference in the provincial average between boys and girls. For the province as a whole, girls (95.31%) are more likely to be in the age-appropriate grade than boys (93.84%).

School District	All respondents (%)	Males (%)	Females (%)
043 Coquitlam	97.79	97.45	98.16
037 Delta	97.51	96.96	98.10
038 Richmond	96.92	96.26	97.62
019 Revelstoke	96.82	96.93	96.70
045 West Vancouver	96.60	96.17	97.05
036 Surrey	96.14	95.64	96.67
041 Burnaby	95.95	95.18	96.79
061 Greater Victoria	95.83	95.41	96.25
067 Okanagan Skaha	95.77	94.58	96.98
072 Campbell River	95.73	95.01	96.48
042 Maple Ridge-Pitt Meadows	95.61	94.95	96.31
068 Nanaimo-Ladysmith	95.50	94.46	96.60
039 Vancouver	95.49	95.11	95.89
081 Fort Nelson	95.39	94.31	96.57
064 Gulf Islands	95.35	95.14	95.56
059 Peace River South	95.32	94.96	95.70
044 North Vancouver	95.13	94.56	95.75
006 Rocky Mountain	95.09	94.22	95.98
034 Abbotsford	95.08	94.53	95.67
057 Prince George	95.01	94.41	95.66
023 Central Okanagan	94.99	93.60	96.47
048 Howe Sound	94.96	94.36	95.63
062 Sooke	94.94	94.31	95.62
022 Vernon	94.91	94.07	95.78
005 Southeast Kootenay	94.61	93.38	95.93
020 Kootenay-Columbia	94.60	93.57	95.74
053 Okanagan Similkameen	94.51	92.44	96.72
010 Arrow Lakes	94.45	93.10	95.92
046 Sunshine Coast	93.98	93.42	94.54
047 Powell River	93.94	92.95	95.05
054 Bulkley Valley	93.90	93.44	94.38
035 Langley	93.79	92.94	94.69
051 Boundary	93.69	93.66	93.73
069 Qualicum	93.49	92.52	94.52
083 North Okanagan-Shuswap	93.36	92.20	94.57
071 Comox Valley	93.35	92.99	93.71
063 Saanich	93.23	93.29	93.17
085 Vancouver Island North	93.11	91.70	94.66
073 Kamloops/Thompson	93.08	91.59	94.64
075 Mission	92.93	91.77	94.15
008 Kootenay Lake	92.44	91.49	93.42
082 Coast Mountains	92.34	91.33	93.46
028 Quesnel	92.08	90.25	94.02
060 Peace River North	92.07	91.20	92.93
070 Alberni	91.80	90.40	93.27
033 Chilliwack	91.51	90.69	92.38
079 Cowichan Valley	91.43	89.97	92.94
040 New Westminster	91.28	91.15	91.42
052 Prince Rupert	91.13	90.10	92.23
092 Nisga'a	91.07	88.89	93.33
027 Cariboo-Chilcotin	90.46	89.70	91.23
084 Vancouver Island West	90.29	87.55	93.18
091 Nechako Lakes	90.03	89.12	90.96
050 Haida Gwaii/Queen Charlotte	88.99	86.94	91.33
078 Fraser-Cascade	88.68	87.18	90.34
058 Nicola-Similkameen	85.88	85.28	86.48
049 Central Coast	84.50	83.02	86.10
074 Gold Trail	83.74	80.80	86.74
087 Stikine	66.27	64.22	68.50
999 Province	**94.56**	**93.84**	**95.31**

This difference was fairly consistent throughout the province, with girls out-performing boys on this measure in most school districts. Geographically, the overall patterns for both males and females were quite similar to the pattern for both sexes combined.

Age-appropriate grade

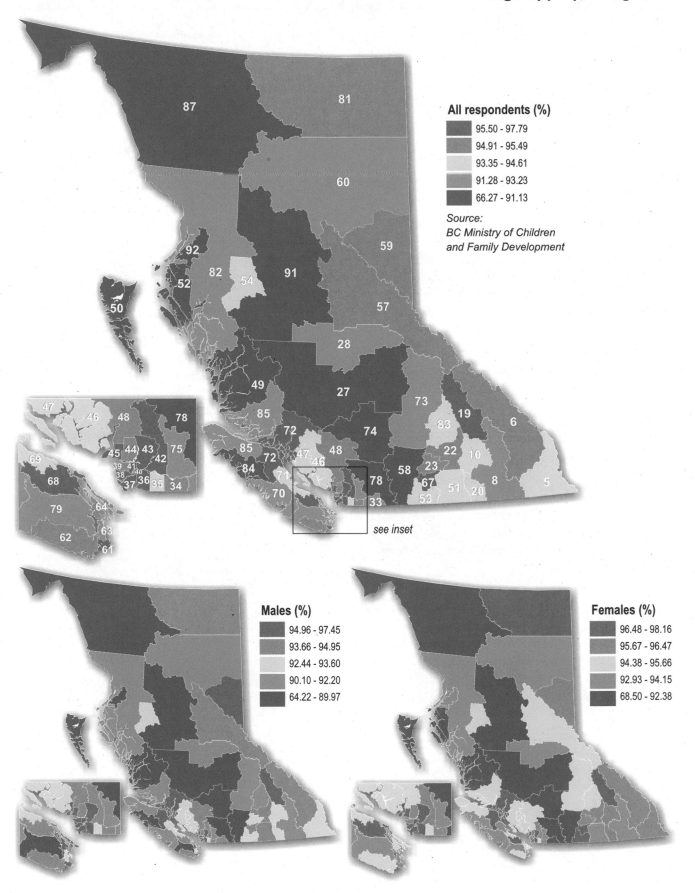

All respondents (%)

- 95.50 - 97.79
- 94.91 - 95.49
- 93.35 - 94.61
- 91.28 - 93.23
- 66.27 - 91.13

Source:
BC Ministry of Children
and Family Development

Males (%)

- 94.96 - 97.45
- 93.66 - 94.95
- 92.44 - 93.60
- 90.10 - 92.20
- 64.22 - 89.97

Females (%)

- 96.48 - 98.16
- 95.67 - 96.47
- 94.38 - 95.66
- 92.93 - 94.15
- 68.50 - 92.38

Age-appropriate grade for Aboriginal students

Research shows that Aboriginal students do not fare as well as the general population on most educational indicators (Ministry of Education, 2001; Cowley and Easton, 2006). This results in poorer average lifetime achievements for this group of students. The age-appropriate grade indicator was no exception to this trend. Only 88.81% of Aboriginal students were in an age-appropriate grade provincially. This compares with 94.56% for all students combined.

Aboriginal students in some school districts did quite well compared to the provincial average. For example, Aboriginal students in Conseil Scolaire Francophone (not shown), Richmond, Delta, Arrow Lakes, Coquitlam, Maple Ridge-Pitt Meadows, and Campbell River all did better than the provincial average of 94.56% for all students combined (see previous page).

In a few cases, Aboriginal students did better than the school district average for all students combined (see, for example, Conseil Scolaire Francophone, Richmond, and Arrow Lakes). In most cases, however, Aboriginal student performance rates were, at best, equivalent to the lowest performing quintile school districts for the general student population.

There was great variation between school districts in the percentage of Aboriginal children that were in an age-appropriate grade. The difference between the highest and the lowest was more than 37 percentage points. This compares with over 30 percentage points for all students combined.

Geographically, Aboriginal students tended to do better in the urban lower mainland school districts and less well in the north and interior districts. Fort Nelson, Prince George, and Peace River South in the northeast, and Arrow Lakes in the southeast were exceptions to this pattern. In an ideal world of equality of opportunity, there would be no variation between either school districts or population groups.

School District	Percent
038 Richmond	97.17
037 Delta	96.68
010 Arrow Lakes	96.67
043 Coquitlam	95.61
042 Maple Ridge-Pitt Meadows	95.36
072 Campbell River	94.80
059 Peace River South	94.25
039 Vancouver	94.03
081 Fort Nelson	93.54
062 Sooke	93.45
057 Prince George	92.92
068 Nanaimo-Ladysmith	92.69
041 Burnaby	92.30
067 Okanagan Skaha	92.05
061 Greater Victoria	91.99
023 Central Okanagan	91.93
045 West Vancouver	91.80
019 Revelstoke	91.67
071 Comox Valley	91.28
051 Boundary	91.14
006 Rocky Mountain	91.12
022 Vernon	91.08
092 Nisga'a	91.05
036 Surrey	90.86
035 Langley	90.83
008 Kootenay Lake	90.67
083 North Okanagan-Shuswap	89.90
034 Abbotsford	89.84
064 Gulf Islands	89.83
046 Sunshine Coast	89.41
047 Powell River	89.04
005 Southeast Kootenay	88.77
048 Howe Sound	88.39
053 Okanagan Similkameen	88.38
020 Kootenay-Columbia	88.36
060 Peace River North	88.26
085 Vancouver Island North	88.17
069 Qualicum	87.71
075 Mission	87.59
082 Coast Mountains	87.54
084 Vancouver Island West	87.21
033 Chilliwack	87.02
052 Prince Rupert	86.63
044 North Vancouver	86.50
073 Kamloops/Thompson	86.17
050 Haida Gwaii/Queen Charlotte	86.04
054 Bulkley Valley	85.87
028 Quesnel	85.84
070 Alberni	83.67
058 Nicola-Similkameen	83.52
063 Saanich	82.97
091 Nechako Lakes	82.61
027 Cariboo-Chilcotin	82.52
049 Central Coast	82.39
040 New Westminster	81.25
079 Cowichan Valley	81.13
074 Gold Trail	78.84
078 Fraser-Cascade	78.11
087 Stikine	60.97
999 Province	**88.81**

Age-appropriate grade for Aboriginal students

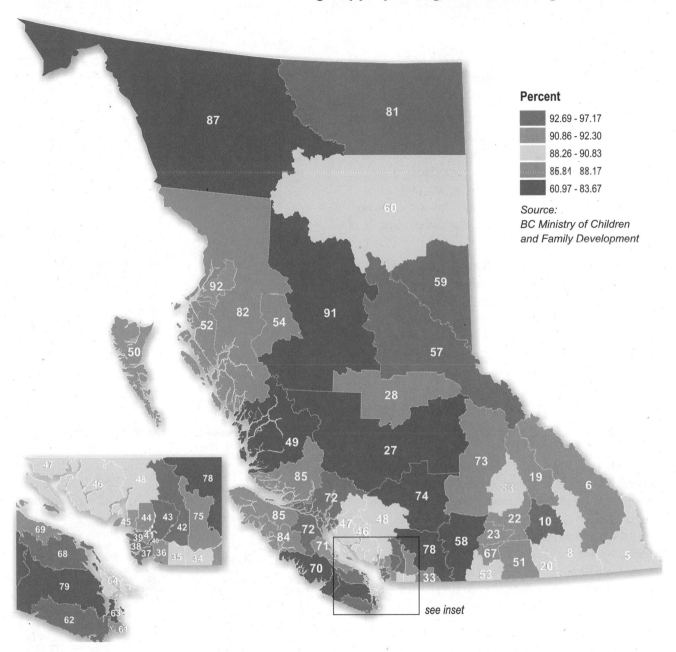

Percent

	92.69 - 97.17
	90.86 - 92.30
	88.26 - 90.83
	85.81 - 88.17
	60.97 - 83.67

Source:
BC Ministry of Children
and Family Development

see inset

High school graduation

Numerous studies have shown how health and wellness improve with the level of education (Canadian Institute for Health Information, 2004; also see Chapter 2).

Within BC for 2004/5, nearly four out of every five students (79%) in Grade 12 successfully graduated from high school. There was a very large range in rates by school district throughout the province, depicting major geographical variation between the regions. The highest percentage of students graduating was 92.95% in Richmond, while the lowest was 58.80% for Vancouver Island West, a range of more than 34 percentage points.

The highest rates were achieved in two regions of the province. The urban lower mainland in the southwest of the province had several school districts achieving graduation rates above 83% (Richmond, West Vancouver, Coquitlam, Burnaby, and Delta). In the southeast of the province, Southeast Kootenay, Kootenay-Columbia, Rocky Mountain, and Revelstoke all achieved rates above 83%, as did neighbouring school districts Boundary and Vernon. Arrow Lakes in the southeast is somewhat of an anomaly in that its graduation rates are considerably lower than its neighbouring school districts.

Graduation rates were much lower among several school districts on Vancouver Island, particularly Vancouver Island West, Alberni, and Sooke, all with rates of 65% or lower. Low graduation rates were also evident throughout northern and interior school districts. For example, Gold Trail, Nicola-Similkameen, Stikine, Nisga'a, Nechako Lakes, and Haida Gwaii/Queen Charlotte all had rates of less than 65%. Peace River North and Bulkley Valley, both northern school districts, out-performed their neighbouring school districts.

Provincially, and for all but five school districts, girls had much higher graduation rates than boys (82% compared to 75%). For Nisga'a, girls graduated at a rate of 83.33% compared to only 42.31% for boys.

The range of 48 percentage points between the highest and lowest districts for boys was much greater than for girls, at 38 percentage points. Both genders showed major geographical variations in graduation rates individually, although patterns were quite similar for the genders combined. The five school districts where boys out-performed girls in graduation rates were all small (Vancouver Island North, Central Coast, Fraser-Cascade, Haida Gwaii/Queen Charlotte, and Stikine). In Central Coast, boys had a rate of 81.15% compared to only 57.77% for girls.

School District	All respondents (%)	Males (%)	Females (%)
038 Richmond	92.95	89.78	96.38
045 West Vancouver	90.95	90.49	91.42
043 Coquitlam	87.73	85.48	90.32
005 Southeast Kootenay	87.07	83.79	90.70
020 Kootenay-Columbia	86.56	82.90	90.02
041 Burnaby	85.65	81.69	89.88
051 Boundary	85.01	78.20	92.60
037 Delta	84.84	81.06	89.08
006 Rocky Mountain	83.98	79.00	89.95
019 Revelstoke	83.69	78.15	89.80
022 Vernon	83.24	82.23	84.36
067 Okanagan Skaha	81.87	79.43	84.56
036 Surrey	81.84	76.05	88.17
053 Okanagan Similkameen	81.25	75.36	88.50
044 North Vancouver	81.09	79.24	83.08
008 Kootenay Lake	80.98	79.57	82.37
046 Sunshine Coast	80.42	77.35	83.44
083 North Okanagan-Shuswap	80.20	78.72	82.01
039 Vancouver	80.07	75.99	84.31
060 Peace River North	78.98	74.23	84.48
054 Bulkley Valley	77.99	75.94	80.79
068 Nanaimo-Ladysmith	77.40	75.25	79.71
048 Howe Sound	77.22	71.41	84.07
040 New Westminster	77.10	72.36	82.11
035 Langley	77.01	73.84	80.23
042 Maple Ridge-Pitt Meadows	76.36	71.68	81.27
072 Campbell River	75.83	72.04	80.11
052 Prince Rupert	75.80	71.37	79.78
047 Powell River	75.68	74.68	76.78
023 Central Okanagan	75.64	72.59	78.96
073 Kamloops/Thompson	75.64	70.86	80.86
061 Greater Victoria	75.53	73.61	77.54
082 Coast Mountains	74.49	72.88	76.27
034 Abbotsford	73.88	70.55	77.79
069 Qualicum	73.50	68.84	78.20
085 Vancouver Island North	73.38	78.30	68.05
075 Mission	73.21	66.02	81.57
010 Arrow Lakes	72.80	72.16	73.19
081 Fort Nelson	72.62	66.52	79.20
063 Saanich	71.70	71.59	71.82
071 Comox Valley	70.69	69.53	71.91
049 Central Coast	70.62	81.15	57.77
028 Quesnel	70.51	66.68	74.53
078 Fraser-Cascade	69.88	70.69	69.19
059 Peace River South	69.84	66.36	73.96
033 Chilliwack	69.42	64.59	74.63
079 Cowichan Valley	69.38	66.22	72.65
057 Prince George	69.34	63.99	74.97
027 Cariboo-Chilcotin	68.57	64.06	74.00
064 Gulf Islands	67.70	67.70	67.71
062 Sooke	65.09	59.34	71.93
050 Haida Gwaii/Queen Charlotte	63.26	65.14	60.64
091 Nechako Lakes	63.03	62.35	63.79
070 Alberni	63.02	62.80	63.25
092 Nisga'a	62.98	42.31	83.33
087 Stikine	61.87	65.32	58.77
058 Nicola-Similkameen	60.03	53.73	66.44
074 Gold Trail	59.98	45.35	73.93
084 Vancouver Island West	58.80	49.19	69.69
999 Province	**79.00**	**75.00**	**82.00**

High school graduation

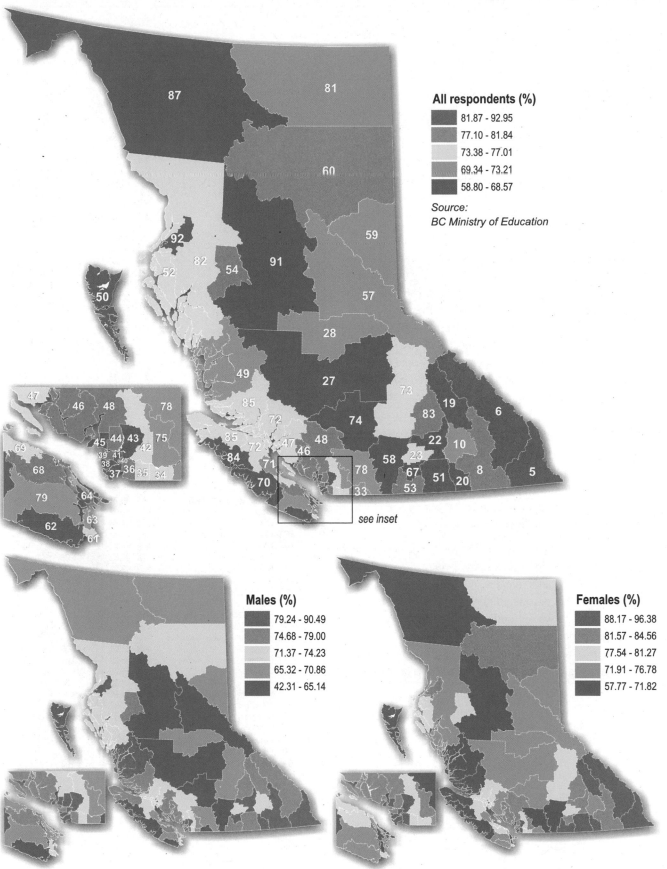

All respondents (%)

- 81.87 - 92.95
- 77.10 - 81.84
- 73.38 - 77.01
- 69.34 - 73.21
- 58.80 - 68.57

Source:
BC Ministry of Education

see inset

Males (%)

- 79.24 - 90.49
- 74.68 - 79.00
- 71.37 - 74.23
- 65.32 - 70.86
- 42.31 - 65.14

Females (%)

- 88.17 - 96.38
- 81.57 - 84.56
- 77.54 - 81.27
- 71.91 - 76.78
- 57.77 - 71.82

High school graduation for Aboriginal students

Graduation rates for Aboriginal students were substantially lower than for the Grade 12 student population as a whole. Less than half (48%) of all Aboriginal students graduated from high school in 2004/5, thus putting them at a severe developmental disadvantage over their life course when compared to the large majority of students in the province. It must be remembered that we are dealing with small numbers and it is not possible to show the percentage graduation rates for several school districts because of these small numbers (Arrow Lakes and West Vancouver for both genders, Stikine for males, and Gulf Islands for females).

There was major geographic variation in graduation rates, and a range among school districts of nearly 60 percentage points. The highest rate was 74.12% in Revelstoke, which would put it in the bottom part of the middle quintile for provincial students as a whole. The graduation rates for all but four school districts (Revelstoke, Kootenay-Columbia, Rocky Mountain, and Peace River North) would be in the lowest quintile group of school districts when compared with the provincial Grade 12 graduation rates for all students.

School districts with graduation rates above 60% were in the northeast and southeast parts of the province, with outliers in the southern Okanagan (Okanagan Similkameen and Okanagan Skaha), central (Central Coast) and north coast (Nisga'a), and southwest (Sunshine Coast and Coquitlam). On Vancouver Island, only Comox Valley and Nanaimo-Ladysmith had graduation rates above 50%.

As for all Grade 12 students in the province, Aboriginal girls out-performed Aboriginal boys provincially (51% compared to 44%). All Aboriginal females in Revelstoke graduated, while only 15.77% graduated in New Westminster. For 13 school districts, boys out-performed girls in graduation rates. The range among school districts for boys was 55 percentage points, with Okanagan Skaha graduating nearly 70% of Aboriginal boys and Vancouver Island North graduating only 13.80%.

School District	All respondents (%)	Males (%)	Females (%)
019 Revelstoke	74.12	37.39	100.00
020 Kootenay-Columbia	73.05	67.10	79.57
006 Rocky Mountain	72.06	66.73	79.91
060 Peace River North	68.61	61.88	75.19
053 Okanagan Similkameen	65.85	55.96	71.47
067 Okanagan Skaha	64.67	69.75	61.15
043 Coquitlam	63.09	56.67	73.58
046 Sunshine Coast	62.39	65.52	57.91
092 Nisga'a	61.58	42.31	81.94
008 Kootenay Lake	61.44	50.28	72.85
049 Central Coast	60.84	75.52	36.20
081 Fort Nelson	59.95	61.41	58.94
071 Comox Valley	59.83	56.64	63.73
035 Langley	59.27	57.68	60.90
022 Vernon	59.17	56.45	61.63
051 Boundary	57.66	60.34	54.83
034 Abbotsford	57.17	51.10	65.13
083 North Okanagan-Shuswap	56.98	52.61	60.24
052 Prince Rupert	56.71	50.76	62.46
054 Bulkley Valley	56.17	49.18	67.32
069 Qualicum	55.80	35.91	74.96
082 Coast Mountains	55.25	57.28	53.05
037 Delta	54.27	62.07	46.28
005 Southeast Kootenay	52.88	55.36	49.26
087 Stikine	51.87	Msk	42.78
068 Nanaimo-Ladysmith	51.47	48.66	54.37
042 Maple Ridge-Pitt Meadows	51.15	44.70	57.36
036 Surrey	49.51	47.39	51.37
075 Mission	49.16	35.53	60.82
023 Central Okanagan	48.98	41.22	57.27
047 Powell River	48.92	47.88	50.01
033 Chilliwack	47.75	44.62	51.13
074 Gold Trail	47.49	34.96	60.26
044 North Vancouver	46.59	45.17	47.79
028 Quesnel	46.50	42.25	52.47
072 Campbell River	46.25	41.61	52.05
085 Vancouver Island North	46.24	50.21	41.04
078 Fraser-Cascade	46.01	53.03	42.11
058 Nicola-Similkameen	44.86	39.69	50.22
073 Kamloops/Thompson	44.42	31.46	58.19
091 Nechako Lakes	43.22	34.98	50.16
038 Richmond	42.52	34.86	48.98
041 Burnaby	42.29	34.51	52.79
059 Peace River South	41.81	38.40	45.89
048 Howe Sound	38.81	40.41	37.13
070 Alberni	38.75	48.17	31.72
057 Prince George	37.54	36.52	38.60
061 Greater Victoria	37.40	36.76	38.30
050 Haida Gwaii/Queen Charlotte	37.34	37.37	37.30
062 Sooke	36.06	37.07	35.19
027 Cariboo-Chilcotin	35.29	33.08	38.49
079 Cowichan Valley	35.25	31.77	39.16
064 Gulf Islands	33.33	37.51	Msk
039 Vancouver	31.21	28.60	33.10
063 Saanich	27.97	25.44	30.32
084 Vancouver Island West	23.82	13.80	37.41
040 New Westminster	17.77	19.65	15.77
010 Arrow Lakes	Msk	Msk	Msk
045 West Vancouver	Msk	Msk	Msk
999 Province	**48.00**	**44.00**	**51.00**

High school graduation for Aboriginal students

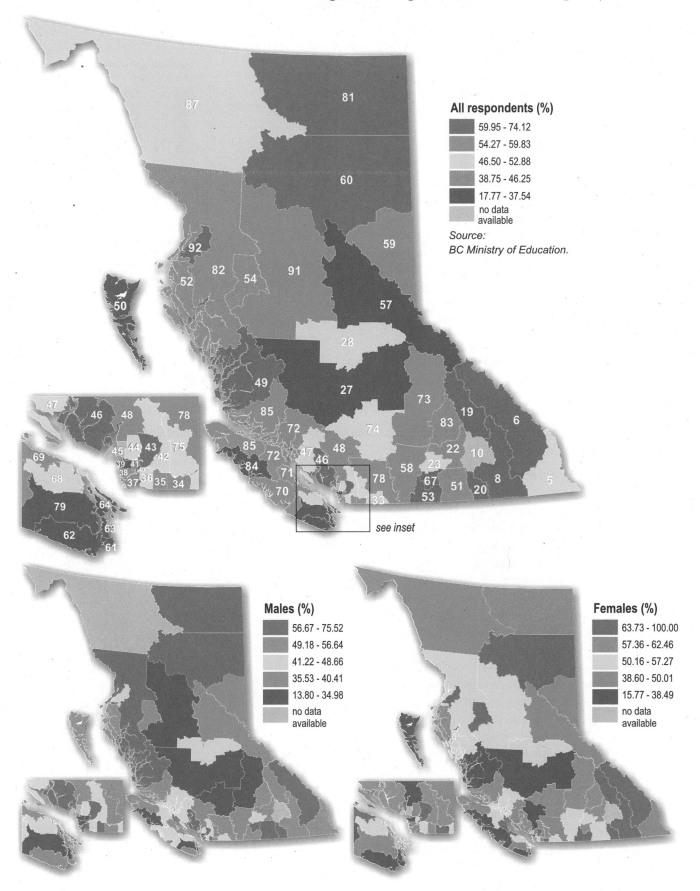

All respondents (%)
- 59.95 - 74.12
- 54.27 - 59.83
- 46.50 - 52.88
- 38.75 - 46.25
- 17.77 - 37.54
- no data available

Source:
BC Ministry of Education.

Males (%)
- 56.67 - 75.52
- 49.18 - 56.64
- 41.22 - 48.66
- 35.53 - 40.41
- 13.80 - 34.98
- no data available

Females (%)
- 63.73 - 100.00
- 57.36 - 62.46
- 50.16 - 57.27
- 38.60 - 50.01
- 15.77 - 38.49
- no data available

see inset

Adult educational achievement

People not completing high school are more likely to rate their health only fair or poor, to report problems with functional health, and to be smokers (Canadian Institute for Health Information, 2004). Completion of post-secondary education goes a long way to getting a good, well-paying job, which also improves health and wellness. "The effects of education extend beyond the economic sphere. Most agree that the total benefits to society from education are greater than the sum of what individuals earn as a result of their educational attainment...the schooling system is the primary agent of socialization in modern societies" (Desjardins and Schuller, 2006, p. 11). Higher levels of schooling contribute to better levels of civic and social engagement, both important wellness assets (Campbell, 2006).

The two maps opposite provide information on key educational achievements related to graduation from high school and completion of post-secondary education. Both sets of data are from the 2001 Canada Census.

High school graduates

For BC as a whole, more than four out of every five residents (82.84%) between the ages of 25 and 54 had successfully completed their high school education in 2001. There were major regional differences throughout the province, however, and the range between the highest and lowest levels of completion was 16 percentage points. The lower mainland and South Vancouver Island regions had the highest completion rates: North Shore/Coast Garibaldi, South Vancouver Island, Fraser North, Vancouver, and Richmond all had more than 85% high school completion rate among their residents aged 25 to 54. By contrast, the northern HSDAs and interior areas of the province were lower than the provincial average completion rates. Northeast had only 73.44% of its population with high school completion, while Northwest, North Vancouver Island, and Northern Interior all had rates below 76%.

Post-secondary graduates

For the province as a whole, more than half of the population (57.7%) between the ages of 25 and 54 had completed some type of post-secondary education in 2001. The range between the highest and lowest

Health Service Delivery Area	High school graduates (%)	Post-secondary graduates (%)
033 North Shore/Coast Garibaldi	89.47	66.76
041 South Vancouver Island	86.59	61.82
022 Fraser North	86.22	60.87
032 Vancouver	85.55	64.96
031 Richmond	85.25	60.54
012 Kootenay Boundary	82.38	56.88
023 Fraser South	81.31	53.93
013 Okanagan	80.89	54.93
042 Central Vancouver Island	80.67	54.05
011 East Kootenay	79.26	53.70
014 Thompson Cariboo Shuswap	77.61	50.86
021 Fraser East	76.65	48.93
051 Northwest	75.94	48.09
043 North Vancouver Island	75.93	48.13
052 Northern Interior	75.60	46.98
053 Northeast	73.44	47.54
999 Province	**82.84**	**57.70**

regions was 19 percentage points. Similar to the pattern for high school completion, the highest rates for post-secondary completion occurred in the lower mainland, North Shore/Coast Garibaldi, Vancouver, Fraser North, and Richmond, as well as South Vancouver Island. All had rates in excess of 60% with post-secondary education completion in their population aged 25 to 54. Again, the northern HSDAs, Northern Interior, Northeast, and Northwest, and North Vancouver Island, had the lowest rates (around 48% or less). This is 10 percentage points or more below the provincial average.

Adult educational achievement

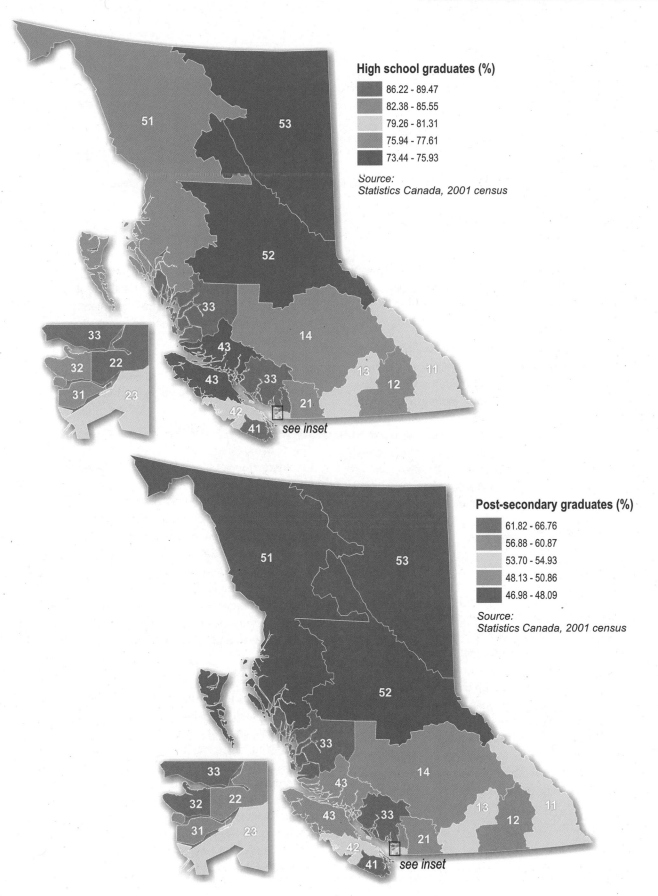

High school graduates (%)

- 86.22 - 89.47
- 82.38 - 85.55
- 79.26 - 81.31
- 75.94 - 77.61
- 73.44 - 75.93

Source:
Statistics Canada, 2001 census

Post-secondary graduates (%)

- 61.82 - 66.76
- 56.88 - 60.87
- 53.70 - 54.93
- 48.13 - 50.86
- 46.98 - 48.09

Source:
Statistics Canada, 2001 census

Composite learning index: Lifelong learning

Learning affects all areas of life, including physical, emotional, and spiritual components of living. A Composite Learning Index (CLI) developed by the Canadian Council on Learning combines several data sets to develop a single score that represents the state of lifelong learning for 2006. Four key elements, described below, are combined to create a composite learning index (see *www.ccl-cca. ca/ccl* for more information). Each of the four elements has a value of five for Canada as a whole. For mapping purposes, only three divisions are used, rather than the normal quintile range. This is because there are only eight economic development regions.

	Economic Development Region	Overall CLI score	Learning to know	Learning to do	Learning to live together	Learning to be
1	Vancouver Island and Coast	80	5.1	6.7	5.5	5.7
2	Lower Mainland-Southwest	79	5.9	6.8	4.4	5.0
4	Kootenay	72	4.4	6.5	4.5	5.0
3	Thompson-Okanagan	70	4.5	6.4	4.5	4.3
5	Cariboo	70	4.3	6.3	3.5	5.6
8	Northeast	61	2.8	6.4	3.3	4.9
6	North Coast	61	2.7	6.4	3.4	5.0
7	Nechako	60	2.7	6.3	3.6	4.3

Overall CLI score

The overall range in values of the Index was from 60 for the Nechako economic development region to a high of 80 (out of a possible score of 100) for the Vancouver Island and Coast region. Generally, the north and interior parts of the province scored lower than the lower mainland and Vancouver Island. By comparison, the highest value across Canada was Calgary, with a value of 88, and the lowest were Campbellton-Miramichi in New Brunswick and Gaspesie-Iles-de-la-Madeleine in Quebec, both with a value of 47. For Canada overall, the index had a value of 73.0 for 2006, with BC's score of 76.6 second only to Alberta at 80.1.

Learning to know

This element is based on developing a foundation of knowledge and skills that are required to function in today's world, including literacy, numeracy, general knowledge, and the ability for critical thinking. Key components are: student skills in reading, math, and problem solving; high school drop out rates; young adults' participation in post-secondary education; and post-secondary achievement among working age adults. The scores within BC ranged from 5.9 for Lower Mainland-Southwest to 2.7 for Nechako and North Coast. Across Canada, Montreal had the highest value at 6.4, while Yorkton, Saskatchewan had a low of 2.1.

Learning to do

Included in this aspect is acquisition of applied skills, involving technical as well as "hands on" skills and knowledge, which is closely related to employment success. Key components are job-related training, availability of employment training, and access to learning institutions. Overall, there was little geographical variation, with Lower Mainland-Southwest scoring 6.8 (highest of all economic regions in Canada), while Nechako and Cariboo scored 6.3; this compares with the lowest value across Canada of 3.0 for both South Coast-Burin Peninsula in Newfoundland and Gaspesie-Iles-de-la-Madeleine in Quebec.

Learning to live together

The development of values of respect and concern for others around us are the basis of this element. It involves the acquisition of social and interpersonal skills and an appreciation of diversity within society. It helps develop and support a cohesive society. Attributes include charitable giving, volunteerism, participation in social and other organizations, and access to community institutions. BC values ranged from a high of 5.5 for Vancouver Island and Coast to 3.3 for Northeast. By contrast, the high and low scores across Canada were 7.5 for Regina-Moose Mountain in Saskatchewan and 1.9 for the North region in Manitoba.

Learning to be

Learning to be helps develop the whole individual—mind, body, and spirit—and involves personal discovery, self-awareness, creativity, and a healthy and well-balanced life. Key attributes include exposure to media, sports and recreation, cultural events and activities, festivals, performing arts, and resources such as libraries. The range across the province was from 5.7 for Vancouver Island Coast to 4.3 for Thompson-Okanagan and Nechako. Across Canada, Calgary with a score of 6.9 and Bas-Saint-Laurent in Quebec with 1.3 are the highest and lowest regions.

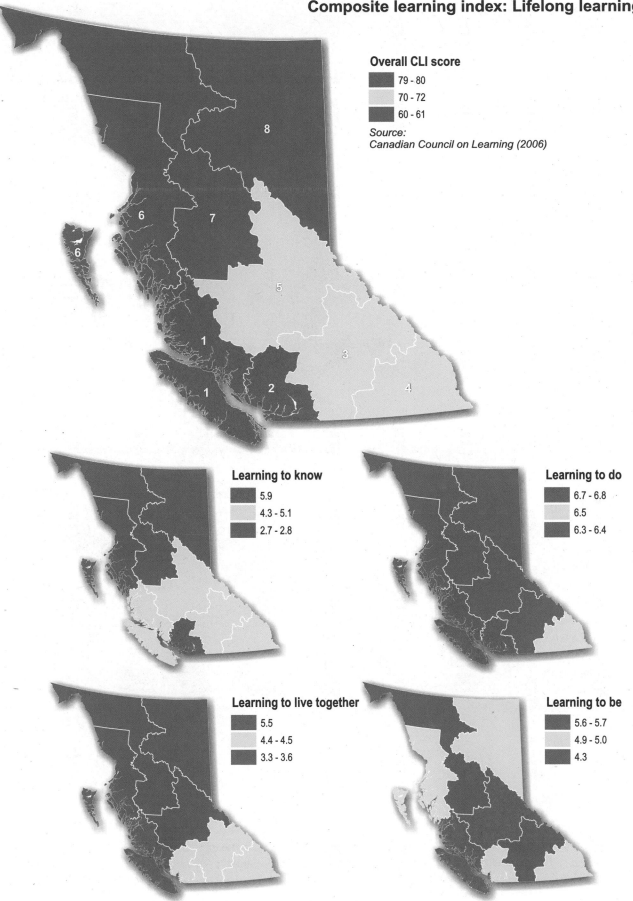

Composite learning index: Lifelong learning

Overall CLI score
- 79 - 80
- 70 - 72
- 60 - 61

Source:
Canadian Council on Learning (2006)

Learning to know
- 5.9
- 4.3 - 5.1
- 2.7 - 2.8

Learning to do
- 6.7 - 6.8
- 6.5
- 6.3 - 6.4

Learning to live together
- 5.5
- 4.4 - 4.5
- 3.3 - 3.6

Learning to be
- 5.6 - 5.7
- 4.9 - 5.0
- 4.3

Libraries and literacy

There are 31 public library systems in BC, each of which has a number of branches. In addition, there are 40 small libraries run by library associations that rèly on over 1,200 volunteers to assist in their daily operations. Overall, there are approximately 240 separate public library service outlets. The largest libraries are run by municipalities (26), and there are also three regional library systems serving the Fraser Valley, Okanagan, and Vancouver Island regions, and two integrated public library systems serving participating municipalities and electoral areas in the Cariboo and Thompson-Nicola regional districts of the province. Finally, there is the InterLINK Federated Public Library System, which links all of the lower mainland libraries together (Ministry of Education, 2006).

Libraries vary greatly in terms of the resident cardholders as a percentage of the population served. For the province as a whole, in 2005-2006, approximately 53% of the population served were resident cardholders of libraries. Rossland in the southeast of the province had the highest percentage of population

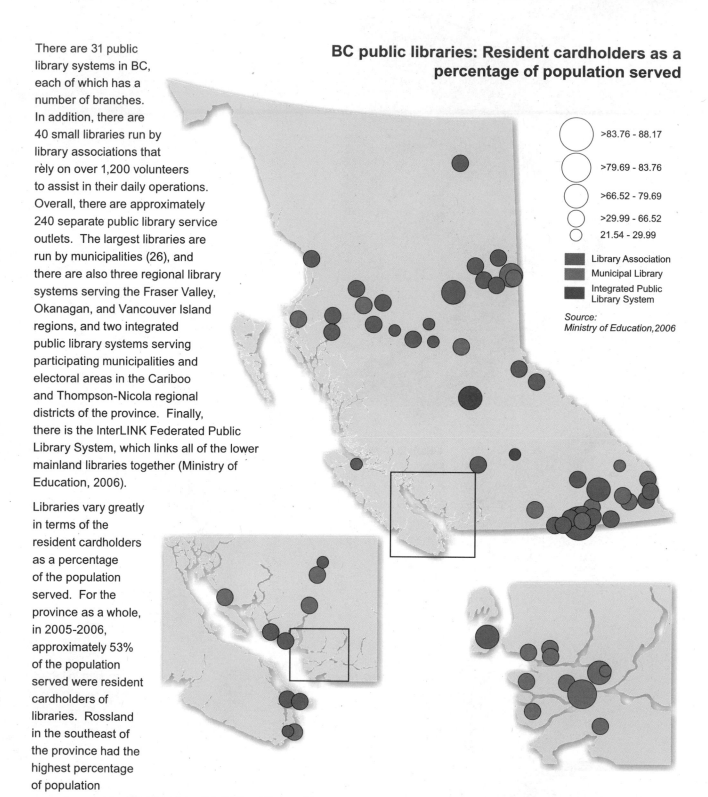

BC public libraries: Resident cardholders as a percentage of population served

>83.76 - 88.17
>79.69 - 83.76
>66.52 - 79.69
>29.99 - 66.52
21.54 - 29.99

Library Association
Municipal Library
Integrated Public Library System

Source:
Ministry of Education, 2006

served as resident cardholders (88.17%). Others with high percentages included New Westminster (83.76%), Bowen Island (79.69%), and Port Moody (70.44%) in the lower mainland of the province, Dawson Creek (72.82%)

in the northeast, Cariboo (74.99%) and Mackenzie (73.68%) in the interior, and Kaslo and District (77.35%) in the southeast. Several systems had relatively few resident cardholders as a percentage of population

BC public libraries: Circulation per capita

served: Vanderhoof, View Royal, Burns Lake, Pemberton and District, Fort St. James, Alert Bay, Thompson-Nicola, Coquitlam, and Invermere (all less than 30%).

A second measure of the importance of a library to the local community is circulation (or borrowing of items) per capita. On an annual basis, the average for the province was 12.61 items per capita for 2005-2006. The highest circulation rates tended to be in the urban lower mainland part of the province and southern Vancouver Island. West Vancouver, Richmond, and North Vancouver District all had rates in excess of 20 per capita. Others with high rates included Port Moody, Gibson's and District, Burnaby, Vancouver, and Greater Victoria, all with annual borrowing rates between 15 and 20 per capita.

Higher levels of literacy are associated with greater involvement with community groups, better employment prospects, and better income and overall health and wellness. 2010 Legacies Now is supporting a series of Literacy Now projects around the province. The focus is on community development strategies to stimulate literacy initiatives, alliances, and planning within communities. Pilot projects around the province reflect the diversity of BC, and in 2006 there were more than 50 literacy task groups around the province representing more than 100 communities.

Legend:
- >20.66 - 22.43
- >14.93 - 20.66
- >13.25 - 14.93
- >2.16 - 13.25
- 1.13 - 2.16

Library Association
Municipal Library
Integrated Public Library System

Source: Ministry of Education, 2006

Feels safe at school

The BC Ministry of Education defines safe schools as "ones in which members of the school community are free of the fear of harm, including potential threats from inside or outside the school" (Ministry of Education, 2004, p. 11). In order to measure feelings of safety, the School Satisfaction Survey asks students in Grades 3/4, 7, 10, and 12 the simple question *"Do you feel safe at school?"*. The three maps included here provide a picture of the percentage of students by school district who answered "many times, or always" for all of the four grades combined. Maps for males and females are also provided.

Overall, only 77% of all students in the sampled grades felt safe at school in the 2005-2006 survey (a percentage that has remained fairly consistent over the 5 years that the survey has been used), although there was a relatively large variation (more than 20 percentage points) among school districts. There were several groupings within the province with higher percentages of feeling safe. These included a group of school districts in the lower mainland and the southern part of Vancouver Island, as well as in the southern interior of the province. Geographical outliers included the smaller Central Coast and Fort Nelson school districts. Those scoring lower on the safety scale were located in the northern and western part of Vancouver Island and in the central part of the province, with outliers in the extreme southeast.

By gender, females generally had a higher percentage of students feeling safe compared to males, although this was not the case for every school district. For example, the Nisga'a school district had a much higher percentage of males feeling safe than females (80.49% compared with 68.97%). The geographical patterns were quite similar to those for the sampled students as a whole.

While not mapped here, among the four grade groups, Grades 3/4 felt the safest (83%), followed by Grade 7 (78%), Grade 12 (76%), and Grade 10 (70%). Rates showed a very modest improvement over time (except for Grades 3/4), with the largest improvement occurring for Grade 7, which went from 64% feeling safe in 2001-2002 to 70% in 2005-2006.

School District	All respondents (%)	Males (%)	Females (%)
049 Central Coast	86.36	87.88	84.85
045 West Vancouver	85.44	82.92	88.10
051 Boundary	81.71	81.19	82.27
081 Fort Nelson	81.61	80.41	82.67
038 Richmond	81.01	78.60	83.46
010 Arrow Lakes	80.38	77.48	83.67
075 Mission	80.35	79.90	80.81
022 Vernon	80.33	78.02	83.14
037 Delta	79.91	76.63	83.23
035 Langley	79.46	77.98	80.98
064 Gulf Islands	79.41	74.75	84.39
061 Greater Victoria	79.31	77.13	81.53
008 Kootenay Lake	79.26	77.74	80.99
046 Sunshine Coast	78.77	74.89	82.36
044 North Vancouver	78.77	77.50	80.12
023 Central Okanagan	78.64	76.65	80.59
078 Fraser-Cascade	78.48	78.67	78.22
079 Cowichan Valley	78.45	76.94	79.76
068 Nanaimo-Ladysmith	78.05	76.38	79.59
039 Vancouver	77.82	75.63	80.28
020 Kootenay-Columbia	77.52	74.32	81.40
053 Okanagan Similkameen	77.36	73.85	80.54
063 Saanich	77.16	74.26	80.14
071 Comox Valley	77.05	73.18	81.03
073 Kamloops/Thompson	77.01	76.22	77.79
067 Okanagan Skaha	76.90	74.34	79.33
069 Qualicum	76.82	70.75	83.22
043 Coquitlam	76.61	74.20	79.08
019 Revelstoke	76.56	75.27	77.84
036 Surrey	76.31	73.90	78.91
083 North Okanagan-Shuswap	76.24	74.45	78.43
040 New Westminster	76.22	75.65	76.83
058 Nicola-Similkameen	76.20	74.05	78.43
057 Prince George	76.07	74.65	77.64
034 Abbotsford	75.84	72.55	79.43
092 Nisga'a	75.71	80.49	68.97
006 Rocky Mountain	75.64	75.00	76.89
082 Coast Mountains	75.62	72.58	78.08
042 Maple Ridge-Pitt Meadows	75.42	74.62	76.51
048 Howe Sound	74.93	72.59	77.27
033 Chilliwack	74.81	72.07	77.64
091 Nechako Lakes	73.72	73.32	74.30
052 Prince Rupert	73.64	74.41	72.78
041 Burnaby	73.60	71.96	75.43
050 Haida Gwaii/Queen Charlotte	73.58	71.25	75.64
059 Peace River South	73.25	71.46	75.33
072 Campbell River	72.96	70.09	76.01
028 Quesnel	72.79	72.44	73.01
027 Cariboo-Chilcotin	72.75	69.46	76.33
054 Bulkley Valley	72.54	72.27	72.78
060 Peace River North	71.10	70.32	71.80
070 Alberni	70.63	67.55	74.40
062 Sooke	70.55	69.52	71.44
005 Southeast Kootenay	70.22	70.53	70.19
084 Vancouver Island West	70.21	66.67	76.47
074 Gold Trail	69.70	70.44	68.15
047 Powell River	68.54	68.97	68.06
085 Vancouver Island North	65.18	65.76	64.76
087 Stikine	N/A	N/A	N/A
999 Province	76.97	74.92	79.13

Feels safe at school

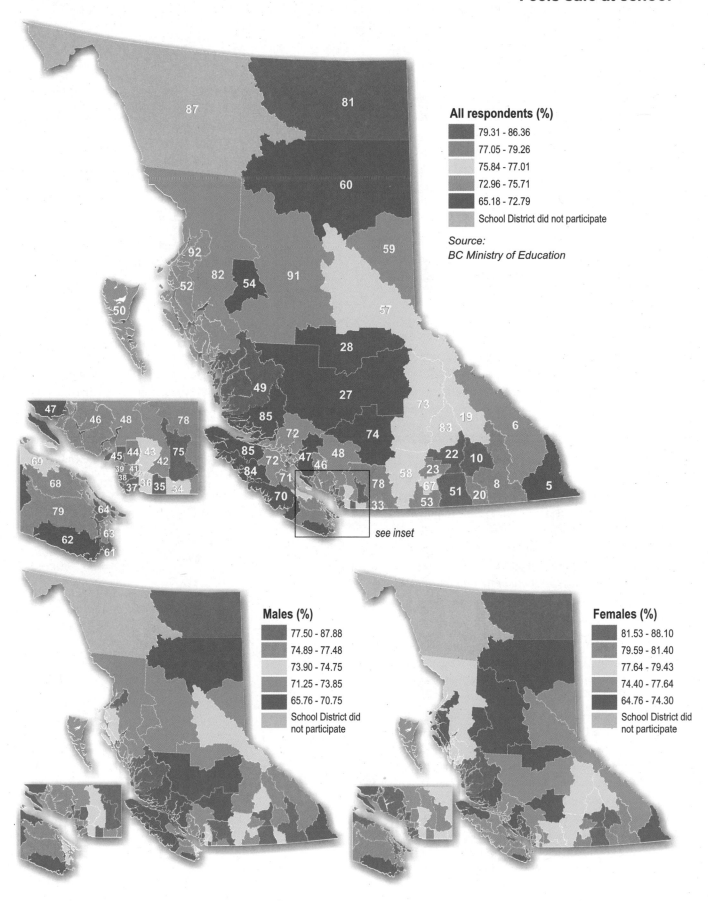

All respondents (%)
- 79.31 - 86.36
- 77.05 - 79.26
- 75.84 - 77.01
- 72.96 - 75.71
- 65.18 - 72.79
- School District did not participate

Source:
BC Ministry of Education

see inset

Males (%)
- 77.50 - 87.88
- 74.89 - 77.48
- 73.90 - 74.75
- 71.25 - 73.85
- 65.76 - 70.75
- School District did not participate

Females (%)
- 81.53 - 88.10
- 79.59 - 81.40
- 77.64 - 79.43
- 74.40 - 77.64
- 64.76 - 74.30
- School District did not participate

Crime rates

Communities with lower crime rates are generally healthier communities. Three different indicators of crime are included here, expressed as the 3 year average of the number of offences per 1,000 population for 2002-2004. The change in the crime rate is the percentage change in the serious crime rate average for the 3 year period 2002-2004 over the rate for the previous 3 year period (1999-2001). The serious violent crime rate is based on reporting within the crime categories of homicide, attempted murder, sexual and non-sexual assault resulting in bodily harm, and robbery and abduction. The serious property crime rate includes breaking and entering, but excludes motor vehicle theft, bicycle theft, and pick-pocketing.

Health Service Delivery Area	Change in total serious crime (%)	Serious violent crime	Serious property crime
032 Vancouver	-15.7	5.5	17.2
041 South Vancouver Island	-12.1	2.3	7.7
023 Fraser South	-9.2	2.9	12.3
043 North Vancouver Island	-7.6	2.5	11.8
013 Okanagan	-7.3	2.0	11.3
042 Central Vancouver Island	-6.6	1.8	11.3
033 North Shore/Coast Garibaldi	-4.5	1.8	9.6
014 Thompson Cariboo Shuswap	-3.2	2.3	12.2
011 East Kootenay	-2.2	1.3	9.4
022 Fraser North	1.5	3.1	13.4
012 Kootenay Boundary	3.9	1.2	7.5
052 Northern Interior	6.3	3.6	15.3
051 Northwest	6.7	3.0	11.2
021 Fraser East	11.1	2.4	14.9
031 Richmond	11.4	1.7	11.5
053 Northeast	17.9	3.7	13.6
999 Province	**-5.1**	**2.9**	**12.6**

Change in total serious crime rate

Overall, the province-wide serious crime rate decreased by 5.1% between the 1999-2001 and 2002-2004 periods. Most of this reduction is related to property crimes, which were 5.9% lower in the latter period, compared to only a 1.8% reduction for violent crime. Geographically, the reduction was far from even. The greatest decreases occurred in Vancouver, South Vancouver Island, and Fraser South, which all saw reductions of close to 10% or more. However, large increases occurred in several HSDAs. Northeast, Richmond, and Fraser East all saw increases in excess of 10%. For the Northeast and Fraser East, this increase was equally distributed between violent and property crimes. For Richmond, there was a much greater increase in violent crime (16.4%) than in property crime (10.7%).

Serious violent crime rate

For the province as a whole, the rate for violent crime was quite low when compared to other types of crime, at 2.9 per 1,000 population. Vancouver, at 5.5, was nearly twice the provincial average, while high rates also occurred in Northeast and Northern Interior. The lowest crime rates were in the southeast of the province, East Kootenay and Kootenay Boundary both with rates less than half the provincial average. Despite the recent large percentage increase in violent crime rates in Richmond, it still had one of the lowest rates in the province at 1.7 per 1,000 population. Overall, the southeast part of the province had the lowest rates, while the north had the highest, along with Vancouver in the south.

Serious property crime rate

Serious property crimes outnumbered violent crimes by a factor of more than four to one. The highest rates occurred in Vancouver (17.2 per 1,000), Northern Interior, and Fraser East. Other lower mainland HSDAs had higher than average rates (Fraser North and South). The HSDAs with the lowest rates were again in the southeast of the province (East Kootenay and Kootenay Boundary) and on South Vancouver Island.

Crime rates

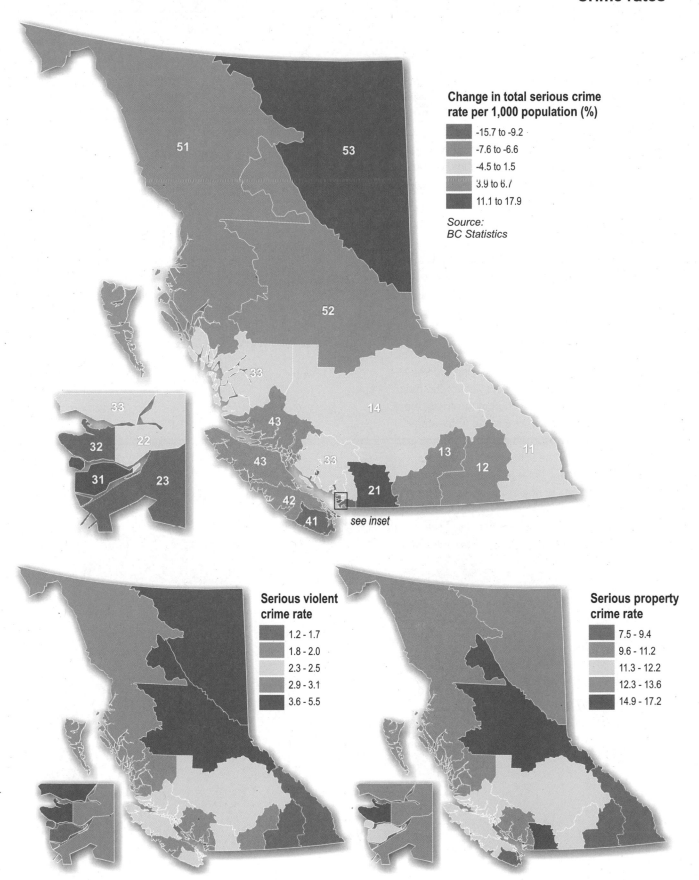

Change in total serious crime rate per 1,000 population (%)

- -15.7 to -9.2
- -7.6 to -6.6
- -4.5 to 1.5
- 3.9 to 6.7
- 11.1 to 17.9

Source:
BC Statistics

Serious violent crime rate

- 1.2 - 1.7
- 1.8 - 2.0
- 2.3 - 2.5
- 2.9 - 3.1
- 3.6 - 5.5

Serious property crime rate

- 7.5 - 9.4
- 9.6 - 11.2
- 11.3 - 12.2
- 12.3 - 13.6
- 14.9 - 17.2

Civic engagement: Voting in the 2005 BC provincial election

Not all individuals who can vote, provincially, actually register to vote, so the data presented here probably over-estimate the percent of individuals voting who can vote. Voting has properties of civic and political engagement and is a measure of interest in, trust of, and the desire to influence civil institutions that affect public policies and our way of living. For many, voting is viewed as a civic obligation (Campbell, 2006).

The map opposite provides the pattern of voter turnout for the May, 2005 provincial election. It should be noted that, overall, there are 79 ridings for which these data are available. Data were obtained at the poll station level and converted to HSDAs so that there would be an opportunity for users of the Atlas to compare this measure with other measures of wellness that are available at the HSDA level.

For the province as a whole in the 2005 provincial election, nearly 6 out of every 10 registered voters (58.19%) actually voted. As with many of the other variables included in this section of the Atlas, there are major regional differences in the percentage of registered voters who turned out to vote in the last provincial election. The three HSDAs on Vancouver Island had the highest voter turnout, all with rates in excess of two-thirds of registered voters. Other HSDAs with relatively high turnout rates included North Shore/ Coast Garibaldi and Fraser South in the lower mainland, and Thompson Cariboo Shuswap in the interior of the province.

Much lower rates were evident in the extreme northeast (Northeast) and southeast (East Kootenay) of the province, along with Richmond and Vancouver in the lower mainland, all of which had turnout rates of about 56% or less.

Health Service Delivery Area	Registered voters that voted (%)
042 Central Vancouver Island	67.70
041 South Vancouver Island	67.67
043 North Vancouver Island	67.35
033 North Shore/Coast Garibaldi	65.23
023 Fraser South	62.80
014 Thompson Cariboo Shuswap	62.62
022 Fraser North	61.13
052 Northern Interior	59.90
012 Kootenay Boundary	59.14
013 Okanagan	58.84
021 Fraser East	57.66
051 Northwest	57.08
032 Vancouver	56.41
011 East Kootenay	55.50
031 Richmond	53.93
053 Northeast	51.63
999 Province	**58.19**

Civic engagement: Voting in the 2005 BC provincial election

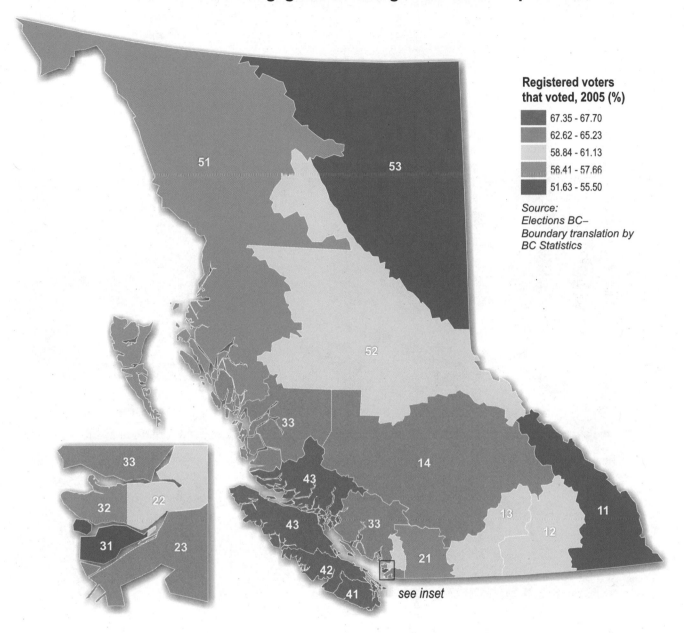

**Registered voters
that voted, 2005 (%)**

- 67.35 - 67.70
- 62.62 - 65.23
- 58.84 - 61.13
- 56.41 - 57.66
- 51.63 - 55.50

*Source:
Elections BC–
Boundary translation by
BC Statistics*

see inset

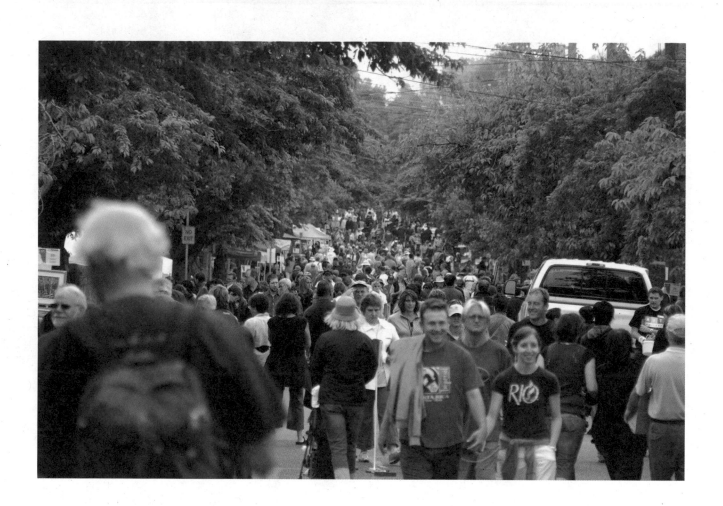

While BC has the lowest smoking rates in Canada, smoking behaviour and second-hand or environmental tobacco smoke are still causes and contributors to many key diseases and illnesses in the province. Tobacco is still the greatest preventable cause of death and illness in Canada (Bridge and Turpin, 2004; Ministry of Health Services, 2005). Annually, the Vital Statistics Agency publishes an estimate of the Smoking Attributable Mortality based on a variety of diagnoses related to smoking.

These include:

- Circulatory system diseases, such as hypertension, ischemic heart diseases, cerebrovascular diseases, other forms of heart diseases, and others;

- Cancers, such as cancers of the trachea, lung, pancreas, esophagus, and bladder, among others;

- Respiratory system diseases, such as chronic obstructive pulmonary disease, pneumonia and influenza, and bronchitis and emphysema.

In both 2004 and 2005, the total number of deaths attributable to smoking and its effects was estimated at nearly 6,000 in BC (Vital Statistics, 2005, 2006), out of a total of almost 30,000 deaths occurring in each of those years. In other words, approximately 20% of deaths in BC can be attributed to smoking. On average, it has been estimated that smokers who quit can realize a reversal of the effects fairly quickly after quitting and could gain back up to 4.2 years of life that would otherwise have been lost through the impacts of continued smoking (Bridge and Turpin, 2004).

Not only are current smokers at risk of ill health and premature mortality, but so are non-smokers who inhale other people's exhaled smoke, known as "mainstream" smoke, and/or substances from cigarettes, known as "sidestream" smoke. The latter is likely the more dangerous of the two. Effects can be felt not only by those in the immediate vicinity of a smoker, but also those who may be in neighbouring apartments or housing units in multi-unit buildings. Smoke from one unit can enter a neighbouring unit through a variety of mechanisms, such as neighbouring patio, common ventilation systems, electrical outlets, and cracks and gaps around sinks and countertops (see *www. cleanaircoalitionbc.com*).

A recent report by the US Office of the Surgeon General (2006) has extensively reviewed the health effects of second-hand smoke and concluded that there is no risk-free level of exposure. Children in particular are vulnerable, because their bodies are still developing. There is evidence indicating that babies exposed to second-hand smoke have a much higher probability of dying from sudden infant death syndrome (Foster, Kierans, and Macdonald, 2002), as well as suffering from several ailments related to second-hand smoke.

While many premature deaths result from tobacco smoke, the health care and other costs associated with smoking-related diseases are very high (Select Standing Committee on Health, 2004). Bridge and Turpin (2004) indicate that, in 2002 dollars, smoking cost British Columbians conservatively approximately $525 million annually in medical care costs and more than $900 million in productivity losses related to excess disability of smokers and premature mortality. In addition, substantially more costs are borne directly by BC employers.

In many ways, BC has been a leader over the past 15 years or so in working to reduce smoking rates, both provincially and locally. The Capital Regional District was the first in Canada to enact a municipal bylaw to ensure that public indoor spaces were completely smoke-free 100% of the time. This action was not without considerable controversy and debate (McLintock, 2004). Many have since followed this lead. Smoking was also banned in all government offices in 1990, and many communities passed smoking restriction bylaws through the 1980s (Hollander, Foster, Curtis, and Galloway, 1992). However, the province has lost some of its leadership in the area of no smoking. There is no province-wide legislation that regulates smoking in all public places, although there is a regulation through the Workers' Compensation Board that regulates smoking in the work place, except for hospitality workers who still can work in Designated Smoking Rooms (see *www. cleanaircoalitionbc.com* for a history of this regulation).

In November 2006, the Premier of the province announced that: "By 2008, smoking will be banned in all indoor public places and starting next September smoking will be banned on all school property, public and private, across British Columbia." In March 2007, the province announced major changes to the Tobacco Sales Act, which will limit both the promotion and sale of tobacco, and ban smoking in public places. The amendments will implement the Premier's November 2006 announcement and ban: smoking in all indoor public spaces; tobacco use in schools and on school grounds; smoking in public doorways, near public doors, windows, and air intakes to protect indoor air quality; and tobacco sales in public hospital and health facilities, public universities and colleges, public athletic and recreational facilities, and all provincial buildings. The amendments will also provide for a ban on the display of tobacco products in all places where tobacco is sold that are accessible to youth under 19. This will include products like lighters and caps with tobacco brands on them and certain other tobacco advertising features.

Between 1985 and 2002, smoking rates in BC declined by 51% in those aged 15 and over (Bridge and Turpin, 2004). Some of the above-noted actions have certainly helped achieve this reduction. However, there is still much that can be done to prevent young people from initiating smoking, and to provide individual smokers with access to assistance to quit smoking altogether. The latter is often not easy because of the very addictive properties of tobacco. There are also other opportunities for role modelling in many venues, such as at the community level in public places, by school districts in schools, by employers in work places, and by individuals in their homes and through their own non-smoking behaviour.

In short, being a non-smoker, living in a non-smoking household, having enforced smoking restrictions in your place of work or school, not allowing smoking while driving, and living in a community that enforces restrictions on smoking in public places are all major wellness assets.

While BC does have relatively low rates of smoking, there are substantial variations throughout the province in a variety of key indicators related to non-smoking wellness assets and behaviours. What follows is the presentation of a total of 38 maps that describe eight key indicators related to these wellness assets for BC's population.

The first three maps present indicators related to healthy public policy to encourage non-smoking behaviours. Generally, healthy public policy is characterized by:

- broad emphasis on a healthy lifestyle and a healthy society;
- concern with ecology, the environment, and social justice;

- holistic approach to health;
- public participation in the health of one's community; and
- integrated and multisectoral approach to health (Hollander et al., 1992).

The first map in this series indicates the depth of smoking restriction policies adopted by the province's school districts. This gives an idea of the leadership being provided by the school boards in this important area of healthy public policy. Policies cover a variety of areas that have smoking bans and restrictions, including school grounds, buses, and buildings.

The next two maps provide data related to the adoption and type of no smoking bylaws introduced by municipalities at the community level. Such bylaws can help set the stage for specific restrictions within communities, and set local standards for non-smoking behaviour in the absence of provincial legislation. BC's first bylaw was enacted in 1968 by the City of Burnaby, but its focus was primarily related to preventing fires caused by careless smoking (Hollander et al., 1992). Throughout the 1980s, more than 40 communities adopted some type of smoking restriction that covered diverse public areas such as elevators, escalators and stairways, school buses and taxis, and public areas of local government offices, to name but a few.

The main grouping of maps in this section, using data from the CCHS, consists of 30 maps and depicts six separate indicators, each having five maps to cover age and gender characteristics of responses. The first of this group looks at the degree to which respondents frequent smoke-free public places, usually in leisure time activities. The next set of five maps provides information on the degree to which respondents are able to work in a smoke-free work environment. This is followed by data on choosing to travel in smoke-free vehicles. The next two groups of maps provide responses to two questions related to smoking restrictions in the home environment, while the final indicator looks at the results related to non-smoking by individuals.

All maps are provided at the HSDA level, with the exception of the map on school district policies which is at the school district level.

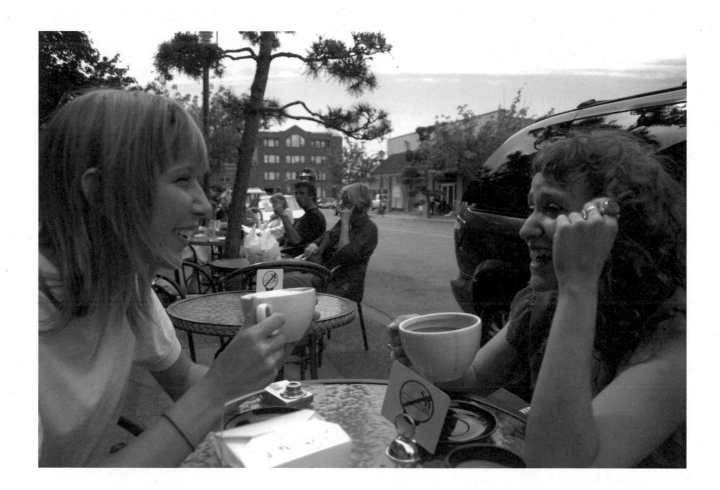

Smoking restrictions in school

Smoking restriction policies by school districts are important in that children do not have to endure second-hand smoke at an early age. In addition, restricting smoking sets a positive example for children, provides a role modelling environment, and helps get the message through to children and youth that not smoking is a positive behavioural attribute, or wellness asset.

In 2005, the Ministry of Health commissioned a review of the status of smoking policies in schools to identify opportunities for improvement (McBride, 2005). The survey, based on information from 58 school districts (Nisga'a and Conseil Scolaire Francophone were not included), indicated a large variation in terms of the type of smoking restrictions in place. All school districts had passed policies, except Kootenay-Columbia (School District 20) which relied on the policies provided by two previous school districts that were combined to create the Kootenay-Columbia district.

The map opposite shows the variation in school district smoking restriction policies based on seven different criteria which prohibited smoking in/on: buildings; grounds; district vehicles; other (e.g., vehicles parked on school grounds, all district functions, or sporting events); community use of school property; transportation; and enforcement provisions of policies.

Overall, no school district had implemented policies with all seven of the criteria. Several had policies in place on all restriction criteria but did not have an enforcement policy. In fact, many school districts had not put together a formal policy on enforcement.

Those with six of the criteria in place in their policies (7 school districts) were scattered around the province, although three were in the lower mainland.

Those with five criteria (15 school districts) tended to be in, or adjacent to, the lower mainland, southern/central Vancouver Island, and central coast/coast mountains. Kamloops/Thompson in the interior was an outlier to this pattern. The school districts with two or less criteria included in policies (9 school districts) tended to cluster in the extreme north and in the southern interior of the province, in addition to parts of Vancouver Island. School District 41 (Burnaby) was something of an outlier in the lower mainland.

The large variety of responses by school districts should disappear in the future based on the Premier's recent announcement on introducing universal smoking restrictions. The key issue, then, will become enforcement.

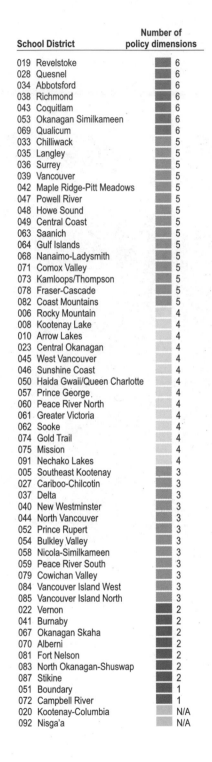

School District	Number of policy dimensions
019 Revelstoke	6
028 Quesnel	6
034 Abbotsford	6
038 Richmond	6
043 Coquitlam	6
053 Okanagan Similkameen	6
069 Qualicum	6
033 Chilliwack	5
035 Langley	5
036 Surrey	5
039 Vancouver	5
042 Maple Ridge-Pitt Meadows	5
047 Powell River	5
048 Howe Sound	5
049 Central Coast	5
063 Saanich	5
064 Gulf Islands	5
068 Nanaimo-Ladysmith	5
071 Comox Valley	5
073 Kamloops/Thompson	5
078 Fraser-Cascade	5
082 Coast Mountains	5
006 Rocky Mountain	4
008 Kootenay Lake	4
010 Arrow Lakes	4
023 Central Okanagan	4
045 West Vancouver	4
046 Sunshine Coast	4
050 Haida Gwaii/Queen Charlotte	4
057 Prince George	4
060 Peace River North	4
061 Greater Victoria	4
062 Sooke	4
074 Gold Trail	4
075 Mission	4
091 Nechako Lakes	4
005 Southeast Kootenay	3
027 Cariboo-Chilcotin	3
037 Delta	3
040 New Westminster	3
044 North Vancouver	3
052 Prince Rupert	3
054 Bulkley Valley	3
058 Nicola-Similkameen	3
059 Peace River South	3
079 Cowichan Valley	3
084 Vancouver Island West	3
085 Vancouver Island North	3
022 Vernon	2
041 Burnaby	2
067 Okanagan Skaha	2
070 Alberni	2
081 Fort Nelson	2
083 North Okanagan-Shuswap	2
087 Stikine	2
051 Boundary	1
072 Campbell River	1
020 Kootenay-Columbia	N/A
092 Nisga'a	N/A

Smoking restrictions in school

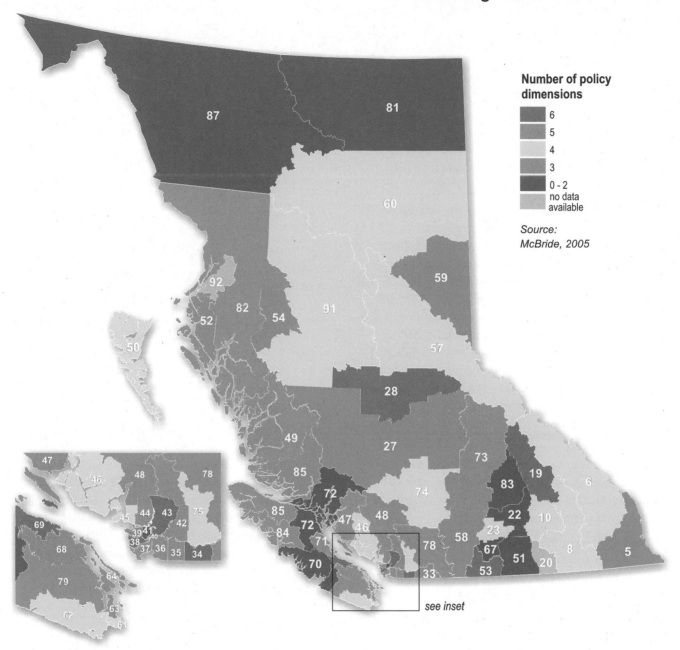

Number of policy dimensions

6
5
4
3
0 - 2
no data available

*Source:
McBride, 2005*

see inset

Municipal smoking restriction bylaws

The main purpose for creating no smoking bylaws in public areas is to protect people from the health hazards of second-hand tobacco smoke. The first map opposite shows the percent of the 2005 population, by HSDA, that is covered by some type of municipal restriction on smoking in public places, based on data provided by the Ministry of Health. Major geographical patterns are evident.

All HSDAs have some municipal no smoking bylaws coverage and, in total, more than three-quarters (76.7%) of the province's population lives, works, and plays in municipalities with some restrictions on smoking in public. Over 80% of the population in the urbanized lower mainland and South Vancouver Island live and work in municipalities that have adopted some smoking restrictions in public places. Thompson Cariboo Shuswap in the central interior has between 80% and 60% population coverage, while the northern half of the province has between 60% and 40% coverage, as does Fraser East. By contrast, the southeast part of the province has less than 40% of its population covered.

Not all bylaws are equally stringent, and some have been, or still are, symbolic rather than extensive in nature. Some have been moderated and reduced in smoking restriction coverage, while many have been made more stringent over time.

For several years, the Non-Smokers' Rights Association (NSRA) has monitored the adoption of smoke-free bylaws by municipalities in terms of their rigour and coverage, and has devised a "Gold, Silver, Bronze" system to categorize municipalities with bylaws that reflect "best practices" (NSRA, 2006). These best practices require 100% smoke-free environments in key public areas 100% of the time.

The Gold Standard prohibits smoking in all public places, including restaurants, bars, billiard halls, bingo halls, bowling alleys, and casinos/slots. No designated smoking rooms are allowed under this standard. Silver prohibits smoking in most public places, including restaurants, but may allow for designated smoking rooms. One exemption is permitted among one of the following: bars, billiard halls, bingo halls, bowling alleys, or casinos/slots. Bronze bans smoking in most public places, including restaurants, and may allow for a designated smoking room. Two or more exemptions are

Health Service Delivery Area	Population protected by municipal bylaw (%)	NSRA standard (%)
031 Richmond	100.0	100
022 Fraser North	100.0	18
041 South Vancouver Island	100.0	100
032 Vancouver	100.0	100
033 North Shore/Coast Garibaldi	84.5	48
023 Fraser South	81.0	81
014 Thompson Cariboo Shuswap	73.8	0
042 Central Vancouver Island	70.5	0
052 Northern Interior	57.4	0
053 Northeast	51.4	0
021 Fraser East	51.0	0
043 North Vancouver Island	49.9	0
051 Northwest	47.6	0
013 Okanagan	29.0	33
012 Kootenay Boundary	28.2	0
011 East Kootenay	23.9	0
999 Province	**76.7**	**46.6**

allowed among the following: bars, billiard halls, bingo halls, bowling alleys, and casinos/slots. These bylaws may include designated smoking rooms or areas. Using these criteria, BC has 17 municipalities with one of these bylaw standards: 5 gold; 8 silver; 4 bronze.

The second map shows that, at the start of 2005, three HSDAs had 100% smoke-free public area coverage that qualify as gold, silver, or bronze. South Vancouver Island and Richmond both had 100% gold coverage. Vancouver had 100% bronze coverage. Fraser South had over 80% coverage with a variety of standards among its municipalities. Three other HSDAs, Fraser North, North Shore/Coast Garibaldi, and Okanagan, had some gold, silver, or bronze standards, but less than half the population was covered. All other HSDAs had no municipalities that qualified for any of the three standard ratings.

More than 46% of the province's population was covered by one of the standards bylaws at the start of 2005 and most of the coverage was in the urbanized southwest of the province.

Municipal smoking restriction bylaws

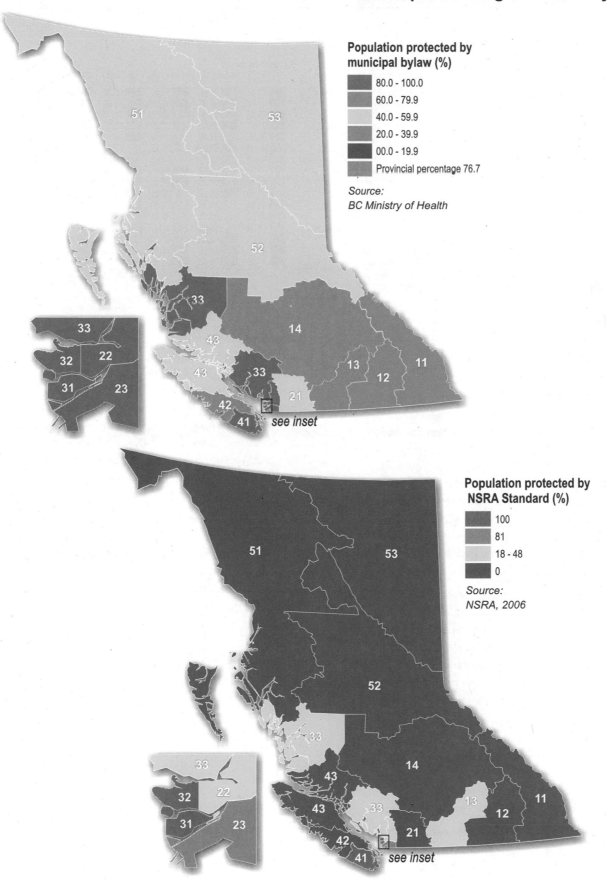

Population protected by municipal bylaw (%)

- 80.0 - 100.0
- 60.0 - 79.9
- 40.0 - 59.9
- 20.0 - 39.9
- 00.0 - 19.9
- Provincial percentage 76.7

Source:
BC Ministry of Health

Population protected by NSRA Standard (%)

- 100
- 81
- 18 - 48
- 0

Source:
NSRA, 2006

Smoke-free environment in public places frequented in the past month

Places where people gather can be smoke free, thus establishing an environmental asset for wellness. In answer to the CCHS question *"In the past month were you exposed to second-hand smoke every day or almost everyday in public places (such as bars, restaurants, shopping malls, arenas, bingo halls, bowling alleys)?"* nearly 9 out of every 10 respondents (89.14%) answered negatively, indicating a large number of residents regularly spent their leisure time in areas that had banned smoking. This percentage is significantly higher than the Canadian average of 84.97%.

Health Service Delivery Area	All respondents (%)	Males (%)	Females (%)	Ages 12-19 (%)	Ages 20-64 (%)	Ages 65+ (%)
042 Central Vancouver Island	92.38	91.10	93.60	90.35	91.23	96.79
051 Northwest	92.31	90.81	93.91	79.96	94.58	98.42
031 Richmond	92.23	92.00	92.43	88.86	91.72	96.96
041 South Vancouver Island	92.17	93.15	91.29	86.62	92.22	95.33
052 Northern Interior	90.55	91.22	89.86	86.74	91.22	92.47
043 North Vancouver Island	90.49	91.23	89.69	82.65	90.73	95.88
033 North Shore/Coast Garibaldi	89.90	88.71	90.94	78.33‡	89.88	97.55‡
012 Kootenay Boundary	89.81	90.53	89.05	66.96‡	92.51	97.65
013 Okanagan	89.10	86.85	91.20	77.39‡	89.19	95.43
032 Vancouver	88.92	88.60	89.21	75.14‡	89.70	93.62
022 Fraser North	88.81	89.25	88.39	69.66‡	90.99	94.04
021 Fraser East	88.80	89.27	88.37	81.01	88.79	96.05‡
014 Thompson Cariboo Shuswap	88.24	89.07	87.45	84.05	86.87	96.30‡
011 East Kootenay	86.04	83.36	88.81	82.51	84.65	94.58
023 Fraser South	85.65	84.96	86.30	82.94	85.00	91.54
053 Northeast	84.95	76.46	92.65	84.45	83.62	95.06
999 Province	**89.14**	**88.73**	**89.53**	**80.30‡**	**89.39**	**94.94‡**

‡ Age group differs significantly from 20-64 group.

The difference between the highest and lowest percentages by HSDA was a little over 7 percentage points. The top map opposite (and table above) shows that Vancouver Island had relatively high values for smoke-free public places, but only South Vancouver Island was significantly higher than the provincial average. Central Vancouver Island and Richmond also had high percentages, as did Northwest. The lowest percentages recorded were in the eastern extremities of the province (Northeast and East Kootenay) and also in Fraser South in the lower mainland. The latter was significantly lower than the provincial average.

While the range in percentages for males, at 17 points, was large, no HSDA was significantly different from the provincial average for males. The large range was very much related to one area, Northeast, which had, relatively speaking, a very low percentage of 76.46%. Geographically, the pattern was very similar to that for the population as a whole.

For females, the geographical pattern was also similar, with one major exception: females in Northeast recorded one of the highest smoke-free public environments, while for both genders combined it had the lowest. The difference, while large, was not significant. The range among females by HSDA was much less than for males.

There were some significant differences in responses by age group. The 12 to 19 age cohort as a whole was statistically significantly lower (only four in every five

frequented smoke-free public places in the past month) than for the 20 to 64 age group. Five HSDAs were also significantly lower for the 12 to 19 age group when compared to the middle age group. On the other hand, seniors were significantly more likely (19 out of 20) to frequent smoke-free public spaces than their younger counterparts. Three HSDAs (North Shore/Coast Garibaldi, Thompson Cariboo Shuswap, and Fraser East) had significantly higher values than the 20 to 64 age group in their areas.

Geographically, there were no significant differences among the seniors or the 12 to 19 age group by HSDA. The overall geographical patterns, however, were quite different among the separate age groups. For example, Kootenay Boundary, North Shore/Coast Garibaldi, and Vancouver HSDAs were lower for the 12- to 19-year-olds than for the other age groups.

Smoke-free environment in public places frequented in the past month

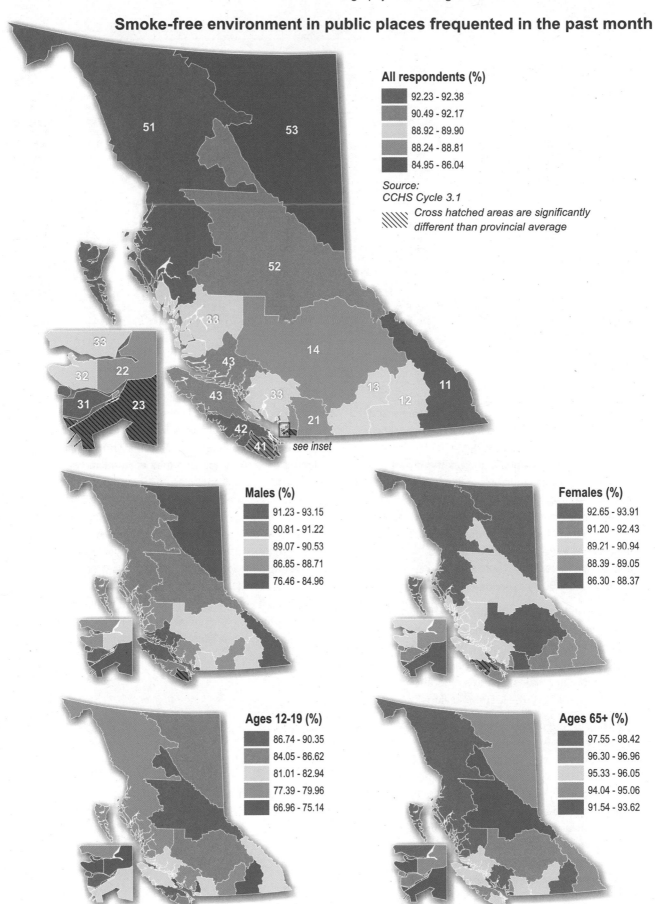

All respondents (%)

- 92.23 - 92.38
- 90.49 - 92.17
- 88.92 - 89.90
- 88.24 - 88.81
- 84.95 - 86.04

Source:
CCHS Cycle 3.1

Cross hatched areas are significantly different than provincial average

see inset

Males (%)

- 91.23 - 93.15
- 90.81 - 91.22
- 89.07 - 90.53
- 86.85 - 88.71
- 76.46 - 84.96

Females (%)

- 92.65 - 93.91
- 91.20 - 92.43
- 89.21 - 90.94
- 88.39 - 89.05
- 86.30 - 88.37

Ages 12-19 (%)

- 86.74 - 90.35
- 84.05 - 86.62
- 81.01 - 82.94
- 77.39 - 79.96
- 66.96 - 75.14

Ages 65+ (%)

- 97.55 - 98.42
- 96.30 - 96.96
- 95.33 - 96.05
- 94.04 - 95.06
- 91.54 - 93.62

Smoke-free work environment

Working individuals, especially those in full time employment, spend a considerable amount of time at their work place. As such, having a work place completely free of environmental tobacco smoke is an important wellness asset. The CCHS asked the question *"At your place of work, what are the restrictions on smoking?"* For the province as a whole, fully two-thirds of the 7,264 respondents aged 15 to 74 who worked indicated that smoking was completely restricted in their work place. For Aboriginal respondents, the percentage was 50.19%, significantly lower statistically than for BC as a whole.

Health Service Delivery Area	All respondents (%)	Males (%)	Females (%)	Ages 15-19 (%)	Ages 20-64 (%)	Ages 55-74 (%)
032　Vancouver	76.92	73.06	81.18	F	77.89	80.37
031　Richmond	75.72	70.25	81.93	F	76.51	79.71
041　South Vancouver Island	73.14	65.64†	81.21†	F	73.45	84.97‡
033　North Shore/Coast Garibaldi	72.24	65.01†	81.09†	F	72.39	84.79
022　Fraser North	68.82	64.40	73.88	F	68.79	70.75
023　Fraser South	65.65	59.09†	74.25†	56.55	66.21	79.87‡
043　North Vancouver Island	65.54	50.80†	80.78†	F	65.97	78.35
051　Northwest	65.38	56.98	76.15	F	65.73	80.35
012　Kootenay Boundary	61.96	47.85†	77.55†	F	61.57	F
013　Okanagan	61.25	53.47†	69.98†	41.72	63.32	68.38
021　Fraser East	58.82	53.76	65.59	F	60.33	69.77
014　Thompson Cariboo Shuswap	58.01	45.56†	72.47†	F	57.82	64.76
052　Northern Interior	57.78	42.28†	77.10†	F	56.80	52.47
042　Central Vancouver Island	55.25	41.16†	71.10†	F	56.62	64.70
053　Northeast	54.03	44.61†	66.68	F	53.75	44.80
011　East Kootenay	49.22	38.71E	63.10	F	49.89	64.17
999　Province	**66.64**	**59.01†**	**75.62†**	**56.02‡**	**67.42**	**74.19‡**

‡ Age group differs significantly from 20-64 group.
† Males differ significantly from females.
E Interpret data with caution (16.77< coefficient of variation <33.3).
F Data suppressed due to Statistics Canada sampling rules.

Within the province, however, as the table above and maps opposite show, there is considerable variation in smoking restrictions in the work place by region. The urbanized lower mainland and southern part of Vancouver Island were much more likely to have work place smoking restrictions than the average for the province, especially Vancouver, Richmond, and South Vancouver Island (statistically significant), while much of the central and extreme northeast and southeast parts of the province, as well as Central Vancouver Island, had statistically significantly lower percentages than average.

Female workers were significantly more likely than males to indicate they work in smoke-free environments. Not only did this difference hold at the provincial level, but geographically all regions had higher values for females than for males, and this difference was significant for 10 of the 16 HSDAs individually.

Geographically, the patterns evident for males and for females separately were quite similar to that of the population as a whole. The range in values for males, however, was much greater than for females. Among males, Vancouver and Richmond were significantly better than the average for males, while Thompson Cariboo Shuswap, Northern Interior, Central Vancouver Island, Northeast, and East Kootenay had significantly lower values than the male average. Only Vancouver was statistically significantly different from the provincial value for females.

Provincially, the 15- to19-year-old youths who work were significantly less likely to work in a smoke-free environment than workers in the 20 to 64 age cohort, while those workers aged 55 to 74 were significantly more likely to do so. Because of small numbers, it is not possible to map the 15 to 19 age group, but for the highest age cohort the pattern was very similar to that for the province as a whole. The range in values for the 55 to 74 age group was much greater than for the 20 to 64 age cohort. South Vancouver Island and Fraser South seniors had significantly higher values than their 20- to 64-year-old counterparts. Geographically, Northeast and Northern Interior had significantly lower values than the provincial average for seniors, while South Vancouver Island and Vancouver had significantly higher ones.

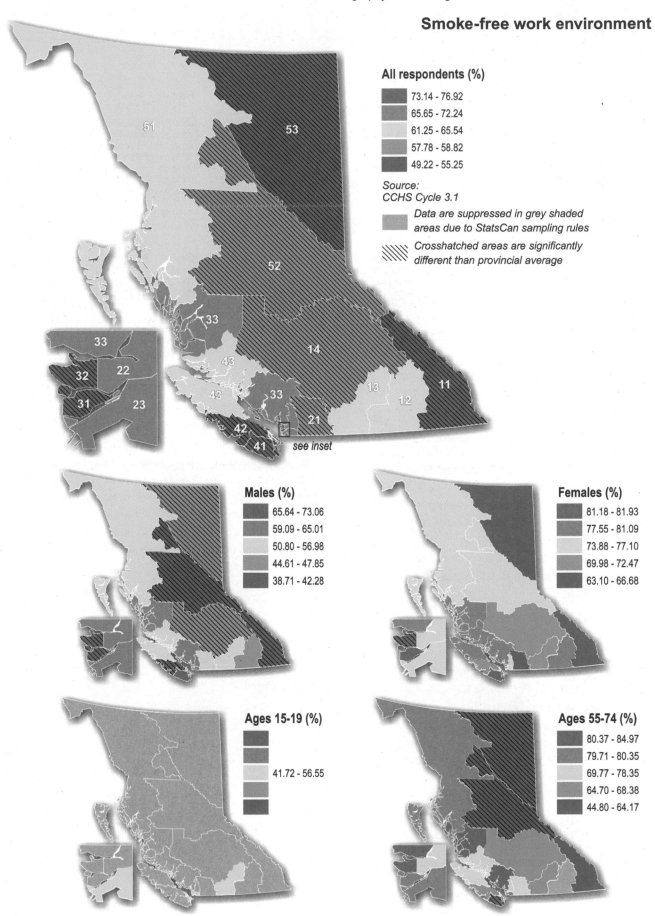

Smoke-free work environment

All respondents (%)

- 73.14 - 76.92
- 65.65 - 72.24
- 61.25 - 65.54
- 57.78 - 58.82
- 49.22 - 55.25

Source:
CCHS Cycle 3.1

Data are suppressed in grey shaded areas due to StatsCan sampling rules

Crosshatched areas are significantly different than provincial average

Males (%)

- 65.64 - 73.06
- 59.09 - 65.01
- 50.80 - 56.98
- 44.61 - 47.85
- 38.71 - 42.28

Females (%)

- 81.18 - 81.93
- 77.55 - 81.09
- 73.88 - 77.10
- 69.98 - 72.47
- 63.10 - 66.68

Ages 15-19 (%)

- 41.72 - 56.55

Ages 55-74 (%)

- 80.37 - 84.97
- 79.71 - 80.35
- 69.77 - 78.35
- 64.70 - 68.38
- 44.80 - 64.17

Smoke-free vehicle environment

Many Canadians commute by car and use a vehicle to undertake errands and other activities, particularly in the suburbs or in communities that have little mixed land use. The environment of a vehicle is very confined and so a smoke-free vehicle environment is an asset that can maintain present and future wellness. When asked, as part of the CCHS, the question *"In the past month were you exposed to second-hand smoke every day or almost every day in a car or private vehicle?"* nearly 19 out of 20 respondents (94.03%) in BC answered in the negative, a statistically significantly higher percentage than for Canada as a whole (91.76%).

Health Service Delivery Area	All respondents (%)	Males (%)	Females (%)	Ages 12-19 (%)	Ages 20-64 (%)	Ages 65+ (%)
031 Richmond	97.08	96.13	97.89	92.88	97.18	99.51
033 North Shore/Coast Garibaldi	96.60	96.81	96.42	88.75‡	97.04	100.00‡
041 South Vancouver Island	96.38	97.11	95.73	86.26‡	97.57	98.44
032 Vancouver	95.30	94.98	95.58	90.43	95.43	97.64
022 Fraser North	95.27	94.94	95.58	88.35	95.71	99.14
042 Central Vancouver Island	94.24	92.72	95.69	85.53	94.26	98.95‡
023 Fraser South	93.65	92.63	94.63	90.00	93.41	98.51‡
012 Kootenay Boundary	93.64	94.82	92.41	83.29	95.04	96.64
013 Okanagan	93.38	92.07	94.59	79.59‡	94.60	97.86
014 Thompson Cariboo Shuswap	92.66	92.30	93.00	83.98	93.70	95.16
011 East Kootenay	91.59	88.24	95.05	87.47	91.30	96.36
051 Northwest	91.02	87.54	94.73	94.78	88.67	100.00‡
021 Fraser East	90.71	89.33	91.95	81.93	91.38	96.29
052 Northern Interior	90.05	88.12	92.04	88.37	90.19	91.95
043 North Vancouver Island	88.41	85.01	92.04	90.55	85.58	97.01‡
053 Northeast	84.67	83.45	85.77	64.87‡	88.07	98.23
999 Province	**94.03**	**93.20†**	**94.80†**	**86.96‡**	**94.39**	**98.00‡**

‡ Age group differs significantly from 20-64 group.
† Males differ significantly from females.

For the total population aged 12 and over, the range in values was more than 12 percentage points, and the values were highest in the urbanized lower mainland (with the exception of Fraser South) and South Vancouver Island, and lowest in the north (Northern Interior and Northeast) and North Vancouver Island. Richmond, North Shore/Coast Garibaldi, and South Vancouver Island were all significantly higher, while Northeast and Fraser East (in the southwest of the province) were significantly lower than the provincial average.

At the provincial level, while the difference was quite small, females were significantly more likely than males to ride in smoke-free vehicles, but at the individual HSDA level there was no significant difference. For males only, South Vancouver Island and North Shore/Coast Garibaldi had significantly higher values than the provincial average for males, while Northeast had a significantly lower value. For females only, Richmond had a significantly higher value and Northeast a significantly lower value than the provincial female average.

Overall, the geographical patterns were very similar to the patterns for the population as a whole.

Ridership in smoke-free vehicles increased with age. The 12 to 19 age cohort was significantly lower than the 20 to 64 age group, while the 65 and over age group was significantly higher. Provincially, 98% of seniors rode in relatively smoke-free cars. There were some dramatic geographical differences. While Northwest overall had relatively low smoke-free ridership, the youngest age cohort was statistically significantly high. Young people in North Vancouver Island also had relatively high rates compared to the 20 to 64 age group in that HSDA, but not significantly so. For the seniors group, Northwest also had a statistically significantly high value, as did North Shore/Coast Garibaldi. In both cases, 100% of respondents rode in smoke-free vehicles.

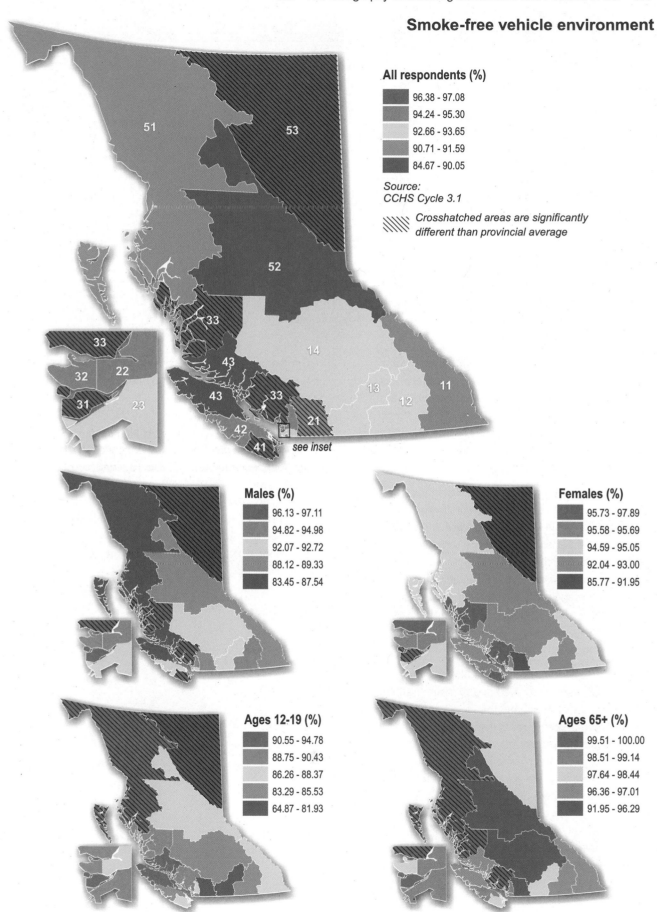

Smoke-free vehicle environment

All respondents (%)

- 96.38 - 97.08
- 94.24 - 95.30
- 92.66 - 93.65
- 90.71 - 91.59
- 84.67 - 90.05

Source:
CCHS Cycle 3.1

Crosshatched areas are significantly different than provincial average

Males (%)

- 96.13 - 97.11
- 94.82 - 94.98
- 92.07 - 92.72
- 88.12 - 89.33
- 83.45 - 87.54

Females (%)

- 95.73 - 97.89
- 95.58 - 95.69
- 94.59 - 95.05
- 92.04 - 93.00
- 85.77 - 91.95

Ages 12-19 (%)

- 90.55 - 94.78
- 88.75 - 90.43
- 86.26 - 88.37
- 83.29 - 85.53
- 64.87 - 81.93

Ages 65+ (%)

- 99.51 - 100.00
- 98.51 - 99.14
- 97.64 - 98.44
- 96.36 - 97.01
- 91.95 - 96.29

Smoke-free home environment

Individuals and families spend more than one-third of their time in their homes. Home environments can be either healthy or less so, depending on behaviours within the home. Because of relatively small spaces within the home, tobacco smoke-free home environments are important from a wellness perspective, for all inhabitants. As noted earlier, there is no risk-free level of exposure, and babies and younger children are particularly at risk to the ill effects of second-hand smoke in the home (Kendall and Morley, 2006).

Health Service Delivery Area	All respondents (%)	Males (%)	Females (%)	Ages 12-19 (%)	Ages 20-64 (%)	Ages 65+ (%)
032 Vancouver	95.20	96.23	94.22	85.75	95.96	96.85
041 South Vancouver Island	94.73	94.25	95.16	84.12‡	96.16	95.65
031 Richmond	93.22	93.98	92.51	92.56	93.54	92.01
022 Fraser North	92.22	91.58	92.85	82.11‡	93.21	95.57
023 Fraser South	91.99	91.56	92.41	87.10	92.27	95.48
013 Okanagan	91.47	91.63	91.31	87.93	90.73	95.91
042 Central Vancouver Island	90.96	90.08	91.80	81.06	91.14	96.56‡
033 North Shore/Coast Garibaldi	90.66	89.38	91.89	84.35	90.12	97.91‡
021 Fraser East	89.85	90.38	89.34	81.55	90.41	95.18
012 Kootenay Boundary	89.57	91.54	87.62	78.10	91.20	91.65
043 North Vancouver Island	88.53	90.68	86.40	77.08	89.70	93.65
014 Thompson Cariboo Shuswap	86.92	87.27	86.58	71.92	88.66	91.73
051 Northwest	86.60	84.68	88.62	84.19	85.96	95.28
011 East Kootenay	86.14	86.21	86.08	82.55	85.62	91.78
052 Northern Interior	85.25	84.02	86.57	81.63	86.15	84.01
053 Northeast	79.10	79.54	78.63	77.53	78.27	89.21
999 Province	**91.40**	**91.30**	**91.50**	**83.46‡**	**91.96**	**95.08‡**

‡ Age group differs significantly from 20-64 group.

In answer to the CCHS question "*Including both household members and regular visitors, does anyone smoke inside your home every day or almost every day?*" 91.40% answered negatively. This is significantly higher than the Canadian average of 84.04%, indicating healthier tobacco smoke-free home environments for provincial residents.

The urbanized lower mainland and South Vancouver Island had the highest percentage of smoke-free home environments, while moving northward and eastward to the more rural parts of the province saw a reduction in smoke-free home environments. Both Vancouver and South Vancouver Island had statistically significantly higher percentages, while Northeast, Northern Interior, East Kootenay, and Thompson Cariboo Shuswap HSDAs had significantly lower smoke-free home environments when compared to the provincial average.

Vancouver had the greatest percentage of male respondents with smoke-free home environments (96.23%) and Northeast had the lowest (79.54%). Both of these percentages are statistically significantly different from the provincial value of 91.30% for males. Overall, the geographic pattern is similar to that for the population. For female respondents, South Vancouver Island had the highest percentage with a smoke-free home environment (95.16%), while Northeast again had the lowest (78.63%). Both of these HSDAs had values that were significantly different from the provincial average for females (91.50%). The overall geographic pattern of variation was similar to that of the population as a whole.

Comparisons among age groups indicate that seniors have a statistically significantly better smoke-free environment than those in the 20 to 64 age group, and Central Vancouver Island and North Shore/Coast Garibaldi were both individually significantly better than the younger age cohorts. The opposite was the case for the youngest age cohort (12 to 19), for which provincially a significantly lower percentage had a tobacco smoke-free home environment than the 20 to 64 age group, and two HSDAs, South Vancouver Island and Fraser North, both had significantly lower percentages. Among teens, Richmond was significantly higher than the provincial teen average.

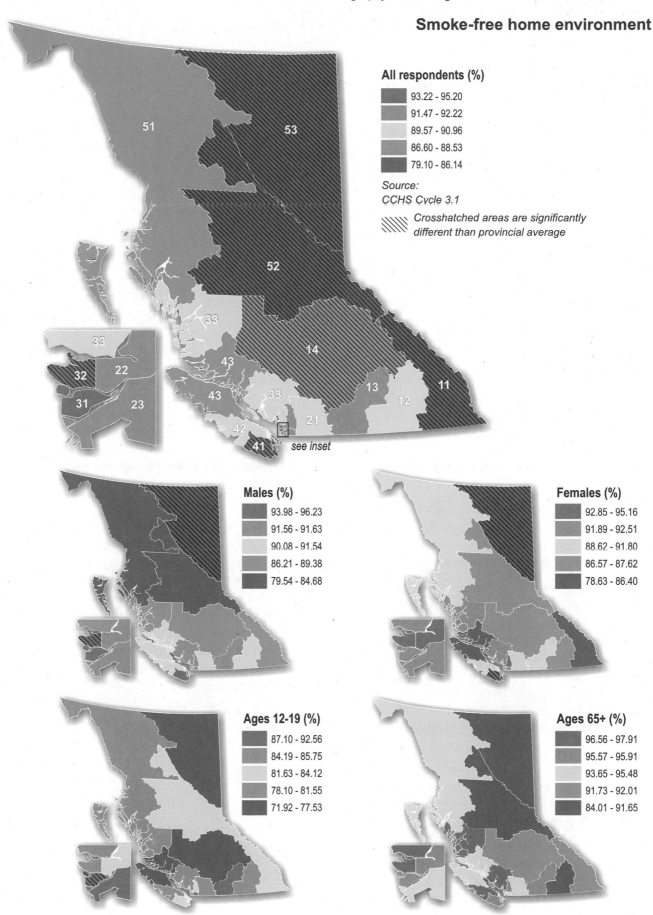

Smoke-free home environment

All respondents (%)

- 93.22 - 95.20
- 91.47 - 92.22
- 89.57 - 90.96
- 86.60 - 88.53
- 79.10 - 86.14

Source:
CCHS Cycle 3.1

Crosshatched areas are significantly different than provincial average

Males (%)

- 93.98 - 96.23
- 91.56 - 91.63
- 90.08 - 91.54
- 86.21 - 89.38
- 79.54 - 84.68

Females (%)

- 92.85 - 95.16
- 91.89 - 92.51
- 88.62 - 91.80
- 86.57 - 87.62
- 78.63 - 86.40

Ages 12-19 (%)

- 87.10 - 92.56
- 84.19 - 85.75
- 81.63 - 84.12
- 78.10 - 81.55
- 71.92 - 77.53

Ages 65+ (%)

- 96.56 - 97.91
- 95.57 - 95.91
- 93.65 - 95.48
- 91.73 - 92.01
- 84.01 - 91.65

Some restriction against smoking cigarettes in home

A previous CCHS question asked about smoke-free home environments. A second question asked: *"Are there any restrictions against smoking cigarettes in your home?"* Nearly four out of five (79.37%) respondents indicated that there were restrictions at home, significantly higher than the Canadian average of 69.75%, but the responses were considerably lower than to the previous question for both BC and Canadian respondents.

Health Service Delivery Area	All respondents (%)	Males (%)	Females (%)	Ages 12-19 (%)	Ages 20-64 (%)	Ages 65+ (%)
043 North Vancouver Island	86.52	86.19	86.84	78.22	89.21	81.61
041 South Vancouver Island	84.23	83.99	84.45	75.89‡	86.90	78.89
021 Fraser East	83.34	80.51	86.10	80.82	83.81	83.56
042 Central Vancouver Island	82.89	79.46	86.19	78.92	84.62	79.52
013 Okanagan	82.48	82.43	82.52	79.36	82.86	83.04
033 North Shore/Coast Garibaldi	81.92	80.94	82.86	82.93	83.02	76.17
023 Fraser South	80.65	79.02	82.25	79.97	81.15	78.51
051 Northwest	79.87	77.60	82.31	82.33	79.41	79.42
014 Thompson Cariboo Shuswap	79.72	82.49	76.98	73.28	81.85	75.65
011 East Kootenay	79.05	76.34	81.82	79.35	81.35	68.23
031 Richmond	78.97	82.07	76.07	89.50	79.29	69.84
022 Fraser North	77.58	75.61	79.49	79.03	78.05	73.39
012 Kootenay Boundary	77.29	75.67	78.91	73.22	79.20	72.65
032 Vancouver	72.63	70.72	74.48	69.05	75.04	66.84
052 Northern Interior	72.47	68.21	76.95	75.79	74.68	51.81‡
053 Northeast	69.90	67.88	72.07	76.18	70.59	52.70
999 Province	**79.37**	**78.04†**	**80.67†**	**78.12**	**80.38**	**75.52‡**

‡ Age group differs significantly from 20-64 group.
† Males differ significantly from females.

Most restrictions on smoking in the home occurred on Vancouver Island, particularly in North and South Vancouver Island. The lower mainland, with the key exception of Fraser East, and to a lesser extent North Shore/Coast Garibaldi, had relatively low levels of restrictions, and Vancouver was significantly lower than the provincial average. Northern Interior and Northeast also had significantly lower levels of restrictions on smoking in the home.

For the province as a whole, female respondents had a statistically significantly higher percentage, indicating greater restrictions than males. However, there was no significant difference between the genders for any of the individual HSDAs.

The geographical patterns for each gender were similar to that for the total population, although males in Thompson Cariboo Shuswap, and to a lesser extent Richmond, had higher, and Fraser East lower, restrictions than the population in their HSDAs as a whole. South and North Vancouver Island males also had significantly higher restrictions, while Vancouver and Northeast had significantly lower restrictions than the male population as a whole.

For females, North and Central Vancouver Island and Fraser East were significantly higher, while again Vancouver and Northeast were significantly lower than for the female population as a whole.

Overall, both the 12 to 19 and 65 and over age groups had lower restrictions than the 20 to 64 age group, but only seniors were statistically significant. Among seniors, Fraser East and Okanagan had significantly higher smoking restrictions, while Northeast and Northern Interior had significantly lower restrictions, with one out of every two respondents indicating relatively limited restrictions on smoking in the home. Northern Interior was also significantly lower than the 20 to 64 age population in its HSDA. Overall, the geographical pattern was quite similar to the pattern for the population as a whole.

There are some interesting differences between the 12 to 19 age group and the 20 to 64 age group. Richmond was statistically significantly high and also had the most restrictive home no smoking conditions for the youth group. At the other extreme, South Vancouver Island teens had significantly lower smoking restrictions than their 20 to 64 age counterparts. North and Central Vancouver Island also had lower percentages for youth when compared to the 20 to 64 age cohort, but not significantly so.

Some restriction against smoking cigarettes in home

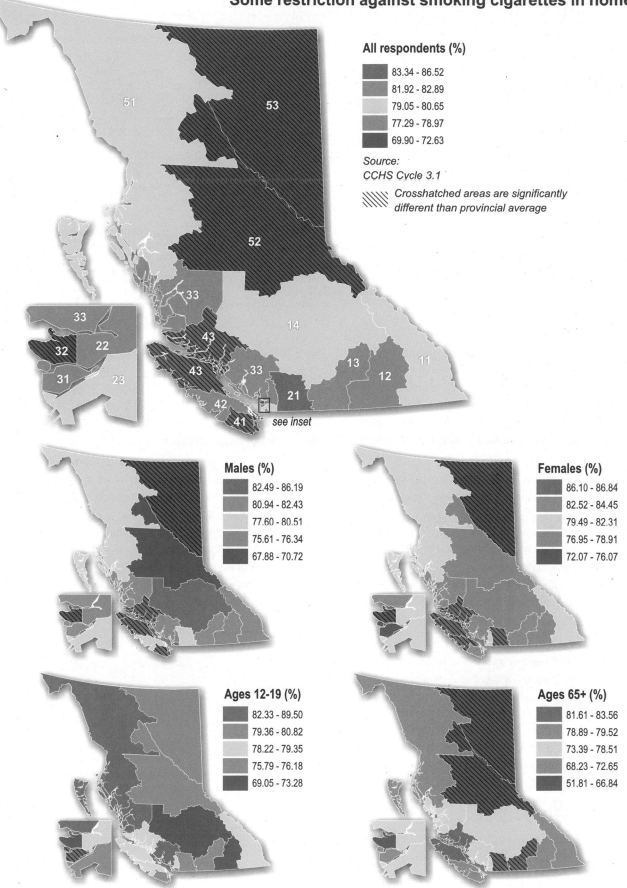

All respondents (%)

- 83.34 - 86.52
- 81.92 - 82.89
- 79.05 - 80.65
- 77.29 - 78.97
- 69.90 - 72.63

Source:
CCHS Cycle 3.1

Crosshatched areas are significantly
different than provincial average

Males (%)

- 82.49 - 86.19
- 80.94 - 82.43
- 77.60 - 80.51
- 75.61 - 76.34
- 67.88 - 70.72

Females (%)

- 86.10 - 86.84
- 82.52 - 84.45
- 79.49 - 82.31
- 76.95 - 78.91
- 72.07 - 76.07

Ages 12-19 (%)

- 82.33 - 89.50
- 79.36 - 80.82
- 78.22 - 79.35
- 75.79 - 76.18
- 69.05 - 73.28

Ages 65+ (%)

- 81.61 - 83.56
- 78.89 - 79.52
- 73.39 - 78.51
- 68.23 - 72.65
- 51.81 - 66.84

Presently non-smoker

As indicated earlier, tobacco smoke and smoking is related to many major diseases. Being a non-smoker is an important asset for wellness. The CCHS shows that 82.24% of respondents in BC indicated they were presently a non-smoker, a significantly higher percentage than for Canada as a whole (78.21%). For Aboriginal CCHS respondents in BC, only 60.63% were presently non-smokers, statistically significantly lower than the provincial average.

Health Service Delivery Area	All respondents (%)	Males (%)	Females (%)	Ages 12-19 (%)	Ages 20-64 (%)	Ages 65+ (%)
031 Richmond	87.69	83.87	91.25	91.39	85.92	94.20‡
022 Fraser North	85.90	83.99	87.77	91.88	84.33	90.03
033 North Shore/Coast Garibaldi	84.12	80.55	87.54	86.57	81.55	94.19‡
041 South Vancouver Island	84.06	83.64	84.43	94.94‡	80.63	90.83‡
023 Fraser South	82.65	81.15	84.13	91.07‡	79.52	91.82‡
032 Vancouver	82.18	78.44†	85.81†	92.68‡	79.85	88.82‡
021 Fraser East	81.68	78.33	84.95	91.09‡	77.79	90.41‡
042 Central Vancouver Island	81.52	81.41	81.62	81.76	78.56	91.29‡
013 Okanagan	81.27	80.74	81.76	89.98‡	76.35	91.90‡
051 Northwest	79.83	79.42	80.26	94.43‡	75.72	87.97
011 East Kootenay	79.45	79.74	79.15	92.95‡	74.96	88.72‡
043 North Vancouver Island	79.21	82.16	76.28	85.48	75.05	92.44‡
012 Kootenay Boundary	78.70	80.37	77.02	92.98‡	73.75	88.10‡
014 Thompson Cariboo Shuswap	77.55	75.55	79.54	80.84	74.54	87.99‡
052 Northern Interior	75.92	75.25	76.64	92.67‡	72.39	77.61
053 Northeast	70.68	64.49	77.33	86.10‡	66.01	82.94
999 Province	**82.24**	**80.40†**	**84.03†**	**90.06‡**	**79.26**	**90.45‡**

‡ Age group differs significantly from 20-64 group.
† Males differ significantly from females.

Within the province, there was a 17 percentage point difference between the HSDA with the highest percentage and the one with the lowest. The highest non-smoking percentages occurred in the urban southwest of the province, with values decreasing as one moves east and north. Richmond and Fraser North had significantly higher percentages of non-smokers, while Northern Interior and Northeast had significantly lower values.

For the province as a whole, females had significantly higher rates of non-smoking behaviour than did males, although among HSDAs only Vancouver shows a significant difference between the two genders. In a couple of instances, some HSDAs, notably North Vancouver Island and Kootenay Boundary, had higher non-smoking rates for males than for females, but the difference was not statistically significant. For Aboriginal respondents, there was no significant difference between the genders.

The pattern for males generally reflected the geographical pattern for the population as a whole, with the exception of Vancouver which, as previously noted, had a significantly lower non-smoking percentage. Only Northeast was significantly different than the others, and was nearly 30 percentage points lower than the highest HSDAs. For females, the geographical pattern is also similar to that for the population as a whole, although only Northern Interior was significantly different from the provincial average for females.

Among the three major age cohorts, both the 12 to 19 age group and seniors aged 65 and over had statistically significantly higher percentages of no smoking behaviours than the 20 to 64 age group. The youngest age group showed significantly higher values for 10 of the 16 HSDAs individually, while 12 HSDAs had significantly higher no smoking behaviour for seniors than the middle 20 to 64 age group.

The geographical pattern for seniors was quite similar to that for the population as a whole, although North Vancouver Island seniors had a much higher percentage of non-smokers than that HSDA's population as a whole. The pattern for the 12 to 19 age group varied quite substantially from that for the population as a whole, with the highest no smoking rates occurring outside of the urban southwest of the province, with the exception of South Vancouver Island, and to a lesser extent, Vancouver.

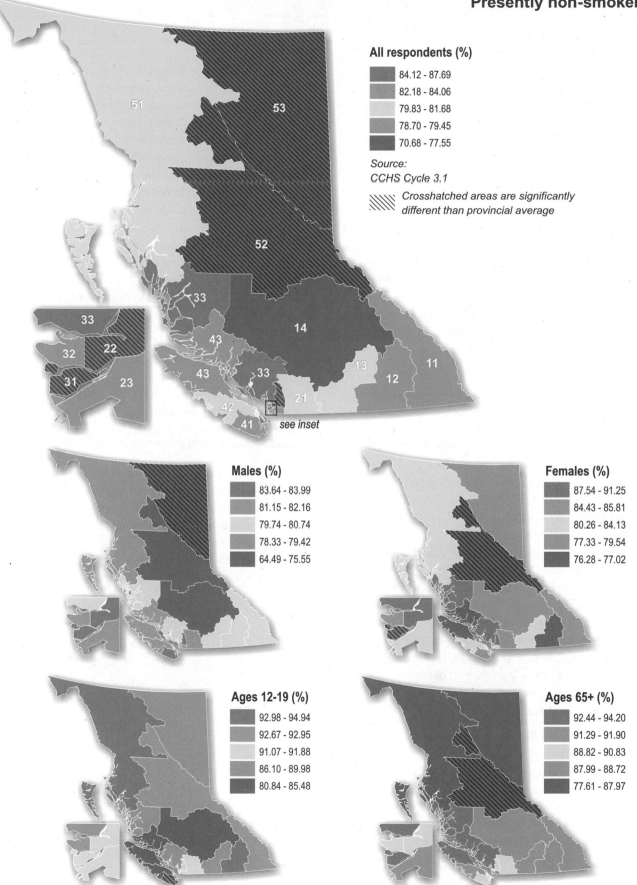

Presently non-smoker

All respondents (%)

- 84.12 - 87.69
- 82.18 - 84.06
- 79.83 - 81.68
- 78.70 - 79.45
- 70.68 - 77.55

Source:
CCHS Cycle 3.1

Crosshatched areas are significantly different than provincial average

Males (%)

- 83.64 - 83.99
- 81.15 - 82.16
- 79.74 - 80.74
- 78.33 - 79.42
- 64.49 - 75.55

Females (%)

- 87.54 - 91.25
- 84.43 - 85.81
- 80.26 - 84.13
- 77.33 - 79.54
- 76.28 - 77.02

Ages 12-19 (%)

- 92.98 - 94.94
- 92.67 - 92.95
- 91.07 - 91.88
- 86.10 - 89.98
- 80.84 - 85.48

Ages 65+ (%)

- 92.44 - 94.20
- 91.29 - 91.90
- 88.82 - 90.83
- 87.99 - 88.72
- 77.61 - 87.97

Summary

While BC residents continue to do significantly better than their Canadian counterparts on many of the indicators presented here, there are major variations or inequities within the province indicating that wellness in terms of no smoking is far from being shared equally. For most of the indicators, smoke-free environments are substantially more common in the urbanized southwest part of the province—the lower mainland and South Vancouver Island—while there is a fall-off in wellness assets as one moves geographically away from this area into the more rural and less densely populated central, eastern, and northern parts of the province. Wellness on this dimension is least developed in the extreme northeast of the province. These variations suggest that there are substantial opportunities for improvements, and it may be useful to consider targeting specific segments of the population in specific regions, as well as universal healthy public policy strategies.

School districts can positively influence children and youth by implementing more restrictive no smoking policies and enforcing existing policies. Schools can play a significant role in deterring early initiation of smoking behaviour among children and youth (Kendall, 2003). Avoiding early onset of smoking behaviour will go a very long way to improving the wellness of not only children, but also future adults. While the Premier of BC committed to a ban on smoking on all school property in every public and private school across BC by September 2007, appropriate enforcement will be required as this has not been a strong point of past school district smoking-related policies (McBride, 2005). More than 90% of youth are non-smokers, but many are still exposed to second-hand smoke as indicated by the data from the CCHS. For example, youth travelling in vehicles are less likely than the rest of the population to travel in a smoke-free environment. This also holds true for the home and work environments.

Municipalities can also set a broad, community-wide example by restricting smoking in public places. While many local governments have implemented various types of no smoking bylaws, only about one-half of the population is covered by the Gold, Silver, or Bronze standards devised by the Non-Smokers' Rights Association. In the neighbouring province of Alberta, approximately 70% of the population live, work, play, and learn in municipalities that have implemented bylaws that meet the standards developed by the Non-Smokers' Rights Association, and the great majority of the population (approximately 65%) have the Gold Standard protection (NSRA, 2006). Most other provinces have implemented legislation that ensures their populations live, work, play, and learn in smoke-free public environments. As indicated earlier, a commitment to phase out smoking in all indoor public spaces by 2008 was made by the Premier of BC in the fall of 2006. It was noted nearly 15 years ago that it will be a challenging task to get smaller, more rural municipalities to adopt no smoking bylaws (Hollander et al., 1992). Time will tell whether all municipalities will actively embrace and enforce the initiative announced by the Premier.

Finally, health authorities in the province are responsible for developing their own Tobacco Control Strategy and have performance agreements with the Ministry of Health to achieve reductions in the smoking rates. Careful monitoring and utilization of the data presented here can result in targeting programs to help improve wellness.

While, overall, BC fares better than Canada as a whole on many indicators, there is still some way to go, especially with respect to restricting outdoor smoking, and smoking in vehicles when small children and youth are present. Some jurisdictions in North America have already adopted such measures.

According to Bellows and Hamm (2003): "Community food security exists when all citizens obtain a safe, personally acceptable, nutritional diet through a sustainable food system that maximizes healthy choices, community self-reliance, and equal access for everyone. This definition implies:

- The ability to acquire food is assured;
- Food is obtained in a manner that upholds human dignity;
- Food is safe, nutritionally adequate, and personally and culturally acceptable;
- Food is sufficient in quality and quantity to sustain healthy growth and development and to prevent illness and disease; and
- Food is produced, processed, and distributed in a manner that does not compromise the land, air, or water for future generations" (Food Security Standing Committee, 2004).

The UN Food and Agriculture Organization (FAO) defines food security as existing "when all people, at all times, have physical and economic access to sufficient, safe, and nutritious food to meet their dietary needs and food preferences for an active and healthy life" (FAO, 1996). The BC Ministry of Health has adopted this broad approach to food security and encourages "local, provincial, and national policies to support local food systems" (Ministry of Health Planning, 2003).

Today public interest in nutrition and food security (ranging from worries broadly about the sustainability and safety of systems of agricultural production to the desire for information on the links between vitamin intake and specific diseases) is very high (Ostry, 2006). With growing concerns about a host of food security issues that have emerged in the past decade (e.g., "mad cow" disease cases in Western Canada and bird flu, both with major potential for health and economic impacts), and with increasing publicity and concern about an obesity epidemic, especially among children, government and regional health authorities have also begun to pay attention to food security (Rideout and Ostry, 2006).

As part of the process of monitoring the changing nutrition and food security situation in BC, we have developed baseline indicators against which the nature and extent of future changes in food security can be assessed in different regions of the province. A suite of indicators for nutrition and food security has been selected and these have been mapped to illustrate how nutrition and food security varies across the province and, for some indicators, by gender and age.

What follows is the presentation of 26 maps that describe select indicators of nutrition and food security for much of BC's population. As breastfeeding is a key to good infant health and health in later life, it is appropriate to begin this section of the Atlas with a map of the regional variation in breastfeeding initiation rates.

The following nine maps focus on children and youth, as it is well known that healthy eating as a child promotes optimal growth and development while helping to prevent various nutrition-related diseases (Kendall, 2003). Six of these nine maps focus on the nutritional policy and learning environment in the school system because children on average consume one-third of their daily food intake while at school (Wechsler, Brener, Kuester, and Miller, 2001). Schools are, therefore, in an excellent position to promote healthy food habits by enacting policies that encourage healthy eating at the school district level and in individual schools (Kendall, 2003).

Several unique surveys have been conducted in the BC school system over the past 3 years. As noted earlier, the McCreary Centre Society conducted surveys in 1992, 1998, and more recently in 2003. This latter survey was conducted in 47 (78.3%) school districts in the province. A total of 1,500 public school Grade 7 to 12 classrooms were randomly selected from the 47 participating school districts. Approximately 30,000 students in these classes completed questionnaires for the 2003 survey. The survey was not conducted in independent schools or among institutionalized youth or those not attending schools. Respondents can be considered to represent about 90% of BC's high school students.

Several other surveys have been undertaken in the school system. In 2005/06, the Ministry of Education's School Satisfaction Survey assessed the extent to which Grades 3/4, 7, 10, and 12 students were learning about healthy eating and exercise at school. Maps provided here deal only with Grades 3/4. Two other surveys, one directed to school districts and the other to schools, were conducted in a joint project by the ministries of Education and Health in the spring of 2005 to determine the types of food sales outlets, the types of more healthy versus less healthy (as defined by nutritional experts) foods and beverages offered for sale in all BC school food outlets, and the extent of nutrition policy implementation in BC school districts and in schools (Ostry, Rideout, Levy-Milne, and Martin, 2005; Rideout, Martin, Levy-Milne, and Ostry, in press). The maps based on results from these school-system-based surveys are described in this section of the Atlas.

Given that BC has, over the past year or so, introduced healthy eating guidelines for schools and several programs to improve the nutritional environment in schools, these indicators provide an important baseline for assessing progress over the next few years.

These school-focused maps are followed by 15 maps based on three questions from the Canadian Community Health Survey (CCHS) illustrating the variation in dietary quality and food availability by region, age, and gender. The first two questions speak fairly directly to the ability of people in BC to access foods that they want to eat and that constitute a balanced diet. The third question assesses the extent to which people in the province are eating according to one of the most important of Health Canada's Dietary Guidelines. Access to balanced meals and preferred foods and the extent to which people eat according to these guidelines will likely depend on some mix of an individual's knowledge about healthy eating as well as their access to income and/or home-grown foods, and the cost of food in local stores. The maps based on these three questions provide a rough snapshot of the quality of the diet of British Columbians.

Finally, in keeping with our desire to move to a broader framing of nutrition and food security, we provide a map of farmers markets, which are scattered throughout the province. These markets are outlets where local farmers sell their produce directly to consumers. The development of farmers markets may be important in establishing more direct contact between producers and consumers leading to several advantages, including better pricing for consumers, direct access to consumers for farmers which may lower their costs making their operations more viable, and increased opportunities for basic public education about food production.

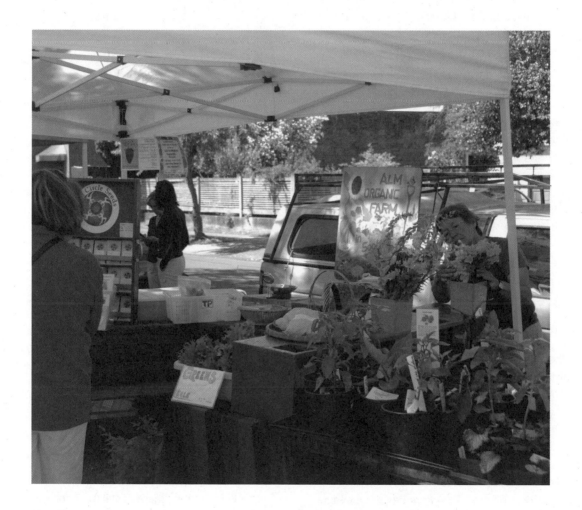

Breastfed baby on discharge from hospital

In Canada, the long-term health advantages of breastfeeding have been well recognized for over a century (MacMurchy, 1923; Ostry, 2005). Recently, breastfed babies have been shown to be less likely to become obese in later life (Canadian Institute for Health Information, 2004, 2006a). Nutritionists and public health professionals have advocated for breastfeeding consistently over the decades (Arnup, 1994; Ostry, 2006). Nonetheless, breastfeeding initiation rates have varied considerably both over time and across the regions of Canada. For example, in the 1920s approximately 90% of women in Canada breastfed. But, in spite of early nutrition programs encouraging breastfeeding, from the 1930s to the 1960s the majority of Canadian women moved away from breastfeeding so that by the late 1960s only about one-third of women were breastfeeding on discharge from hospital. However, during the 1970s, breastfeeding initiation rates increased rapidly, particularly in Quebec. Since the early 1980s, rates have risen only slowly. As well, since the 1960s there has been an east/west gradient in breastfeeding initiation, with the highest rates observed in BC and the lowest in the maritime provinces (McNally, Hendricks, and Horowitz, 1985).

Besides these regional and temporal trends, studies indicate that women who are well educated and from higher income families are more likely to breastfeed compared to their poorer, less educated sisters (Arnup, 1994). Other factors that influence whether or not a woman initiates breastfeeding are social and cultural (in some cultures breastfeeding is more common than others). Finally, it is well known that women are more likely to breastfeed on discharge from those hospitals with policies that encourage breastfeeding and with staff and a culture that actively support and promote the practice (Breastfeeding Committee for Canada, 2003; Myres, 1988).

In order to measure breastfeeding initiation in BC, we obtained data from the BC Perinatal Data Registry. This database records information on each birth in the province, including whether or not the mother was breastfeeding at the time of discharge from hospital. We have obtained data, based on this question, for the 4 year period from April 2000 to March 2004, on approximately 150,000 babies who were discharged from BC's hospitals during this time.

Health Service Delivery Area	Mothers who breastfed (%)
033 North Shore/Coast Garibaldi	96.48
041 South Vancouver Island	94.75
022 Fraser North	93.66
013 Okanagan	92.97
042 Central Vancouver Island	92.82
023 Fraser South	92.68
031 Richmond	92.41
012 Kootenay Boundary	92.38
043 North Vancouver Island	92.17
011 East Kootenay	91.57
032 Vancouver	89.89
021 Fraser East	89.78
051 Northwest	88.78
014 Thompson Cariboo Shuswap	88.75
053 Northeast	88.55
052 Northern Interior	85.73
999 Province	**91.89**

Over this period, the proportion of women breastfeeding on discharge from BC's hospitals ranged from a low of 85.73% in Northern Interior to a high of 96.48% in North Shore/Coast Garibaldi. The map opposite shows:
1) that breastfeeding rates on discharge were high;
2) that the differences in breastfeeding rates on discharge across the 16 HSDAs were fairly large (about 10 percentage points); and 3) that rates for HSDAs located in the more urban southwest corner of the province were generally higher than they were for those in the north and in the interior. The results for the CCHS question about this practice indicated that for women between 15 and 55 who had had children, 85.19% in BC had breastfed or tried to breastfeed with their last baby. This was significantly higher, statistically, than the 77.96% of all Canadian respondents to this question.

These results indicate that, for this indicator of basic food security for infants, there is still room for improvement, particularly in the north central and northeast regions of the province. While most women in BC are breastfeeding on discharge from hospital, several studies indicate that relatively few women breastfeed for the 6 month period now recommended by public health authorities in Canada.

Breastfed baby on discharge from hospital

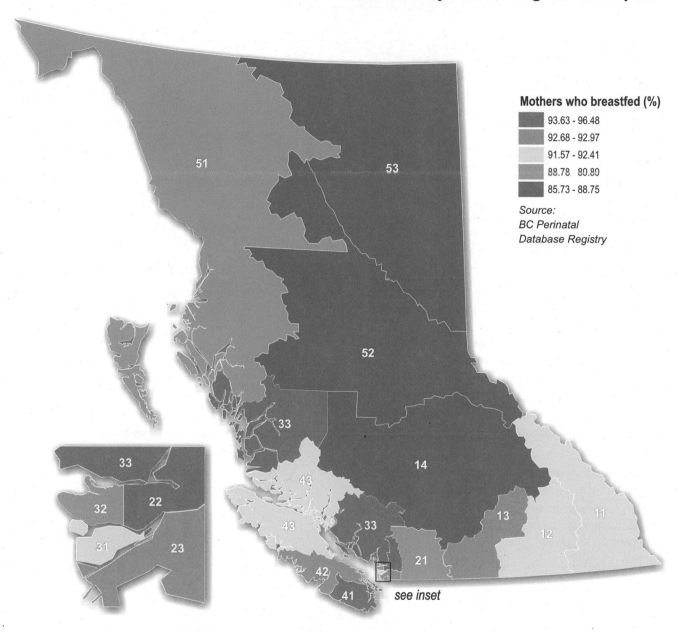

Mothers who breastfed (%)

- 93.63 - 96.48
- 92.68 - 92.97
- 91.57 - 92.41
- 88.78 80.80
- 85.73 - 88.75

Source:
BC Perinatal
Database Registry

Youth who always eat breakfast on school days

Approximately half (49.56%) of the Grade 7 to 12 students who responded to the McCreary Centre survey in 2003 "always ate breakfast on school days." (Note: as shown on the map, data for this question were available from only 13 of the 16 HSDAs.) The difference between the region with the highest (52.57%) and the lowest (46.01%) proportion of students who always eat breakfast was quite small, but more than a 6 percentage point difference. Only one HSDA, Okanagan (52.57%), was significantly higher, statistically, than the provincial average. However, even in this "best" region, almost one-half of BC students stated that they did not "always eat breakfast on school days."

When the two genders are examined separately, female students were much more likely to skip breakfast on school days. At 44.83% for all female students, this is significantly lower than the 54.36% of male students who always ate breakfast. Not only was this difference statistically significant at the provincial level, but the significant difference occurred for 10 of the 13 HSDAs for which we have data, denoting a very strong trend.

Among males, only Okanagan was statistically different from the provincial average, and there were no significant differences among the female respondents by HSDA. It is worth noting that the highest (best) HSDA for female students (48.52% for North Shore/Coast Garibaldi) was below the lowest male value (49.63% for Richmond).

It is clear that many high school youths in BC were not eating breakfast regularly, and that this trend was found fairly equally across all regions of the province. Given the importance of this meal in healthy eating, it is necessary to better understand why so many youths in BC are not eating breakfast regularly. Is this related to economic need, time pressures on parents and children, or some combination of these factors? As well, it may be important to know more about when this trend begins. While we know that lower grades are less likely than higher grades to skip breakfast (McCreary Centre Society, 2006), does it start in Grade 2 or 3, or is it mainly a high school phenomenon? It also raises broader questions about the potential role schools might play in feeding children in the mornings, and perhaps dealing with issues of body image.

Health Service Delivery Area		All respondents (%)	Males (%)	Females (%)
013	Okanagan	52.57	60.27†	45.66†
041	South Vancouver Island	52.30	58.48†	46.18†
033	North Shore/Coast Garibaldi	51.64	54.52	48.52
051	Northwest	50.50	55.54†	45.67†
014	Thompson Cariboo Shuswap	50.33	56.78†	44.53†
022	Fraser North	49.70	52.87†	46.32†
032	Vancouver	49.54	51.56	47.46
042	Central Vancouver Island	48.95	54.95†	43.32†
012	Kootenay Boundary	48.78	55.70†	42.11†
031	Richmond	48.33	49.63	46.89
011	East Kootenay	47.63	53.50†	41.13†
052	Northern Interior	47.41	54.84†	40.81†
043	North Vancouver Island	46.01	52.91†	38.78†
021	Fraser East	F	F	F
023	Fraser South	F	F	F
053	Northeast	F	F	F
999	**Province**	**49.56**	**54.36†**	**44.83†**

† Males differ significantly from females.
F Schools in this region did not participate in the survey.

Youth who always eat breakfast on school days

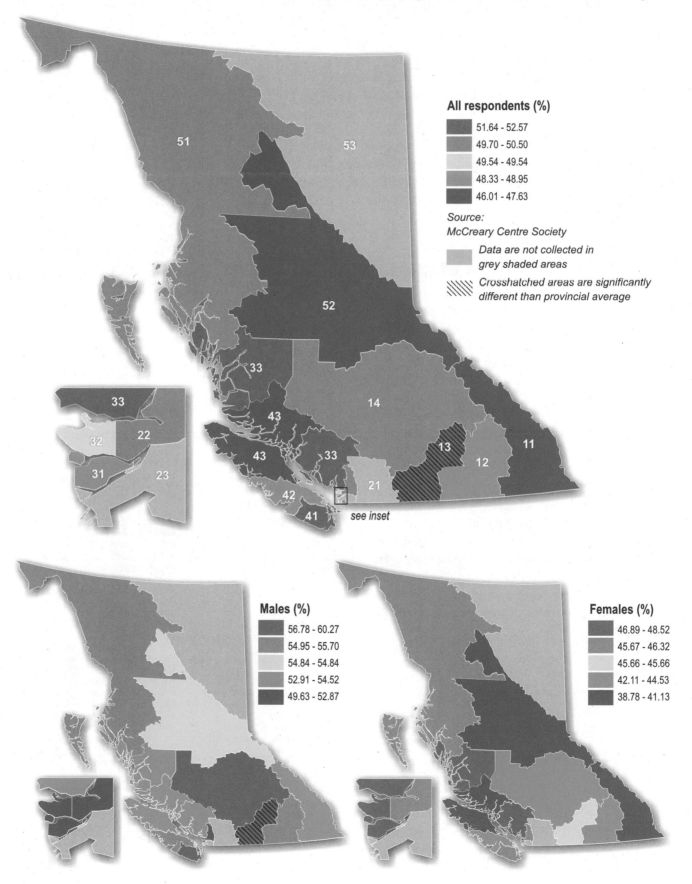

All respondents (%)

- 51.64 - 52.57
- 49.70 - 50.50
- 49.54 - 49.54
- 48.33 - 48.95
- 46.01 - 47.63

Source:
McCreary Centre Society

Data are not collected in grey shaded areas

Crosshatched areas are significantly different than provincial average

Males (%)

- 56.78 - 60.27
- 54.95 - 55.70
- 54.84 - 54.84
- 52.91 - 54.52
- 49.63 - 52.87

Females (%)

- 46.89 - 48.52
- 45.67 - 46.32
- 45.66 - 45.66
- 42.11 - 44.53
- 38.78 - 41.13

Learning about healthy food and exercise at school

The 2005-2006 School Satisfaction Survey was undertaken to assess a series of factors, including the extent to which Grade 3/4 students were learning about healthy eating and exercise at school. According to this survey, school districts in BC reported that 51.32% of girls and boys in Grade 3/4 were learning this important wellness information. There were large variations across school districts in the proportion of boys and girls who reported learning about these subjects. For example, in the Alberni school district a low of 39.18%, and in the francophone school system (not shown here as it is a non-geographic-based school district) a high of 80.6% of students reported learning about healthy eating and exercise.

Systematic (but generally fairly small) differences were noted in the proportion of girls compared to boys who reported learning about healthy eating and exercise. For example, in 50 school districts (83.3%), the proportion of girls who reported learning about healthy eating and exercise was higher than for boys. Across school districts, 54.51% of girls compared to 49.13% of boys reported learning about these subjects. Even at this young age, girls appear to be learning more about healthy food and exercise than boys in BC's school system.

In terms of broad regional trends, the school districts with the lowest proportion of Grade 3/4 students learning about healthy eating and exercise were found in northern Vancouver Island and the southern coast region. The francophone and Haida Gwaii/Queen Charlotte school districts had the greatest proportion of schools with Grade 3/4 students who reported learning about healthy eating and exercise.

School District	All respondents (%)	Males (%)	Females (%)
050 Haida Gwaii/Queen Charlotte	68.75	69.57	68.00
078 Fraser-Cascade	65.82	60.00	69.89
045 West Vancouver	65.22	59.47	72.19
071 Comox Valley	64.91	63.25	66.67
092 Nisga'a	64.71	54.55	83.33
049 Central Coast	64.29	70.59	54.55
063 Saanich	60.66	55.93	65.75
082 Coast Mountains	60.66	60.16	61.21
053 Okanagan Similkameen	58.70	54.55	62.50
008 Kootenay Lake	58.69	58.74	58.62
052 Prince Rupert	57.93	51.25	66.15
027 Cariboo-Chilcotin	57.43	56.63	58.15
067 Okanagan Skaha	57.01	54.95	58.85
036 Surrey	56.13	53.30	59.06
074 Gold Trail	55.21	50.91	60.98
034 Abbotsford	55.00	51.98	58.50
081 Fort Nelson	54.67	52.38	57.58
054 Bulkley Valley	54.49	63.95	42.86
019 Revelstoke	53.76	46.81	60.87
062 Sooke	53.12	50.49	55.99
079 Cowichan Valley	52.30	49.82	55.02
006 Rocky Mountain	52.10	50.71	53.42
038 Richmond	51.63	49.09	54.43
041 Burnaby	51.11	45.85	56.17
059 Peace River South	50.33	48.61	51.92
057 Prince George	50.32	48.10	52.90
023 Central Okanagan	50.25	47.23	53.24
043 Coquitlam	50.05	48.84	51.40
073 Kamloops/Thompson	49.65	48.47	50.92
068 Nanaimo-Ladysmith	49.40	46.80	51.92
022 Vernon	49.37	45.52	53.21
047 Powell River	49.24	45.71	53.23
033 Chilliwack	48.70	45.96	51.80
042 Maple Ridge-Pitt Meadows	48.28	49.33	47.15
058 Nicola-Similkameen	48.13	49.54	46.67
005 Southeast Kootenay	47.38	49.10	45.57
083 North Okanagan-Shuswap	47.31	45.45	49.19
061 Greater Victoria	47.29	46.31	48.33
060 Peace River North	47.12	42.93	51.55
091 Nechako Lakes	47.11	50.53	43.43
040 New Westminster	46.68	42.86	51.31
051 Boundary	46.60	39.62	54.00
035 Langley	46.59	44.17	49.24
069 Qualicum	46.45	38.82	55.38
010 Arrow Lakes	46.34	52.00	37.50
039 Vancouver	46.19	44.54	47.89
075 Mission	45.77	43.85	48.19
072 Campbell River	45.43	44.79	46.01
064 Gulf Islands	45.26	38.46	53.49
037 Delta	45.18	42.12	48.47
044 North Vancouver	45.03	44.08	45.97
048 Howe Sound	43.82	46.76	40.97
028 Quesnel	43.08	38.60	46.76
085 Vancouver Island North	40.17	33.33	49.02
046 Sunshine Coast	39.60	37.40	41.73
070 Alberni	39.18	34.50	44.59
020 Kootenay-Columbia	35.40	36.91	33.60
084 Vancouver Island West	N/A	N/A	N/A
087 Stikine	N/A	N/A	N/A
999 Province	**51.32**	**49.13**	**54.51**

Learning about healthy food and exercise at school

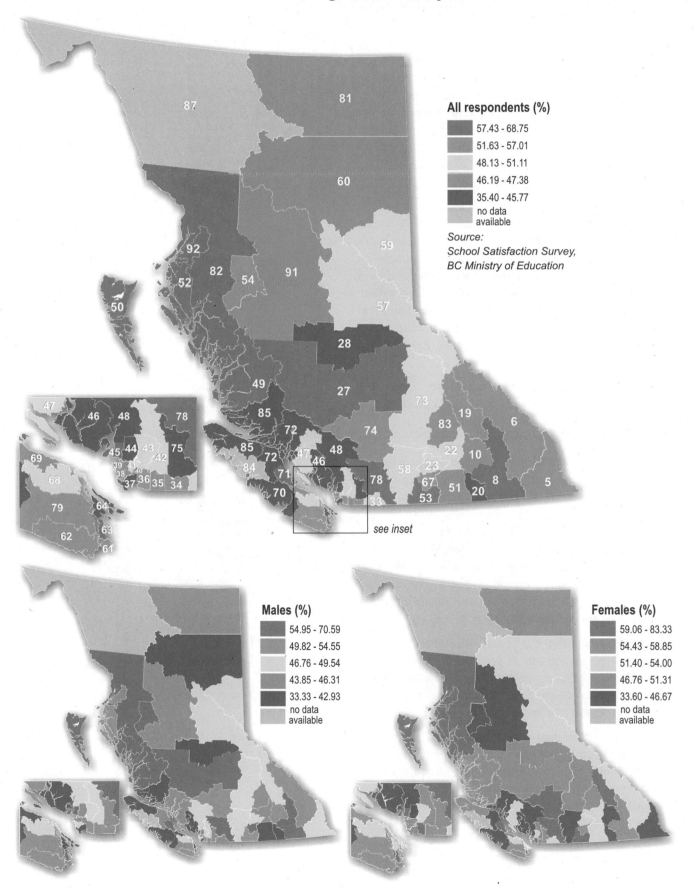

All respondents (%)

- 57.43 - 68.75
- 51.63 - 57.01
- 48.13 - 51.11
- 46.19 - 47.38
- 35.40 - 45.77
- no data available

Source:
School Satisfaction Survey,
BC Ministry of Education

see inset

Males (%)

- 54.95 - 70.59
- 49.82 - 54.55
- 46.76 - 49.54
- 43.85 - 46.31
- 33.33 - 42.93
- no data available

Females (%)

- 59.06 - 83.33
- 54.43 - 58.85
- 51.40 - 54.00
- 46.76 - 51.31
- 33.60 - 46.67
- no data available

Nutrition policy development at the school district level

As noted earlier, two surveys, one of school districts and the other of schools, were conducted in a joint project by the ministries of Education and Health to determine the number and types of different food sales outlets, the types of foods offered for sale in all school food outlets, and the extent of nutrition policy implementation in school districts and in schools in BC (Ostry et al., 2005; Rideout et al., in press).

In the spring of 2005, the two ministries sent each school district a questionnaire. The district superintendent (or a representative) filled out the questionnaire which, among other things, requested information about the extent to which nutrition policies had been planned, established, or, if established, upgraded in each school district. (Note: This questionnaire assesses the extent to which school districts, not individual schools, have taken leadership to improve the nutritional environment by providing guidance for the schools within their district. A second survey that went to individual schools is described on the next page.)

Specifically, each school district was asked: *"Does your school board have nutrition policies and/or guidelines: 1) planned; 2) established; or, if established, 3) do you have plans to upgrade them?"*

Forty-eight school districts (80.0%) responded to the survey. Of those, 29 school districts (60.4%) had no nutrition policies or guidelines in place. Nine of these school districts had no nutrition policies in place and were not planning to develop any, but 20 school districts were planning nutrition policies or guidelines at the time of survey. Nineteen (39.6%) responding school districts had a nutrition policy in place. Seven of these school districts had nutrition policies or guidelines in place but had no plans to upgrade them, and 12 school districts had policies in place and also had plans to upgrade them.

On Vancouver Island, 6 of 11 school districts (54.5%) had policies in place, and 9 of 11 school districts (81.8%) in the lower mainland had policies in place. Of the 26 responding school districts outside Vancouver Island and the lower mainland, 13 (50.0%) had a policy in place.

There was a great deal of variation in the extent to which school districts had developed nutrition policies and were planning them. School districts in the lower mainland, Greater Victoria, and in the Okanagan regions appear to have been more proactive in nutrition policy development than those located in other parts of the province.

School District	Response category
023 Central Okanagan	5
035 Langley	5
068 Nanaimo-Ladysmith	5
091 Nechako Lakes	5
044 North Vancouver	5
059 Peace River South	5
047 Powell River	5
019 Revelstoke	5
038 Richmond	5
006 Rocky Mountain	5
036 Surrey	5
033 Chilliwack	4
037 Delta	4
061 Greater Victoria	4
092 Nisga'a	4
052 Prince Rupert	4
039 Vancouver	4
022 Vernon	4
051 Boundary	3
054 Bulkley Valley	3
041 Burnaby	3
049 Central Coast	3
071 Comox Valley	3
078 Fraser-Cascade	3
074 Gold Trail	3
050 Haida Gwaii/Queen Charlotte	3
048 Howe Sound	3
008 Kootenay Lake	3
020 Kootenay-Columbia	3
042 Maple Ridge-Pitt Meadows	3
075 Mission	3
040 New Westminster	3
083 North Okanagan-Shuswap	3
067 Okanagan Skaha	3
057 Prince George	3
069 Qualicum	3
005 Southeast Kootenay	3
085 Vancouver Island North	3
072 Campbell River	2
082 Coast Mountains	2
079 Cowichan Valley	2
081 Fort Nelson	2
058 Nicola-Similkameen	2
053 Okanagan Similkameen	2
060 Peace River North	2
046 Sunshine Coast	2
084 Vancouver Island West	2
034 Abbotsford	1
070 Alberni	1
010 Arrow Lakes	1
027 Cariboo-Chilcotin	1
043 Coquitlam	1
064 Gulf Islands	1
073 Kamloops/Thompson	1
028 Quesnel	1
063 Saanich	1
062 Sooke	1
087 Stikine	1
045 West Vancouver	1

Nutrition policy development at the school district level

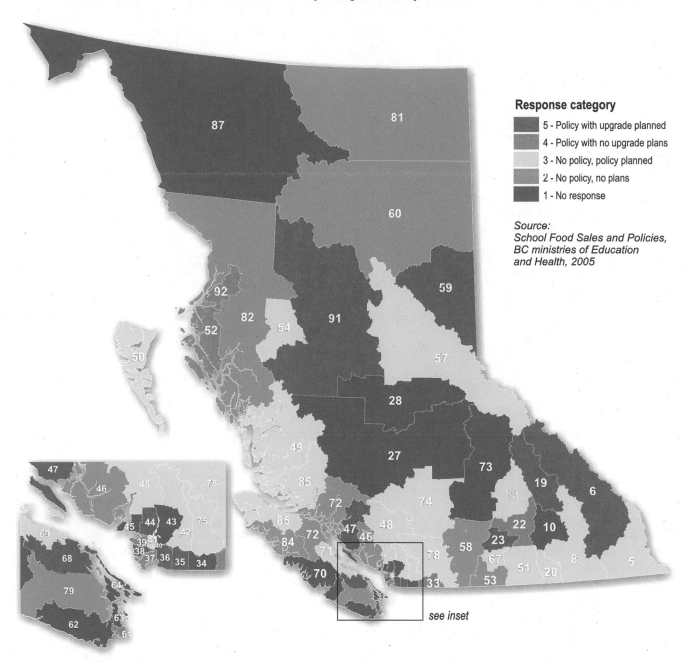

Response category

- 5 - Policy with upgrade planned
- 4 - Policy with no upgrade plans
- 3 - No policy, policy planned
- 2 - No policy, no plans
- 1 - No response

Source:
School Food Sales and Policies,
BC ministries of Education
and Health, 2005

see inset

Nutrition policy development in the schools

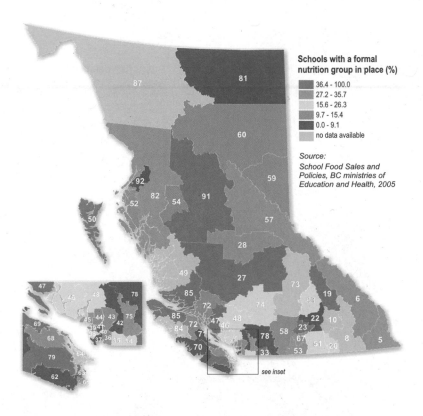

Schools with a formal nutrition group in place (%)
- 36.4 - 100.0
- 27.2 - 35.7
- 15.6 - 26.3
- 9.7 - 15.4
- 0.0 - 9.1
- no data available

Source:
School Food Sales and Policies, BC ministries of Education and Health, 2005

School District		Formal group (%)
085	Vancouver Island North	100.0
023	Central Okanagan	92.3
091	Nechako Lakes	63.2
019	Revelstoke	60.0
050	Haida Gwaii/Queen Charlotte	50.0
063	Saanich	50.0
027	Cariboo-Chilcotin	45.0
079	Cowichan Valley	43.8
069	Qualicum	41.7
047	Powell River	37.5
033	Chilliwack	36.4
006	Rocky Mountain	35.7
005	Southeast Kootenay	35.3
028	Quesnel	33.3
053	Okanagan Similkameen	33.3
075	Mission	33.3
082	Coast Mountains	33.3
067	Okanagan Skaha	31.3
057	Prince George	30.4
061	Greater Victoria	27.5
045	West Vancouver	27.2
083	North Okanagan-Shuswap	26.3
040	New Westminster	22.2
046	Sunshine Coast	22.2
051	Boundary	22.2
048	Howe Sound	21.8
020	Kootenay-Columbia	18.2
034	Abbotsford	18.2
035	Langley	18.2
074	Gold Trail	18.2
038	Richmond	15.6
052	Prince Rupert	15.4
068	Nanaimo-Ladysmith	15.4
054	Bulkley Valley	12.5
059	Peace River South	12.5
072	Campbell River	11.8
036	Surrey	11.4
044	North Vancouver	10.5
060	Peace River North	10.5
058	Nicola-Similkameen	10.0
039	Vancouver	9.7
043	Coquitlam	9.7
078	Fraser-Cascade	9.1
071	Comox Valley	8.3
041	Burnaby	6.4
037	Delta	6.3
022	Vernon	5.9
062	Sooke	4.8
042	Maple Ridge-Pitt Meadows	0.0
070	Alberni	0.0
081	Fort Nelson	0.0
092	Nisga'a	0.0
008	Kootenay Lake	NR
010	Arrow Lakes	NR
049	Central Coast	Msk
064	Gulf Islands	NR
073	Kamloops/Thompson	NR
084	Vancouver Island West	NR
087	Stikine	NR

These two maps show the variation in two indicators related to food policy in schools. While some schools have developed formal groups to promote better nutrition among students, other schools have expanded the role of existing groups within their school (e.g., Parent Advisory Committees, Parent Teacher Associations) to take on a more formal role to improve nutritional quality in the school. These groups have undertaken activities including: reducing the presence of vending machines in schools; increasing the number of healthy choice foods and beverages (e.g., low in fat and sugar, high in fibre) in vending machines and for sale in school tuck shops and cafeterias; and limiting cafeteria contracts with fast food and beverage companies, etc.

Formal groups concerned about nutrition

Analyses from the survey of individual schools, referred to on the previous page, show that schools with formal groups concerned about nutrition had a lower potential for food sales from vending machines and a higher proportion of more healthy snack options in their snack vending machines. They were also more likely to have established nutrition policies and guidelines (Ostry et al., 2005; Rideout et al., in press).

Responses were obtained from 1,169 (71.2%) of BC's 1,643 public schools. Of those responding, 256 (21.9%) reported the presence of a formal group in the school that was concerned with improving nutrition among students. These 256 schools were distributed quite evenly across elementary, middle, and secondary schools (Ostry et al., 2005; Rideout et al., in press).

Given that only 21.9% of responding schools had established a formal group concerned with nutrition, the proportion of schools within most school districts with such a group was quite low. As well, the variation was substantial. There were no groups among schools in four school districts—Maple Ridge-Pitt Meadows, Alberni, Fort Nelson, and Nisga'a—but

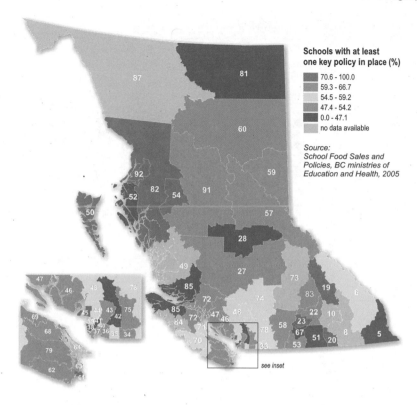

Schools with at least
one key policy in place (%)

■ 70.6 - 100.0
■ 59.3 - 66.7
□ 54.5 - 59.2
■ 47.4 - 54.2
■ 0.0 - 47.1
□ no data available

Source:
School Food Sales and
Policies, BC ministries of
Education and Health, 2005

School District		Key policies (%)
019	Revelstoke	100.0
050	Haida Gwaii/Queen Charlotte	100.0
092	Nisga'a	100.0
023	Central Okanagan	82.1
020	Kootenay-Columbia	81.1
054	Bulkley Valley	75.0
045	West Vancouver	72.7
082	Coast Mountains	71.4
061	Greater Victoria	70.6
046	Sunshine Coast	66.7
053	Okanagan Similkameen	66.7
062	Sooke	66.7
069	Qualicum	66.7
027	Cariboo-Chilcotin	65.0
022	Vernon	64.7
091	Nechako Lakes	63.2
059	Peace River South	62.5
075	Mission	61.9
034	Abbotsford	61.4
057	Prince George	60.1
079	Cowichan Valley	59.3
039	Vancouver	59.2
033	Chilliwack	59.1
035	Langley	59.1
048	Howe Sound	58.3
070	Alberni	58.3
071	Comox Valley	58.3
006	Rocky Mountain	57.1
040	New Westminster	55.6
044	North Vancouver	55.3
078	Fraser-Cascade	54.6
074	Gold Trail	54.5
043	Coquitlam	54.2
072	Campbell River	52.9
068	Nanaimo-Ladysmith	51.3
037	Delta	50.0
047	Powell River	50.0
058	Nicola-Similkameen	50.0
063	Saanich	50.0
036	Surrey	47.7
060	Peace River North	47.4
083	North Okanagan-Shuswap	47.4
005	Southeast Kootenay	47.1
038	Richmond	44.4
051	Boundary	44.4
067	Okanagan Skaha	43.8
081	Fort Nelson	40.0
052	Prince Rupert	38.5
042	Maple Ridge-Pitt Meadows	30.0
028	Quesnel	26.7
041	Burnaby	2.1
085	Vancouver Island North	0.0
008	Kootenay Lake	NR
010	Arrow Lakes	NR
049	Central Coast	Msk
064	Gulf Islands	NR
073	Kamloops/Thompson	NR
084	Vancouver Island West	NR
087	Stikine	NR

all 16 schools in the Vancouver Island North district had established these groups. The 10 school districts in the lower mainland region had among the lowest proportion of schools with a formal group, while the Okanagan and central interior regions had among the highest proportion of schools with formal groups concerned with nutrition.

Schools implementing specific nutrition policies

Respondents were also asked whether or not seven specific nutrition policies had been established in their school. A total of 654 (55.9%) reporting schools had at least one of the following policies in place:

• Restricting the types of food sold in school vending machines, cafeterias, or school stores.

• Restricting the types of food sold at school special events and field trips.

• Fundraising by selling food outside the school.

• Competitive pricing to promote healthy food choices.

• Discouraging the use of food as a reward.

• Limiting access to less nutritious foods during school hours.

• Providing adequate time and pleasant spaces to eat.

Responses were aggregated to the school district level, and the proportion of schools with one of the seven nutrition policies in place at the time of survey is shown on the table accompanying the map above.

There was much regional variation; for example, all the schools in Haida Gwaii/Queen Charlotte and Revelstoke school districts had at least one of the seven nutrition policies, while in the Vancouver Island North school district none of the schools had implemented any of these policies. In terms of geographical trends, the proportion of schools in the lower mainland with one of these policies in place was among the lowest in the province, compared to Northwest, North Shore/Coast Garibaldi, Okanagan, and Central Interior. New surveys are underway and these results will likely change.

Always able to afford to eat balanced meals in the past year

The first three maps opposite show the proportion of survey respondents, over age 12, within each HSDA who, with their household, were "always able to afford to eat balanced meals in the past 12 months." The actual CCHS question asked was: *"You and your household members couldn't afford to eat balanced meals. In the last 12 months was that often true, sometimes true, or never true?"* Approximately 9 out of 10 respondents answered "never," indicating that they were always able to afford a balanced meal. The results for Aboriginal respondents in BC was lower, with 8 out of every 10 (80.99%) responding "never." This difference is significant in a statistical sense.

The top map shows results for all respondents, and there was very little difference across regions of the province. For example, a low of 88.73% of respondents in Fraser East were always able to afford balanced meals compared to a high of 93.74% in Northeast. The next two maps show the results for males and females, age 12 and over, separately. Considering each region, little difference is observed between females and males.

The map at lower left, opposite, shows that teens were less able to afford balanced meals in the past year than their older counterparts. However, these differences were small (e.g., a provincial average of 89.32% for 12- to 19-year-olds, and 90.54% for 20- to 64-year-olds, compared to an average of 92.56% of those over 65 who reported being able to afford balanced meals in the past year). There was virtually no variation across regions for teens and seniors, but Northeast at 94.79% was significantly higher (table above) for 20- to 64-year-olds compared to the average for this age group.

In summary, these five maps indicate that approximately 90% of respondents in all regions of the province were always able to afford balanced meals in the year prior to the survey. Within each region, little variation was noted between males and females or across the three age groups, although teens reported being slightly less able to always afford balanced meals compared to the middle age and senior cohorts, and Aboriginal respondents were significantly less able to afford balanced meals.

Health Service Delivery Area	All respondents (%)	Males (%)	Females (%)	Ages 12-19 (%)	Ages 20-64 (%)	Ages 65+ (%)
053 Northeast	93.74	93.71	93.78	88.09	94.79	94.89
031 Richmond	92.54	94.61	90.61	90.65	92.77	92.68
043 North Vancouver Island	92.16	92.98	91.35	94.52	90.74	96.49
014 Thompson Cariboo Shuswap	91.99	94.07	89.93	92.25	92.56	89.35
022 Fraser North	91.44	93.29	89.64	88.60	92.16	89.66
052 Northern Interior	91.33	89.56	93.20	90.17	91.77	89.81
023 Fraser South	91.21	91.67	90.75	89.87	91.24	92.39
012 Kootenay Boundary	91.17	92.53	89.81	89.35	90.54	94.89
041 South Vancouver Island	91.11	91.89	90.41	92.12	90.15	94.18
011 East Kootenay	91.02	91.31	90.72	94.26	89.39	95.76
033 North Shore/Coast Garibaldi	90.67	91.92	89.49	87.69	90.40	94.03
042 Central Vancouver Island	90.57	89.49	91.60	85.97	90.55	93.43
013 Okanagan	89.95	91.50	88.48	88.99	88.70	94.45
051 Northwest	89.08	88.09	90.14	88.98	88.74	91.76
032 Vancouver	88.88	88.63	89.14	88.44	88.40	91.84
021 Fraser East	88.73	89.28	88.19	85.48	88.90	90.94
999 Province	**90.70**	**91.38**	**90.05**	**89.32**	**90.54**	**92.56**

Always able to afford to eat balanced meals in the past year

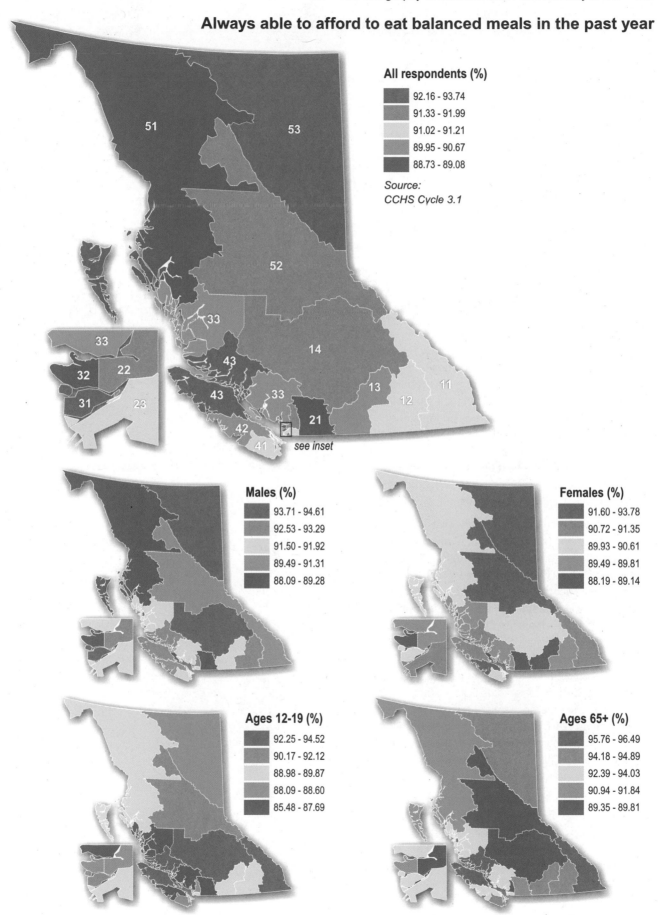

All respondents (%)

- 92.16 - 93.74
- 91.33 - 91.99
- 91.02 - 91.21
- 89.95 - 90.67
- 88.73 - 89.08

Source:
CCHS Cycle 3.1

Males (%)

- 93.71 - 94.61
- 92.53 - 93.29
- 91.50 - 91.92
- 89.49 - 91.31
- 88.09 - 89.28

Females (%)

- 91.60 - 93.78
- 90.72 - 91.35
- 89.93 - 90.61
- 89.49 - 89.81
- 88.19 - 89.14

Ages 12-19 (%)

- 92.25 - 94.52
- 90.17 - 92.12
- 88.98 - 89.87
- 88.09 - 88.60
- 85.48 - 87.69

Ages 65+ (%)

- 95.76 - 96.49
- 94.18 - 94.89
- 92.39 - 94.03
- 90.94 - 91.84
- 89.35 - 89.81

Always had enough of preferred food in the past year

The CCHS asked the following question: *"Which of the following statements best describes the food eaten in your household in the past 12 months? Would you say you always had enough of the kinds of food you wanted to eat, or often you didn't have enough to eat?"* Approximately 85% of all respondents over the age of 12 always had enough of the kinds of foods they wanted to eat in the past 12 months (86.57%). There was no difference from the average of those provinces across Canada that completed this part of the CCHS.

There was little difference across regions of the province, except in Vancouver where the proportion was lower (statistically significantly) than the provincial average. A low of 83.33% of all respondents in Vancouver always had enough preferred foods in the past year compared to a high of 89.36% (virtually next door) in Richmond. The next two maps show little difference in the proportion of males and females who "always had enough preferred foods in the past year."

The bottom two maps opposite show that, on average, 81.73% of respondents aged 12 to 19 always had enough preferred foods, compared to 86.42% of 20- to 64-years-olds (see above table) and 91.09% of those over age 65. These differences were statistically significant. The map at the bottom right shows that the proportion of residents in the North Shore/Coast Garibaldi, East Kootenay, Central Vancouver Island, and North Vancouver Island HSDAs who always had enough preferred foods in the past year was higher for seniors than 20- to 64-year-olds living in these same four regions, and the differences were statistically significant. Finally, among seniors, 96.67% of residents of North Shore/Coast Garibaldi reported having enough of their preferred foods. This was significantly higher than the provincial average for seniors (91.09%).

In summary, these five maps and accompanying table indicate that 80% to 90% of the population (with little variation by region, except for Vancouver) always had enough of their preferred food in 2005. Little variation was noted between males and females. On average, seniors had more and youths had less access to preferred foods than the middle age group.

Health Service Delivery Area	All respondents (%)	Males (%)	Females (%)	Ages 12-19 (%)	Ages 20-64 (%)	Ages 65+ (%)
031 Richmond	89.36	89.18	89.53	86.45	88.63	95.21
012 Kootenay Boundary	89.17	89.64	88.70	83.54	88.21	96.76
053 Northeast	89.10	91.54	86.48	82.23	89.79	95.50
033 North Shore/Coast Garibaldi	88.84	89.41	88.31	78.57	88.74	96.67‡
052 Northern Interior	88.34	86.42	90.36	86.19	88.96	86.95
014 Thompson Cariboo Shuswap	87.58	90.19	84.99	83.64	88.58	86.40
022 Fraser North	87.23	89.81	84.72	80.98	88.08	87.73
023 Fraser South	87.19	86.44	87.93	83.44	87.03	91.90
013 Okanagan	87.03	89.92	84.30	82.76	86.73	90.40
041 South Vancouver Island	86.83	86.77	86.88	84.14	86.23	90.62
042 Central Vancouver Island	86.12	86.22	86.03	80.95	84.71	94.01‡
011 East Kootenay	86.08	86.92	85.22	81.81	84.98	94.75‡
021 Fraser East	85.45	85.50	85.41	77.61	86.24	89.14
051 Northwest	83.84	85.26	82.31	77.71	84.17	91.06
043 North Vancouver Island	83.52	84.82	82.24	80.18	81.44	95.77‡
032 Vancouver	83.33	83.24	83.41	78.88	82.78	89.00
999 Province	**86.57**	**87.24**	**85.93**	**81.73‡**	**86.42**	**91.09‡**

‡ Age group differs significantly from 20-64 group.

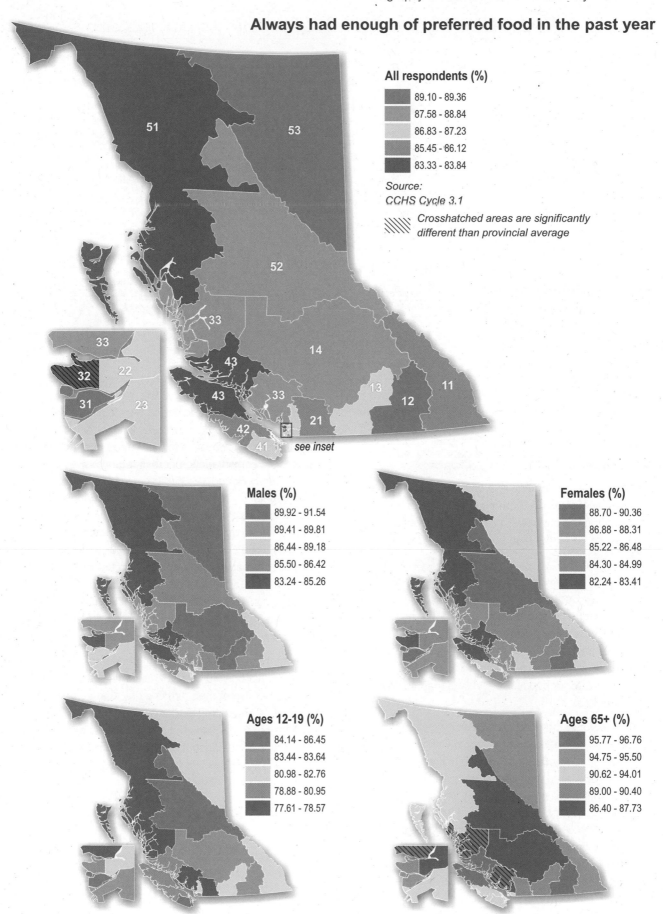

Always had enough of preferred food in the past year

All respondents (%)

- 89.10 - 89.36
- 87.58 - 88.84
- 86.83 - 87.23
- 85.45 - 86.12
- 83.33 - 83.84

Source:
CCHS Cycle 3.1

Crosshatched areas are significantly different than provincial average

Males (%)

- 89.92 - 91.54
- 89.41 - 89.81
- 86.44 - 89.18
- 85.50 - 86.42
- 83.24 - 85.26

Females (%)

- 88.70 - 90.36
- 86.88 - 88.31
- 85.22 - 86.48
- 84.30 - 84.99
- 82.24 - 83.41

Ages 12-19 (%)

- 84.14 - 86.45
- 83.44 - 83.64
- 80.98 - 82.76
- 78.88 - 80.95
- 77.61 - 78.57

Ages 65+ (%)

- 95.77 - 96.76
- 94.75 - 95.50
- 90.62 - 94.01
- 89.00 - 90.40
- 86.40 - 87.73

Eats fruit and vegetables five or more times a day

Approximately 40% of all respondents over the age of 12 ate fruit and vegetables five or more times a day. This was the same percentage for Aboriginal respondents in the province (39.99%).

On average in BC, 46.17% of females compared to 33.74% of males ate fruit and vegetables five or more times daily. In terms of regional differences, a low of 33.87% (statistically significant) of Northern Interior respondents ate fruit and vegetables five or more times a day, as compared to a high of 49.33% of respondents from the East Kootenays (significantly high). South and Central Vancouver Island were also significantly higher than the provincial average.

For males, the range in values was about 20 percentage points. Only in East Kootenay, with the highest value of 48.02%, was the percentage of the population eating fruit and vegetables five or more times a day significantly different than the provincial average. This was an outlier, with a score 10 percentage points higher than the next highest HSDA.

For females, there was some variation across HSDAs, although only South Vancouver Island at 53.88% was significantly different from the provincial average. In Kootenay Boundary, East Kootenay, and all of Vancouver Island, over half the female respondents ate fruit and vegetables five or more times a day, while in Northern Interior and Northeast less than 40% of females did so.

In all 16 regions, the proportion of women eating fruit and vegetables five or more times daily was greater than it was for men. For 8 of the 16 regions these differences were relatively large and statistically significant. The region with the greatest gender difference was Kootenay Boundary, where 53.2% of females compared to 31.1% of males reported eating fruit and vegetables five or more times a day. Interestingly, in East Kootenay (virtually next door to Kootenay Boundary) the differences were quite small: 48.02% for males and 50.67% for females.

Health Service Delivery Area	All respondents (%)	Males (%)	Females (%)	Ages 12-19 (%)	Ages 20-64 (%)	Ages 65+ (%)
011 East Kootenay	49.33	48.02	50.67	F	53.17	44.64
041 South Vancouver Island	45.77	36.80†	53.88†	49.53	45.64	44.12
042 Central Vancouver Island	45.08	38.06†	51.82†	40.07	45.87	45.51
043 North Vancouver Island	44.47	36.32	52.55	F	43.30	50.47
022 Fraser North	42.21	37.44†	46.87†	41.69	43.09	37.41
033 North Shore/Coast Garibaldi	42.20	37.21	46.95	50.12	41.01	41.99
012 Kootenay Boundary	42.12	31.10†	53.20†	65.69‡	38.15	41.31
014 Thompson Cariboo Shuswap	38.80	29.19†	48.35†	45.62	35.77	46.49
051 Northwest	38.44	33.60	43.67	34.07	39.22	39.42E
032 Vancouver	38.38	32.75†	43.87†	44.13	37.80	38.22
023 Fraser South	38.19	31.41†	44.84†	43.19	37.77	35.51
053 Northeast	37.27	36.15	38.48	F	38.08	31.69E
021 Fraser East	37.08	30.91	43.11	40.78	35.81	39.37
031 Richmond	36.39	28.85†	43.44†	38.97	36.03	36.45
013 Okanagan	35.38	30.09	40.38	34.48	33.19	42.88
052 Northern Interior	33.87	28.47	39.57	25.58E	37.22	21.56E‡
999 Province	**40.04**	**33.74†**	**46.17†**	**42.09**	**39.66**	**40.27**

‡ Age group differs significantly from 20-64 group.
† Males differ significantly from females.
E Interpret data with caution (16.77< coefficient of variation <33.3).
F Data suppressed due to Statistics Canada sampling rules.

The bottom two maps (and table above) show that approximately 40% of teens, the middle age group, and seniors ate fruit and vegetables five or more times a day. In other words, there was little variation across age groups. However, within the three age groups there was some variation across regions. For example, in Kootenay Boundary, 65.69% of youths ate fruit and vegetables five or more times daily, compared to 25.58% of youths in Northern Interior (both significantly different from the provincial average for teens). And in East Kootenay, a high of 53.17% of 20- to 64-year-olds were in this category, compared to a low of 33.19% in Okanagan. East Kootenay, along with South and Central Vancouver Island, was significantly higher than the average for this age group. Variability across the 16 regions was less for seniors than for those under age 65.

In summary, these five maps and accompanying table indicate that only 40% of BC residents ate fruit and vegetables five or more times a day. On average, across all regions of the province, this proportion was about 12% higher for females than for males. In general, the proportion of people in the north of the province who ate fruit and vegetables five or more times per day was lower than in the south of the province.

Eats fruit and vegetables five or more times a day

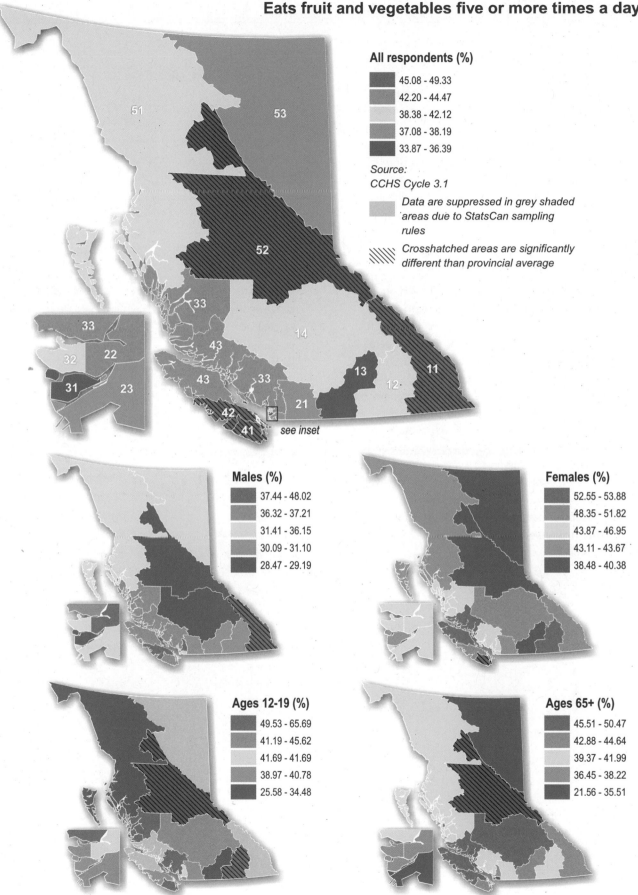

All respondents (%)

- 45.08 - 49.33
- 42.20 - 44.47
- 38.38 - 42.12
- 37.08 - 38.19
- 33.87 - 36.39

Source:
CCHS Cycle 3.1

Data are suppressed in grey shaded areas due to StatsCan sampling rules

Crosshatched areas are significantly different than provincial average

Males (%)

- 37.44 - 48.02
- 36.32 - 37.21
- 31.41 - 36.15
- 30.09 - 31.10
- 28.47 - 29.19

Females (%)

- 52.55 - 53.88
- 48.35 - 51.82
- 43.87 - 46.95
- 43.11 - 43.67
- 38.48 - 40.38

Ages 12-19 (%)

- 49.53 - 65.69
- 41.19 - 45.62
- 41.69 - 41.69
- 38.97 - 40.78
- 25.58 - 34.48

Ages 65+ (%)

- 45.51 - 50.47
- 42.88 - 44.64
- 39.37 - 41.99
- 36.45 - 38.22
- 21.56 - 35.51

Farmers' markets

The Kamloops and Salmon Arm farmers' markets decided in late 1999 to sponsor a conference for all farmers' markets in BC. The first such conference occurred in March 2000 and it was decided to form an association that would represent all the province's farmers' markets. At the conference a steering committee was appointed, and over the next several months preliminary work was undertaken. The Association of Farmers' Markets had a potential membership of more that 60 markets. Of these, 33 markets were represented at the first annual conference and growth has been dramatic since then.

Until 2000, farmers' markets in BC had been operating independently. Many markets had been struggling to stay afloat while others had been very successful. Markets are concerned about increasing their sales by attracting consumers in order to support BC producers of agricultural products, food products, and crafts. Many markets feature produce from local organic food growers. Farmers' markets operate in every type of community across BC, including cities, suburbs, and rural communities. As the BC Association of Farmers' Markets notes, they "vary in size and sophistication, from large sheltered public markets to a few farmers with their trucks parked next to each other in a parking lot or farm field" (*www.bcfarmersmarket.org*). Nine communities have farmers' markets available for more than one day per week.

Listing of Farmers' Markets in BC

1	100 Mile House	41	New Denver
2	Abbotsford	42	North Vancouver
3	Armstrong	43	Oliver
4	Bella Coola	44	Osoyoos
5	Campbell River	45	Peachland
6	Cedar	46	Penticton
7	Chetwynd	47	Port Alberni
8	Chilliwack	48	Port Moody
9	Coquitlam	49	Powell River
10	Courtenay	50	Prince George
11	Creston	51	Quadra Island
12	Dawson Creek	52	Qualicum Beach
13	Delta	53	Queen Charlotte Islands
14	Duncan	54	Quesnel
15	Dunster	55	Revelstoke
16	Errington	56	Richmond
17	Falkland	57	Saanichton
18	Fernie	58	Salmon Arm
19	Fort St. James	59	Saltspring Island
20	Fort St. John	60	Sechelt
21	Gabriola Island	61	Sicamous
22	Grand Forks	62	Silverton
23	Hope	63	Smithers
24	Hornby Island	64	Sooke
25	Invermere	65	Sorrento
26	Jaffray	66	Squamish
27	Kamloops	67	Summerland
28	Kelowna	68	Surrey
29	Ladner	69	Terrace
30	Langley	70	Texada Island
31	Lytton	71	Vancouver
32	Maple Ridge	72	Vancouver (UBC)
33	McBride	73	Vanderhoof
34	Merritt	74	Vernon
35	Metchosin	75	Victoria
36	Mission	76	Victoria (Esquimalt)
37	Mt Lehman	77	West Vancouver
38	Nanaimo	78	Whistler
39	Naramata	79	White Rock
40	Nelson	80	Williams Lake
		81	Winfield

Farmers' markets

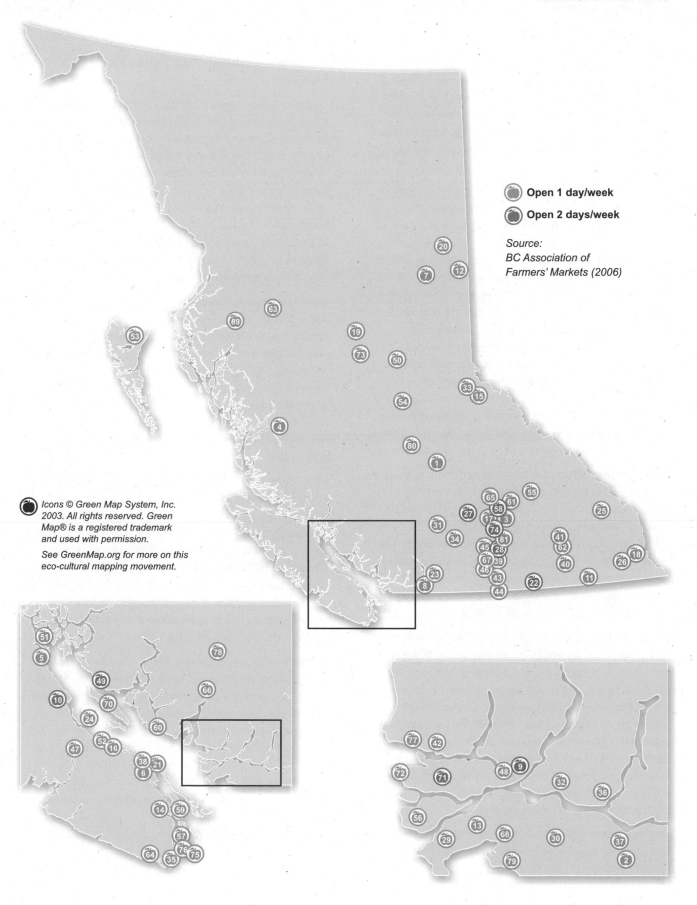

Open 1 day/week

Open 2 days/week

Source:
BC Association of
Farmers' Markets (2006)

Icons © Green Map System, Inc.
2003. All rights reserved. Green
Map® is a registered trademark
and used with permission.

See GreenMap.org for more on this
eco-cultural mapping movement.

Summary

The first part of the nutrition and food section focused on infants and children in BC. The first map indicated that while breastfeeding initiation rates in the province were quite high, they varied, with approximately 10% more women breastfeeding on discharge from hospitals in the urban southwest of the province compared to the north.

The next map showed clearly that high school-aged youth in BC were not eating breakfast regularly and that this trend was found across all parts of the province. These results are cause for concern, and one wonders at what age this trend begins to develop among British Columbian children. Interestingly, according to the School Satisfaction Survey conducted in 2005/06, only about one-half of Grade 3/4 students were learning about healthy eating and exercise at school. Further, there appeared to be small but consistent gender differences, such that girls were more knowledgeable about healthy eating and exercise even at these very young ages. Although in some school districts well over three-quarters of Grade 3/4 students indicated that they were learning about healthy eating and exercise, there is much room for improvement in other school districts.

There are also different levels of commitment to healthy eating at the school district level, as reflected in the leadership taken in developing nutrition guidelines and policy at this level. While 40% had a nutrition policy in place, only about half had plans to upgrade them. The lower mainland, Victoria, and Okanagan school boards were clear leaders. There is room for improvement in other areas of the province, and a survey currently underway may show this in the next edition of the Atlas.

The next survey canvassed schools directly, and these responses were aggregated and mapped at the school district level. Only 21.9% of responding schools had established a formal group concerned with nutrition, so the proportion of schools within most school districts with such a group was quite low. As well, the variation was substantial. In terms of regional patterns, the 10 school districts in the lower mainland region had among the lowest proportion of schools with a group concerned with nutrition, while school districts in the Okanagan and the central interior had a higher proportion.

The proportion of schools in the lower mainland with one of seven specific policies in place was among the lowest compared to the northwest, North Shore/Coast Garibaldi, the Okanagan, and central interior parts of the province.

Comparing the results from the school districts and the school surveys shows an interesting paradox in the lower mainland and northern Vancouver Island. On the one hand, districts in these areas have taken strong leadership at the school district level, but on the other hand, when it comes to schools within each district implementing policies to improve nutrition, they lag behind other districts. In the future, it will be important to explore this apparent disjunction between leadership taken at the district level and lack of progress at the school level in these districts.

Moving to the maps based on the CCHS, it is clear that approximately 90% of respondents in all regions of the province were always able to afford balanced meals and that approximately 80% to 90% of the population always had enough of their preferred food in 2005. Little variation was noted between males and females or between age groups. Looking at access to preferred foods only, on average, seniors had more and youths had less access to preferred foods than the middle age group.

Major differences across gender and region emerged when considering "eating fruit and vegetables five or more times a day." For example, on average, across all regions of the province, the proportion of females who ate fruit and vegetables five or more times a day was about 12% higher than for males. Also, a general north-south gradient was observed, with a higher proportion of males and females of all age groups who ate fruit and vegetables five or more times a day in the south compared to the north of the province.

These trends raise questions about why males, across all regions of the province, were much less likely to eat fruit and vegetables compared to females. As well, one wonders about the north-south gradient. While this gradient had exceptions (e.g., among those over age 65), the proportions who ate fruit and vegetables in parts of the lower mainland were quite low and similar to those in the north of the province, raising questions about the availability and price of fruit and vegetables, especially in the north.

Participation in fitness activities and sports plays an important role in increasing health status and reducing illness and health care costs. As the BC Select Standing Committee on Health (2004) noted, lack of physical exercise is related to many disease risk factors. Although the process is not well understood, physical activity appears to be a protective factor (or wellness asset) for several chronic diseases and illnesses (Kendall, 2006). Mental health is improved because endorphins reduce stress, anxiety, and depression. The strengthening of muscles and enhancement of bone density reduces osteoporosis and improves balance, especially in older people, thus reducing the potential for falls. For seniors, recreation and active living prolong independent functioning by compressing the impairment and disease period typically associated with aging (Torjman, 2004, p. 2). Increasing the metabolic rate can help reduce diabetes. Cardiovascular functions are improved, thus reducing blood pressure and strengthening the heart and lungs. Finally, some cancers are reduced as a result of increased immunity and metabolism rates, among other things.

For young children, physical activity has been found to have an important impact on growth and maturation. Further, recreation and play are key elements for healthy childhood development. They promote the acquisition of key motor skills, social skills, and creativity. For youth, research has shown that recreation reduces boredom and associated risky behaviour (Torjman, 2004).

A recent study by the Canadian Institute for Health Information has noted that physical activity levels are higher among those who have greater contact with friends and family, and those who indicate that their neighbours are active are also likely to be active themselves. In short, social support networks are important. Furthermore, assets such as better street lighting, good sidewalks, and perceived community safety are all associated with greater physical activity, especially walking. Availability of wellness assets such as recreation facilities, parks, and sport grounds are also related to increased physical activity (Canadian Institute for Health Information, 2006a).

It was estimated in a 2000 study that 2.5% of Canada's total health care costs are directly attributable to physical inactivity. Further, a savings of $150 million in health care spending could be achieved by increasing physical activity by 10% (Katzmarzyk, Gledhill, and Shephard, 2000).

In the early 1970s, there was a common belief that the average Swede was in better shape than the average Canadian. In 1972, ParticipACTION introduced the famous comparison between the 60-year-old Swede and the 30-year-old Canadian in a 15-second television commercial. This belief helped contribute to a national emphasis on improving the physical fitness levels of Canadians (Canadian Public Health Association, 2004). While the program was cancelled some time ago, ParticipACTION was one of the best known health promotion branding initiatives worldwide. It is now in the process of being reinvented to focus on not just physical activity, but also on sport and fitness for the entire population.

The World Health Organization (WHO) developed a global strategy in 2004 to promote physical activity and healthy eating. The premise was that this would be an effective strategy for substantially reducing deaths and disease worldwide by improving diet and promoting exercise (World Health Organization, 2004). The strategy has four main thrusts:

- Reduce risk factors for chronic diseases that stem from unhealthy diet and physical inactivity through public health actions.

- Increase awareness and understanding of the influences of diet and physical activity on health and the positive impact of preventive interventions.

- Develop, strengthen, and implement global, regional, and national policies and action plans to improve diet and increase physical activity that are sustainable, comprehensive, and actively engage all sectors.

- Monitor science and promote research on diet and physical activity.

For the school-age population, although 54% of schools in Canada had physical education policies in 2001, only 16% indicated that they had daily physical education classes (Canadian Institute for Health Information, 2006a). The McCreary Adolescent Health Survey undertaken in 2003 showed that less than one in five (18%) students in Grades 7 to 12 exercised every day.

Only 11% of female students exercised daily, compared to 24% of male students, and nearly 1 in 10 students didn't exercise at all (McCreary Centre Society, 2006).

Physical inactivity has been defined by the CCHS as less than 1.5 kcal/kg/day, and in 2003 it was estimated that less than one-third of BC residents aged 12 and older were physically active, and nearly half of the population was not active enough to achieve the health benefits of regular activity (ActNow BC, 2006). Remarkably, the BC Nutrition Survey (Ministry of Health Services, 2004; Forster-Coull, 2004) noted that 80% of adults in BC felt that they were active enough to attain health benefits. More recently, 75% of a suburban population surveyed in BC indicated that they had been physically active during the previous week, but only 39% reported enough physical activity to meet the guidelines for health benefits (Anderson, Snodgrass, and Elliott, 2007). A study conducted in 20 communities (440 sample size per community) throughout BC in 2006 by the BC Recreation and Parks Association determined that 49% of respondents were classified as highly active; Vancouver Island communities led the way with 58% highly active, but only 42% in the lower mainland were categorized as highly active. The average for the Okanagan region was 53%, and 51% for other interior regions (Discovery Research, 2006).

In 2005, there were more than 90,000 individuals who participated in sanctioned road races in BC, and more than 633,000 members were registered in organized sports as reported by member associations of Sports BC, for an overall rate of approximately 150 members for every 1,000 people between the ages of 4 and 74 years in the province. Membership rates were higher for males than females (173 per 1,000 compared to 125 per 1,000). Rates fell from a high of 677 per 1,000 for 4- to 12-year-olds to 58 per 1,000 for 35- to 74-year-olds.

The 48 maps contained in this section of the Atlas are diverse in nature and use a variety of data and information sources. The first three maps provide information related to Action Schools, an initiative promoted by 2010 Legacies Now to encourage schools to increase physical activity among students in Kindergarten to Grade 9. This is followed by four maps that show the increase over time of the percentage of the population that reside in Active Communities, an initiative jointly sponsored by BC Recreation and Parks Association and 2010 Legacies Now to assist communities to encourage their residents to become more physically active.

The next 10 maps provide data from the CCHS for two indicators: physical activity rating and hours walked on a weekly basis, for the total population and for males and females, and also for teens and seniors separately. The next two maps provide information on walking clubs sponsored by the Heart and Stroke Foundation and on public transit use. Research has shown that those using public transit are much more physically active than those who use automobiles. Two maps provide information on assets related to physical activity and show the availability of key recreation and activity facilities and centres.

The next 20 maps, which are provided four to a page, provide information on physical activity assets such as soccer fields and softball diamonds, as well as membership in sports clubs. The final map shows the location of provincial and national park assets in BC.

Caution is required related to the maps of activity centres and sports fields. These data are based on survey data sponsored by the BC Recreaton and Parks Association. As noted previously, only 88% of municipal organizations responded to the questionnaire, thus the data here are for publicly owned and or operated facilities in those municipal organizations that responded.

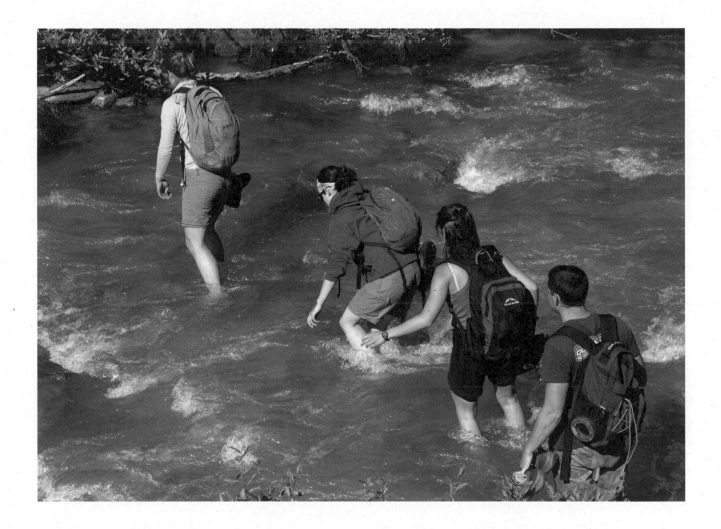

Action schools

Canadian children spend about 30 hours per week in school and about 20 hours per week watching television or playing computer games outside school. In 2003, the Ministry of Health introduced a pilot initiative called Action Schools! BC to 10 schools, promoting "best practices" in physical activity designed to assist elementary schools in creating individualized action plans to promote healthy living. Physical activity and healthy eating were integrated into the school environment. The pilot evaluation showed improvements in physical activity levels, and healthy hearts, weights, eating, bones, and self. Academic performance also improved in the schools using the best practices (McKay, 2004). The voluntary initiative was first made available to all Grade 4 to 7 classes, and more recently expanded to all schools from kindergarten to middle school.

At the end of 2006, nearly 1,150 schools were participating (over 70% of eligible schools), including about 250,000 students. More than 40% of Aboriginal schools and approximately 45% of independent schools had also registered. Action Schools! BC is a framework for action involving six Action Zones: school environment; scheduled physical education; classroom action; family and community; extra-curricular; and school spirit. Registered schools are encouraged to create an Action Team and develop an Action Plan integrating all six Action Zones. All schools are encouraged to book a Classroom Action workshop for their teachers in order to access materials and resources to support teachers in providing more opportunities for more children to be more physically active more often.

The maps opposite show the rapid adoption of the initiative by schools growing from 28% to 51% between December 2004 and December 2005, and to 72% by December 2006. For 2006, this included an expanded target, as all kindergarten to middle schools were included in this initiative. School districts in the southeast (3), Okanagan (3), North Shore/Coast Garibaldi (3), lower mainland (3), and lower Vancouver Island (2) have at least 90% of schools registered. Most school districts have more than half the eligible schools registered, but seven in the central and northern interior of the province and one in the lower Fraser Valley have 50% or less of eligible schools registered. It should be noted that new schools are adopting the initiative on an ongoing basis.

School District	Action Schools in District (%)		
	Dec 31 2006	Dec 31 2005	Dec 31 2004
053 Okanagan Similkameen	100	100	100
050 Haida Gwaii/Queen Charlotte	100	100	0
054 Bulkley Valley	100	50	25
081 Fort Nelson	100	50	0
085 Vancouver Island North	100	33	8
084 Vancouver Island West	100	25	25
019 Revelstoke	100	0	0
042 Maple Ridge-Pitt Meadows	96	100	79
041 Burnaby	95	86	59
028 Quesnel	93	36	13
061 Greater Victoria	90	82	29
052 Prince Rupert	90	70	10
044 North Vancouver	90	55	27
062 Sooke	90	33	5
064 Gulf Islands	89	89	89
051 Boundary	89	50	0
038 Richmond	88	85	69
068 Nanaimo-Ladysmith	88	73	66
022 Vernon	88	65	24
072 Campbell River	88	39	20
063 Saanich	86	67	77
006 Rocky Mountain	86	36	9
079 Cowichan Valley	84	56	46
040 New Westminster	83	75	82
008 Kootenay Lake	83	68	76
075 Mission	83	33	12
048 Howe Sound	82	100	40
078 Fraser-Cascade	80	80	60
067 Okanagan Skaha	80	53	31
073 Kamloops/Thompson	79	67	51
057 Prince George	79	67	18
036 Surrey	75	60	45
087 Stikine	75	50	0
033 Chilliwack	73	46	28
091 Nechako Lakes	72	38	40
045 West Vancouver	71	70	50
069 Qualicum	71	57	46
023 Central Okanagan	68	41	14
037 Delta	67	42	32
039 Vancouver	67	42	31
020 Kootenay-Columbia	64	30	30
027 Cariboo-Chilcotin	63	29	15
035 Langley	63	13	5
070 Alberni	62	46	0
071 Comox Valley	60	44	33
005 Southeast Kootenay	59	20	13
043 Coquitlam	58	47	41
082 Coast Mountains	56	54	25
046 Sunshine Coast	55	45	36
059 Peace River South	55	4	4
047 Powell River	50	63	63
049 Central Coast	50	33	0
092 Nisga'a	50	25	0
074 Gold Trail	45	25	18
034 Abbotsford	44	25	10
060 Peace River North	44	22	12
083 North Okanagan-Shuswap	41	14	0
058 Nicola-Similkameen	38	10	0
010 Arrow Lakes	25	0	0
099 Province	**72**	**51**	**28**

Action schools

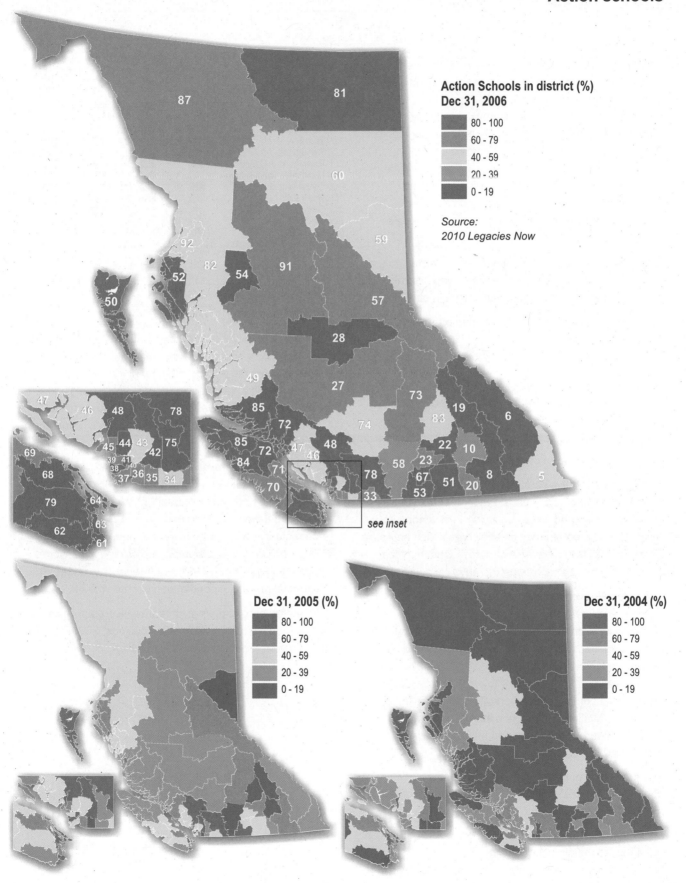

Action Schools in district (%)
Dec 31, 2006

80 - 100
60 - 79
40 - 59
20 - 39
0 - 19

Source:
2010 Legacies Now

see inset

Dec 31, 2005 (%)

80 - 100
60 - 79
40 - 59
20 - 39
0 - 19

Dec 31, 2004 (%)

80 - 100
60 - 79
40 - 59
20 - 39
0 - 19

Active communities

BC Recreation and Parks Association, in cooperation with 2010 Legacies Now, has introduced an initiative called Active Communities to help support the province's plan to increase the physical activity undertaken by the population. There is a recognition that to meet ActNow BC wellness goals it is necessary to have many partners who are committed to improving the health and wellness of the BC population. Local government and communities are very important in this strategy given that people identify with local communities.

The Active Communities initiative has an overall goal of promoting healthy lifestyles and building healthy communities. The initiative has three main objectives:

- supporting communities to develop an Active Community plan;

- increasing local awareness of the benefits of regular physical activity; and

- creating opportunities to increase physical activity levels by 20% by the year 2010.

An Active Community promotes, through an overall strategy, integration of physical activity into daily living.

To become an Active Community, local government must adopt and officially pass a motion to accept the goal of improving physical activity by 20% among its residents. The community must also establish an Active Communities Team, develop an Active Communities plan, and commit to achieving the physical activity goal.

Those local governments that become Active Communities get access to a variety of resources including an Active Communities tool kit, which provides a workbook, fact sheets, a planning guide, and a self assessment checklist. An Active Workplace Workbook is also available for employers to develop physical activity as a component of workplace wellness initiatives. Grants are available to develop an Active Community plan or to improve, develop, and maintain walkways, pathways, bikeways, and trails.

The four maps opposite show the percentage of the population, by HSDA, residing in Active Communities in four different time periods.

By the end of 2005, more than half of the BC population (55.4%) was residing in an Active Community. The greatest coverage was in the urban lower mainland and

Health Service Delivery Areas	Population in active communities (%)			
	Dec 31 2005	Apr 30 2006	Aug 31 2006	Dec 1 2006
031 Richmond	100.0	100.0	100.0	100.0
041 South Vancouver Island	36.6	100.0	100.0	100.0
023 Fraser South	68.5	84.6	99.8	99.8
032 Vancouver	98.3	98.3	98.3	98.3
022 Fraser North	18.1	86.3	86.3	96.6
043 North Vancouver Island	0.3	88.5	93.3	93.3
033 North Shore/Coast Garibaldi	59.3	79.0	85.4	92.0
042 Central Vancouver Island	90.1	90.9	91.6	91.6
021 Fraser East	74.9	79.5	79.5	79.5
013 Okanagan	46.1	58.6	74.3	74.3
051 Northwest	32.6	56.1	59.6	59.6
011 East Kootenay	24.8	48.7	48.7	58.1
014 Thompson Cariboo Shuswap	44.6	48.2	56.8	56.8
053 Northeast	33.3	33.3	40.3	56.7
012 Kootenay Boundary	9.8	30.6	35.8	47.8
052 Northern Interior	8.1	8.6	16.5	16.7
999 Province	**55.4**	**78.6**	**83.8**	**86.2**

Central Vancouver Island. By April 30, 2006, 78.6% of the province's population was residing in a community that had become an Active Community. The adoption of this initiative was most evident in lower mainland, North Shore/Coast Garibaldi, and Vancouver Island communities, with less involvement in the interior, north, and eastern parts of the province.

Four months later, by the end of August 2006, 83.8% of the population was covered, and only Northern Interior and Kootenay Boundary had less than 40% of their populations residing in an Active Community. By December 1, 2006, all HSDAs but one had close to 50% or more of their populations residing in an Active Community, and only Northern Interior was under 20%. The total provincial population covered was 86.2%.

Scattered around the province there were approximately 20 Aboriginal communities (out of almost 200) that had also registered as Active Communities.

Active communities

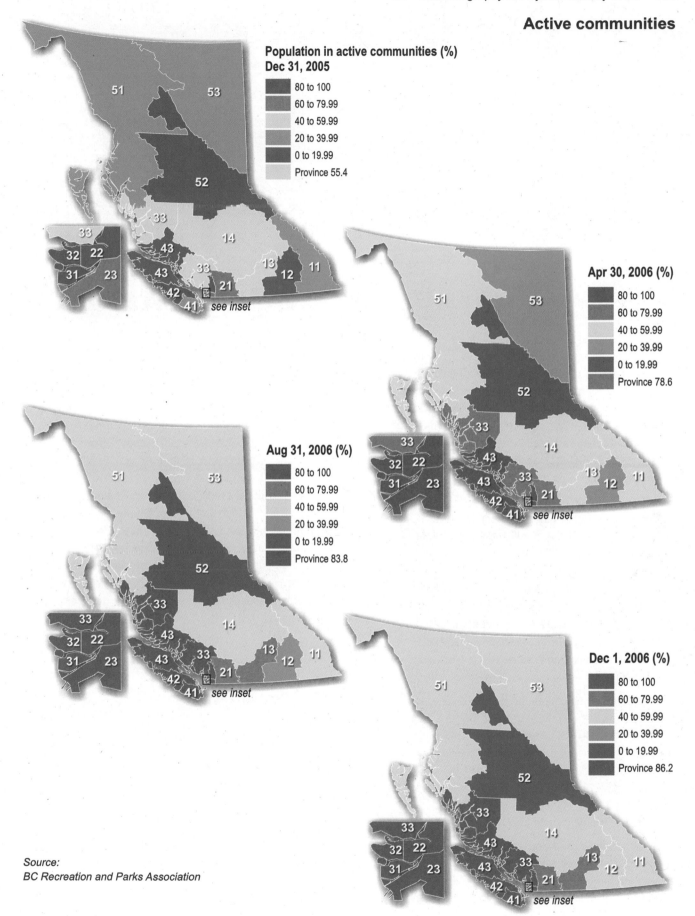

Population in active communities (%)
Dec 31, 2005

- 80 to 100
- 60 to 79.99
- 40 to 59.99
- 20 to 39.99
- 0 to 19.99
- Province 55.4

Apr 30, 2006 (%)

- 80 to 100
- 60 to 79.99
- 40 to 59.99
- 20 to 39.99
- 0 to 19.99
- Province 78.6

Aug 31, 2006 (%)

- 80 to 100
- 60 to 79.99
- 40 to 59.99
- 20 to 39.99
- 0 to 19.99
- Province 83.8

Dec 1, 2006 (%)

- 80 to 100
- 60 to 79.99
- 40 to 59.99
- 20 to 39.99
- 0 to 19.99
- Province 86.2

Source:
BC Recreation and Parks Association

Physical activity index

The CCHS derived a Physical Activity Index based on respondents' answers to several questions related to the frequency, duration, and intensity of their participation in certain activities. For each leisure time activity, an average daily energy expenditure was calculated. Respondents were then classified as Active if their average daily energy expenditure was 3 kcal/kg/day, Moderately Active with an expenditure between 2.9 and 1.5 kcal/kg/day, and Inactive below 1.5 kcal/day. The table on this page and maps opposite are based on the percentage of the population in the Active and Moderately Active categories combined. For BC respondents as a whole, 57.96% were active or moderately active. This was very similar to the result for Aboriginal respondents in the province (55.76%), but significantly higher, statistically, than the average for Canadian respondents as a whole (51.19%).

For all respondents combined, there were major differences throughout the province. The range between the most active and least active regions was 17 percentage points. Geographically, the southeast of the province, South Vancouver Island, and North Shore/Coast Garibaldi areas were the most active, with Richmond and Fraser East in the lower mainland and Northeast the least active. South Vancouver Island, East Kootenay, and North Shore/Coast Garibaldi were all significantly more active, while Northeast was significantly less active than the provincial average.

There was no significant difference between genders, but there was within gender groups. South Vancouver Island and East Kootenay were significantly higher, statistically, and Northeast was significantly lower for males. For females, North Vancouver Island, Kootenay Boundary, and South Vancouver Island were statistically significantly higher. Overall, however, geographical patterns were similar to that for all respondents.

Physical activity diminished significantly with age. Teens, at 72.40%, were significantly more physically active than the middle age cohort of 20- to 64-year-olds (57.15%), which in turn was significantly higher,

statistically, than the seniors group (50.64%). These significant differences occurred not only provincially, but for several individual HSDAs as well. Among teens, six HSDAs were significantly higher than the 20 to 64 year olds in their region: East Kootenay, Fraser North, Vancouver, Fraser South, Richmond, and Fraser East. At 86.94%, East Kootenay was also significantly higher than the provincial average for teens. Seniors in three HSDAs, South Vancouver Island, Okanagan, and Northern Interior, had significantly lower activity levels than their younger counterparts. Northern Interior, Fraser East, and Northeast were also significantly lower among seniors. Caution is required with respect to the Northeast result because of the high coefficient of variation.

Health Service Delivery Area	All respondents (%)	Males (%)	Females (%)	Ages 12-19 (%)	Ages 20-64 (%)	Ages 65+ (%)
041 South Vancouver Island	66.63	67.79	65.58	76.09	68.25	55.00‡
011 East Kootenay	65.84	69.55	62.04	86.94‡	64.92	52.27
012 Kootenay Boundary	65.15	63.49	66.81	80.31	65.13	54.75
033 North Shore/Coast Garibaldi	63.91	64.66	63.20	74.71	63.82	56.83
043 North Vancouver Island	63.64	57.20	70.01	57.58	66.45	56.26
042 Central Vancouver Island	62.14	61.87	62.39	68.13	62.59	56.94
051 Northwest	59.64	62.15	56.92	69.06	59.95	42.32E
014 Thompson Cariboo Shuswap	57.33	56.64	58.02	72.00	56.66	48.61
022 Fraser North	57.32	59.65	55.04	73.29‡	56.28	49.20
013 Okanagan	56.24	60.19	52.51	66.44	58.41	43.54‡
052 Northern Interior	55.88	57.69	53.98	72.17	55.38	36.35‡
032 Vancouver	55.39	57.58	53.26	70.94‡	53.33	57.55
023 Fraser South	54.25	54.43	54.08	75.74‡	51.61	47.47
031 Richmond	53.99	53.94	54.04	74.16‡	51.64	51.88
021 Fraser East	53.02	53.02	53.01	72.39‡	51.75	40.92
053 Northeast	49.66	45.64	53.98	64.68	48.41	33.38E
999 Province	**57.96**	**58.88**	**57.07**	**72.40‡**	**57.15**	**50.64‡**

‡ Age group differs significantly from 20-64 group.
E Interpret data with caution (16.77< coefficient of variation <33.3).

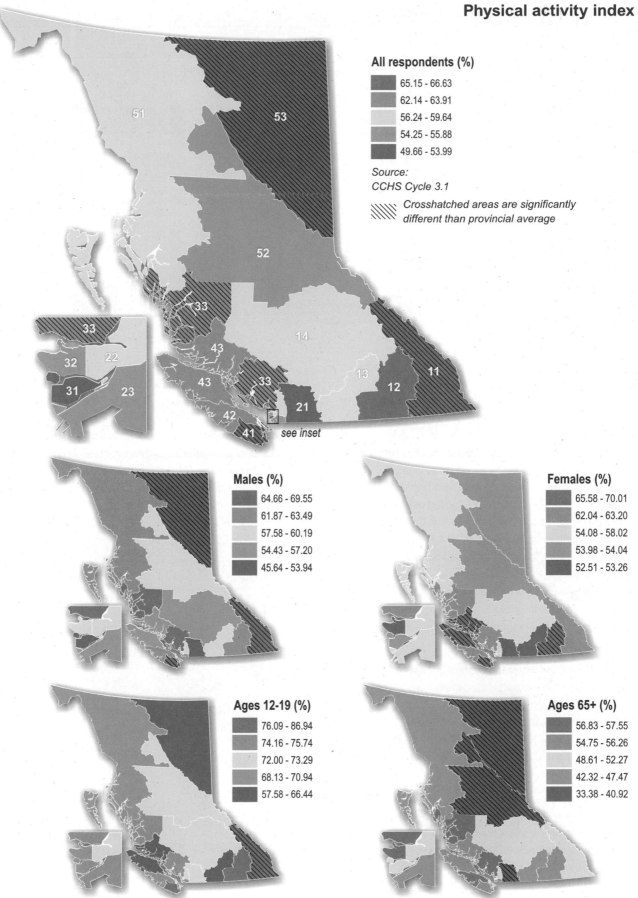

Physical activity index

All respondents (%)

- 65.15 - 66.63
- 62.14 - 63.91
- 56.24 - 59.64
- 54.25 - 55.88
- 49.66 - 53.99

Source:
CCHS Cycle 3.1

Crosshatched areas are significantly
different than provincial average

Males (%)

- 64.66 - 69.55
- 61.87 - 63.49
- 57.58 - 60.19
- 54.43 - 57.20
- 45.64 - 53.94

Females (%)

- 65.58 - 70.01
- 62.04 - 63.20
- 54.08 - 58.02
- 53.98 - 54.04
- 52.51 - 53.26

Ages 12-19 (%)

- 76.09 - 86.94
- 74.16 - 75.74
- 72.00 - 73.29
- 68.13 - 70.94
- 57.58 - 66.44

Ages 65+ (%)

- 56.83 - 57.55
- 54.75 - 56.26
- 48.61 - 52.27
- 42.32 - 47.47
- 33.38 - 40.92

Six or more hours per week walking

The CCHS asked respondents the following question: *"In a typical week in the past three months, how many hours a week did you usually spend walking to work or to school or while doing errands?"* On average, while only 25.30% of BC residents walked six or more hours a week, this is significantly higher, statistically, than for Canadian respondents as a whole (22.85%).

For all respondents, there were major differences throughout the province. The range from highest to lowest was 52.44% for East Kootenay to 18.94% for Richmond. Geographically, this indicator had one of the highest variations among all of the CCHS indicators included in this Atlas. No fewer than 10 HSDAs had significantly different values, statistically, from the provincial average. Generally, the urban southwest part of the province had low percentages of respondents walking six or more hours a week, while the highest percentages walking for this length of time occurred in the southeast of the province and on the southern half of Vancouver Island. Significantly high values occurred in East Kootenay, Central and South Vancouver Island, and Kootenay Boundary. Significantly low levels of walking activity were recorded for Richmond, Fraser East, Vancouver, and Fraser South, all in the lower mainland of the province, Okanagan in the interior, and North Vancouver Island.

There was no appreciable difference between males and females in these patterns, although females walked more than males, but not significantly so. The geographical patterns were very similar to the pattern for all respondents, although males in Northwest (29.43%) were more likely to walk than females (19.30%), but the difference was not statistically significant.

The lower two maps show that there is very incomplete data for this variable because the numbers walking six or more hours a week for both teens and seniors is too low to report for most HSDAs, and several of those that can be reported have relatively unstable values because of low numbers of people who walk six or more

hours a week. What we can say is that teens in East Kootenay are significantly more likely to walk than teens elsewhere in the province. Seniors in East Kootenay and South Vancouver Island are also significantly more likely to walk than are seniors elsewhere in the province. Vancouver seniors are significantly less likely to walk, although because of unstable values, caution should be used in interpreting this result. Overall, seniors in the province are statistically significantly less likely to walk than younger age groups.

Health Service Delivery Area	All respondents (%)	Males (%)	Females (%)	Ages 12-19 (%)	Ages 20-64 (%)	Ages 65+ (%)
011 East Kootenay	52.44	52.49	52.39	55.33	51.79	52.99
042 Central Vancouver Island	38.49	41.79	35.33	32.92	42.92	27.09‡
041 South Vancouver Island	38.17	33.65	42.25	34.06	40.24	32.67
012 Kootenay Boundary	32.63	32.08	33.18	F	34.18	30.25
014 Thompson Cariboo Shuswap	29.93	32.35	27.52	F	32.79	21.28E
022 Fraser North	25.57	22.97	28.12	31.97	26.47	14.43E‡
053 Northeast	25.51	19.55E	31.91	F	26.41	F
033 North Shore/Coast Garibaldi	25.01	25.67	24.38	F	26.61	21.12
051 Northwest	24.56	29.43	19.30	F	27.82	F
052 Northern Interior	23.73	24.17	23.26	F	26.15	F
013 Okanagan	20.83	18.47	23.06	21.93	22.44	15.09E
023 Fraser South	20.59	19.40	21.75	22.80	21.25	14.64
032 Vancouver	19.20	18.75	19.64	F	21.51	12.20E‡
021 Fraser East	19.14	17.02	21.20	F	19.50	19.47
043 North Vancouver Island	19.01	16.93E	21.07E	F	19.92E	F
031 Richmond	18.94	20.87	17.13	F	18.16	F
999 Province	**25.30**	**24.40**	**26.18**	**23.77**	**26.70**	**19.79‡**

‡ Age group differs significantly from 20-64 group.
E Interpret data with caution (16.77< coefficient of variation <33.3).
F Data suppressed due to Statistics Canada sampling rules.

Six or more hours per week walking

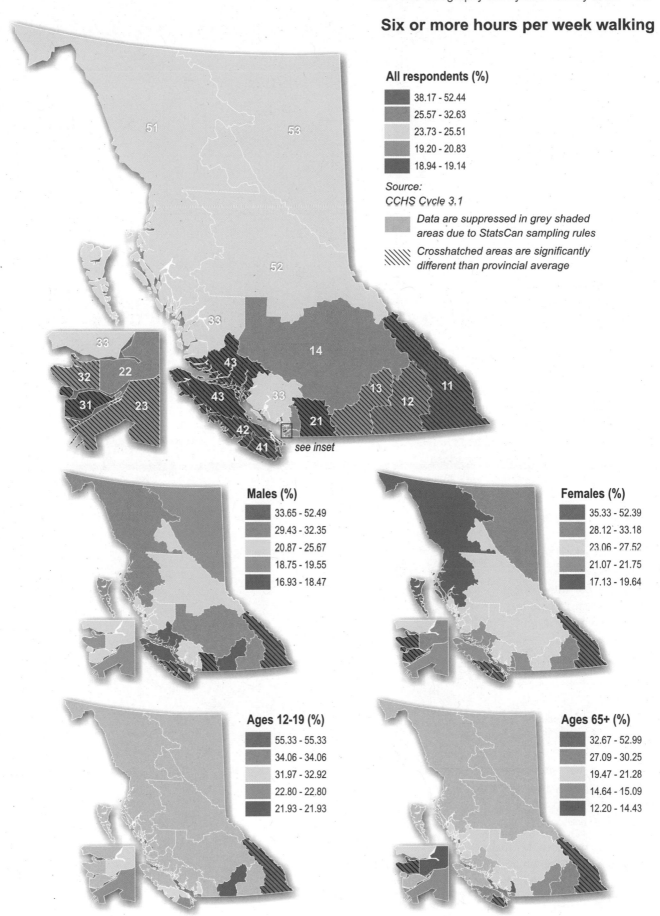

All respondents (%)

- 38.17 - 52.44
- 25.57 - 32.63
- 23.73 - 25.51
- 19.20 - 20.83
- 18.94 - 19.14

Source:
CCHS Cycle 3.1

Data are suppressed in grey shaded areas due to StatsCan sampling rules

Crosshatched areas are significantly different than provincial average

Males (%)

- 33.65 - 52.49
- 29.43 - 32.35
- 20.87 - 25.67
- 18.75 - 19.55
- 16.93 - 18.47

Females (%)

- 35.33 - 52.39
- 28.12 - 33.18
- 23.06 - 27.52
- 21.07 - 21.75
- 17.13 - 19.64

Ages 12-19 (%)

- 55.33 - 55.33
- 34.06 - 34.06
- 31.97 - 32.92
- 22.80 - 22.80
- 21.93 - 21.93

Ages 65+ (%)

- 32.67 - 52.99
- 27.09 - 30.25
- 19.47 - 21.28
- 14.64 - 15.09
- 12.20 - 14.43

Heart and Stroke Foundation Hearts in Motion walking clubs

The Heart and Stroke Foundation of BC and the Yukon is a member of the BC Healthy Living Alliance, which is assisting government to reach its ActNow BC goals. The Heart and Stroke Foundation has reported that Canadians who are dependent on automobiles for transportation are at increased risk of being overweight or obese. Their 2005 Report Card on the Health of Canadians showed a reduction in the likelihood of being obese for every additional kilometre walked each day (Canadian Institute for Health Information, 2006a). Because lack of exercise has been recognized as a major risk factor for heart disease and stroke, the Foundation has helped to create a series of Hearts in Motion walking clubs throughout BC. The clubs have been formed to help get people organized to undertake regular physical activity through walking in groups, which are both social and supportive.

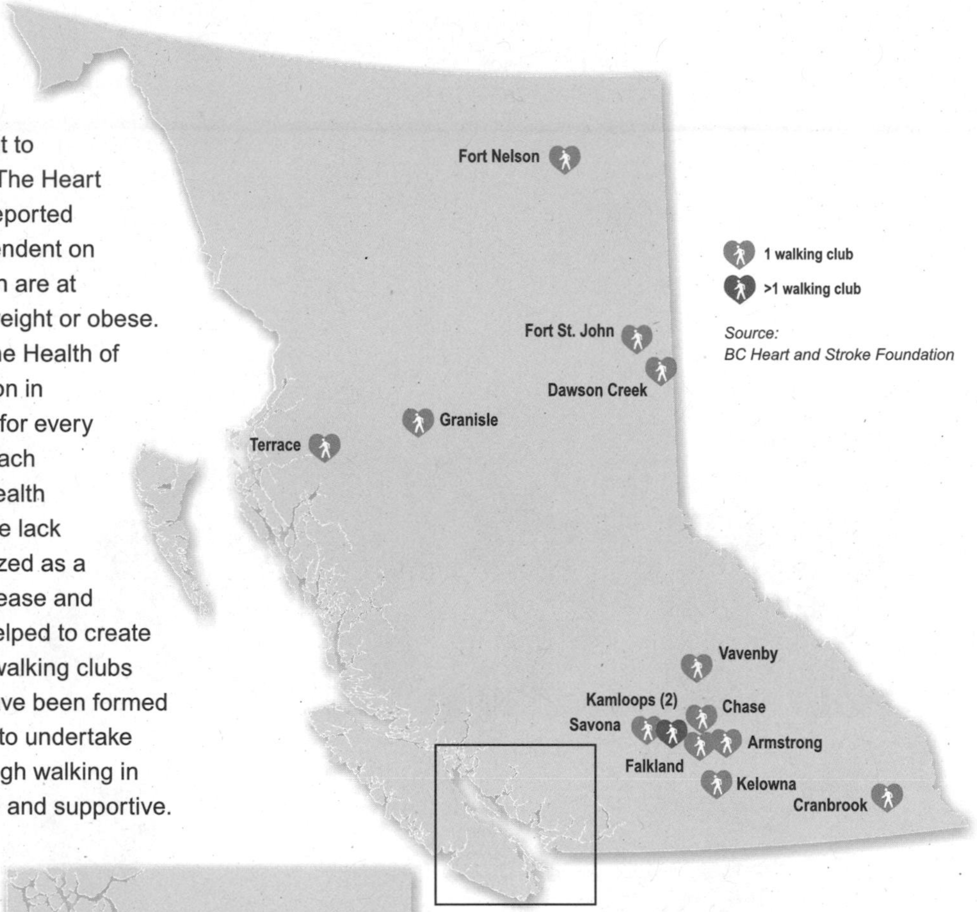

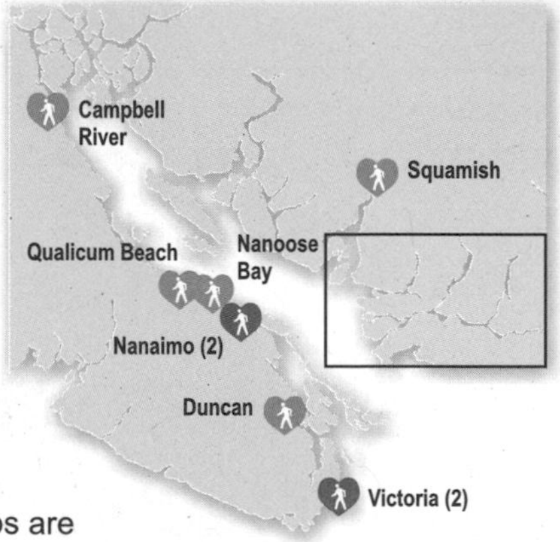

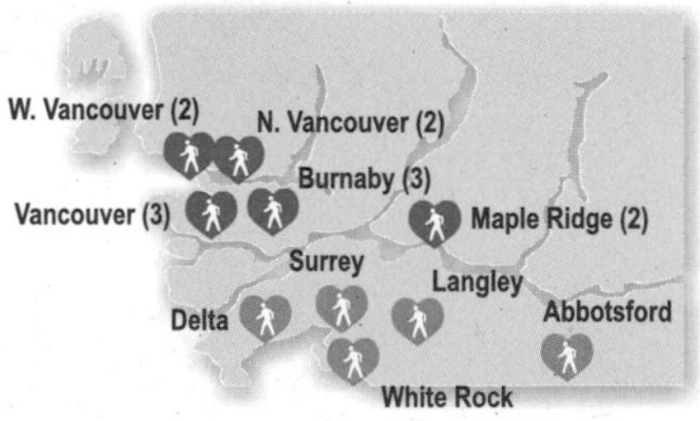

Participants who join one of the clubs throughout BC receive a handbook with tips on getting started in a safe manner, a personal activity card to record distances walked, and awards to recognize personal milestones.

This map indicates where the more than 40 current Hearts in Motion walking clubs are located throughout the province. Several communities have more than one walking club, as indicated above. Burnaby and Vancouver, for example, both have three such walking clubs, while Kamloops, Maple Ridge, Nanaimo, North Vancouver, Victoria, and West Vancouver each have two clubs.

As might be expected, the majority of clubs are located in the lower mainland area of the province, but other clubs can be found in the interior and more northern parts of BC.

Fort Nelson

1 walking club
>1 walking club

Source:
BC Heart and Stroke Foundation

Fort St. John
Dawson Creek
Granisle
Terrace

Vavenby
Kamloops (2)
Chase
Savona
Armstrong
Falkland
Kelowna
Cranbrook

Campbell River
Squamish
Qualicum Beach
Nanoose Bay
Nanaimo (2)
Duncan
Victoria (2)

W. Vancouver (2)
N. Vancouver (2)
Burnaby (3)
Vancouver (3)
Maple Ridge (2)
Surrey
Langley
Delta
Abbotsford
White Rock

Public transit use per capita

The use of public transit can be viewed as an interrupted pedestrian activity. People who use public transit usually walk to the transit stop and then walk from their exit point to their destination. There is much research to suggest that those using public transit are generally healthier than those using the automobile as a travel mode. Those using public transit generally have a lower body mass index (Canadian Institute for Health Information, 2006a).

Within BC, much of the population has access to some type of public transit. The map above shows the location and use per capita of public transit within BC for 2005/6. In total, the population that can be served by municipal systems is over 830,000. In addition, the service in place for the Capital Regional District on South Vancouver Island covers another estimated 340,000 people, while the Translink system covering the Greater Vancouver Regional District has a service population of over two million. In total, about 80% of the provincial population has access to some type of public transit.

As the proportionate circles on the map above show, the ridership per capita varies substantially among the 25 different transit systems mapped (the system for Whistler was not included in this analysis because the data included ridership to and from Vancouver). The annual ridership rates vary from highs of nearly 130 per capita for Translink in the Greater Vancouver Regional District, followed by nearly 60 per capita for the Capital Regional District on Vancouver Island, and over 40 per capita in Kamloops. The ridership rates for Fort St. John in the northeast, Vernon in the Okanagan, and Cowichan Valley on Vancouver Island are all below 10 per capita.

Overall, transit use is much higher in the urban areas of the southwest, where higher population densities make systems a lot more accessible and efficient to operate.

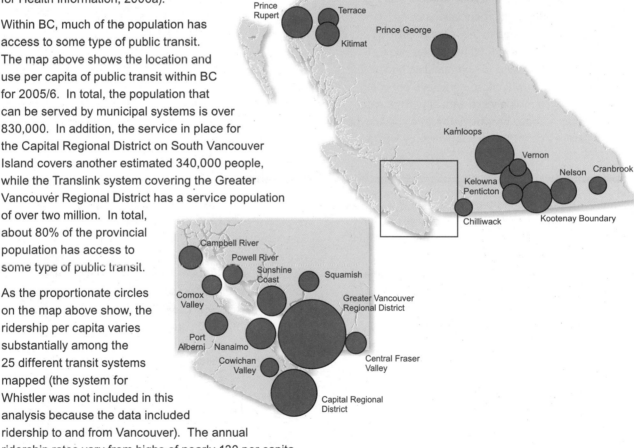

127.9
59.1
28.3
14.3
7.2

Sources:
BC Transit, 2006, Greater Vancouver Regional District, Capital Regional District

Fort St. John
Dawson Creek
Prince Rupert
Terrace
Kitimat
Prince George
Kamloops
Vernon
Nelson   Cranbrook
Kelowna
Penticton
Chilliwack
Kootenay Boundary

Campbell River
Powell River
Sunshine Coast
Squamish
Comox Valley
Greater Vancouver Regional District
Port Alberni   Nanaimo
Cowichan Valley
Central Fraser Valley
Capital Regional District

Community recreation facilities

In early 2004, the BC Recreation and Parks Association published a survey of four major types of publicly owned or operated recreation facilities: indoor pools; outdoor pools; curling rinks; and ice arenas. There was a combined total of 414 facilities. The survey was funded by 2010 Legacies Now, as well as the Ministry of Community, Aboriginal and Women's Services and Pacific Sport. One of the goals of the survey was to ensure that people in BC have access to the facilities they need in order to lead healthy, active lifestyles (BC Recreation and Parks Association, 2004). A total of 185 municipalities, regional districts, and other local government organizations were surveyed, and all responded to the questionnaire. Of the communities surveyed, 65 had no facilities included in the survey, while 15 communities had all four. Of the 292 facilities for which use data were provided, there were nearly 36 million visits annually. The maps opposite and table above provide data by calculating the number of facilities per 100,000 population by HSDA.

Health Service Delivery Area	Indoor pools	Outdoor pools	Curling rinks	Ice arenas
053 Northeast	8.66	2.89	11.55	15.89
043 North Vancouver Island	7.56	1.68	1.68	5.88
012 Kootenay Boundary	4.97	6.21	11.18	12.43
011 East Kootenay	4.83	3.63	8.46	13.29
051 Northwest	4.47	0.00	3.55	9.48
033 North Shore/Coast Garibaldi	3.29	0.37	0.73	3.29
052 Northern Interior	3.25	0.00	5.20	10.39
014 Thompson Cariboo Shuswap	3.15	2.25	3.60	6.75
042 Central Vancouver Island	2.77	1.19	1.98	2.77
041 South Vancouver Island	2.56	0.00	0.85	2.56
021 Fraser East	2.27	1.89	1.51	2.65
013 Okanagan	1.81	2.41	3.02	5.73
022 Fraser North	1.60	3.02	0.71	1.60
032 Vancouver	1.52	1.01	0.17	1.35
023 Fraser South	1.25	1.88	0.63	2.03
031 Richmond	1.15	1.15	0.00	1.15
999 Province	2.44	1.67	1.83	3.78

Indoor pools

Throughout the province there was a total of 103 publicly owned or operated indoor pools for an overall rate for the province as a whole of 2.44 per 100,000 population. Geographically, Northeast, North Vancouver Island, the southeast of the province, and Northwest had the highest number of facilities per 100,000 population. It must be noted that these HSDAs are all rural in nature. The lowest rates were in the urban southwest of the province.

Outdoor pools

There were 72 outdoor pools around the province for an overall rate of 1.67 facilities per 100,000 population for publicly owned or operated outdoor pools. The highest rates were in the southeast part of the province and Fraser North in the lower mainland. Three HSDAs, South Vancouver Island, Northern Interior, and Northwest, did not have any outdoor pools.

Curling rinks

Throughout the province, there were 79 publicly owned or operated curling rinks for a provincial rate of 1.83 facilities per 100,000 population. The highest rates per

100,000 population for these facilities occurred in the extreme northeast and southeast of the province. The lowest rates were in the urban southwest of the province, and Richmond did not have any publicly owned or operated curling rinks.

Ice arenas

There were 161 ice arenas around the province, for a provincial rate of 3.78 facilities per 100,000 population. The highest rates (over 10 per 100,000 population) occurred in Northeast, East Kootenay, Kootenay Boundary, and Northern Interior. The lowest rates were found in the urban southwest of the province, and Vancouver, Richmond, and Fraser North all had rates below 2 per 100,000 population.

Overall, the facilities included in the survey tend to be more available (although not necessarily available to all) in the rural parts of the province and less so in the urban southwest of the province. In some instances, there were no facilities available for some HSDAs.

Community recreation facilities per 100,000 population

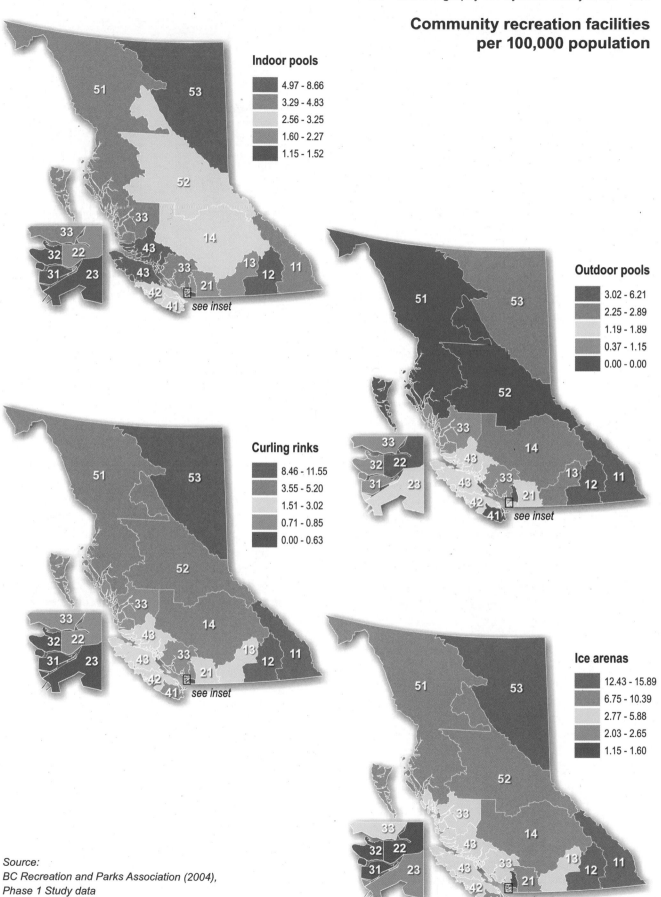

Indoor pools

- 4.97 - 8.66
- 3.29 - 4.83
- 2.56 - 3.25
- 1.60 - 2.27
- 1.15 - 1.52

Outdoor pools

- 3.02 - 6.21
- 2.25 - 2.89
- 1.19 - 1.89
- 0.37 - 1.15
- 0.00 - 0.00

Curling rinks

- 8.46 - 11.55
- 3.55 - 5.20
- 1.51 - 3.02
- 0.71 - 0.85
- 0.00 - 0.63

Ice arenas

- 12.43 - 15.89
- 6.75 - 10.39
- 2.77 - 5.88
- 2.03 - 2.65
- 1.15 - 1.60

Source:
BC Recreation and Parks Association (2004),
Phase 1 Study data

Community centres

In 2006, the BC Recreation and Parks Association released the results of a second major survey of community facilities (BC Recreation and Parks Association, 2006b). The inventory collected information on different types of activity centres. These included publicly funded or operated community halls, community centres, youth centres, and senior centres. Each of these facility types are places where people can gather for different kinds of recreation and other activities. In total, there were 433 centres included in the inventory, with an estimated use of 38 million visits per year. It should be noted that only 88% of the 185 local government organizations who were sent questionnaires responded, and so the rates provided in the maps opposite and the above table are only for those municipalities who participated in the survey. Results must be used cautiously, based on this incomplete information.

Community halls

In total, there were 114 community halls scattered around the province based on the results of those municipalities that responded to the questionnaire. The highest facility rate was found in Kootenay Boundary (26.82 per 100,000 population). This region was far ahead of the next nearest regions, Thompson Cariboo Shuswap and Northwest. At the other extreme, the urban areas of the southwest had very low rates. Richmond had no publicly funded or operated community halls, while Vancouver had 0.67 per 100,000 population.

Community centres

There were 177 publicly operated or owned community centres in BC, based on the survey response. The highest facility rates were in the northwest, northeast, and southeast of the province. Again, Kootenay Boundary with a rate of 21.46 facilities per 100,000 had by far the highest rate of community centres. Low rates were again evident in the urban southwest of the province.

Youth centres

There was a total of 69 publicly owned or operated youth centres around the province. The highest rates were found in the northeast, northwest, and again, Kootenay

Health Service Delivery Area	Community halls	Community centres	Youth centres	Senior centres
012 Kootenay Boundary	26.82	21.46	8.05	10.73
014 Thompson Cariboo Shuswap	10.24	4.78	2.73	3.41
051 Northwest	9.15	12.81	5.49	5.49
042 Central Vancouver Island	4.58	3.75	1.25	0.42
043 North Vancouver Island	4.38	11.38	1.75	2.63
013 Okanagan	4.02	5.87	2.16	3.40
033 North Shore/Coast Garibaldi	3.83	12.04	2.19	1.09
052 Northern Interior	3.28	3.93	1.31	2.62
041 South Vancouver Island	3.20	3.84	1.92	1.92
022 Fraser North	3.17	3.39	2.54	2.12
053 Northeast	3.10	13.97	6.21	4.66
021 Fraser East	1.52	2.28	0.38	0.76
011 East Kootenay	1.44	10.11	1.44	4.33
023 Fraser South	1.29	2.77	1.29	1.66
032 Vancouver	0.67	2.53	1.69	1.01
031 Richmond	0.00	3.46	0.00	0.58
999 Province	**3.05**	**4.73**	**1.84**	**1.95**

Boundary, which had the highest rate of 8.05 facilities per 100,000 population. The lowest rates were found in Richmond, which had no centres at all, and in Fraser East and Central Vancouver Island.

Senior centres

There were 73 senior centres scattered throughout the province. Kootenay Boundary again had the highest rate, with 10.73 facilities per 100,000 population. Northwest and Northeast had relatively high rates, followed by East Kootenay. Central Vancouver Island had the lowest rate, followed by Richmond and Fraser East in the southwest of the province.

In summary, the availability of these four different types of publicly owned and operated activity centres varies substantially throughout the province. The availability in the urban southwest of the province is low, while availability in the more rural parts of the province is much higher, especially in Kootenay Boundary.

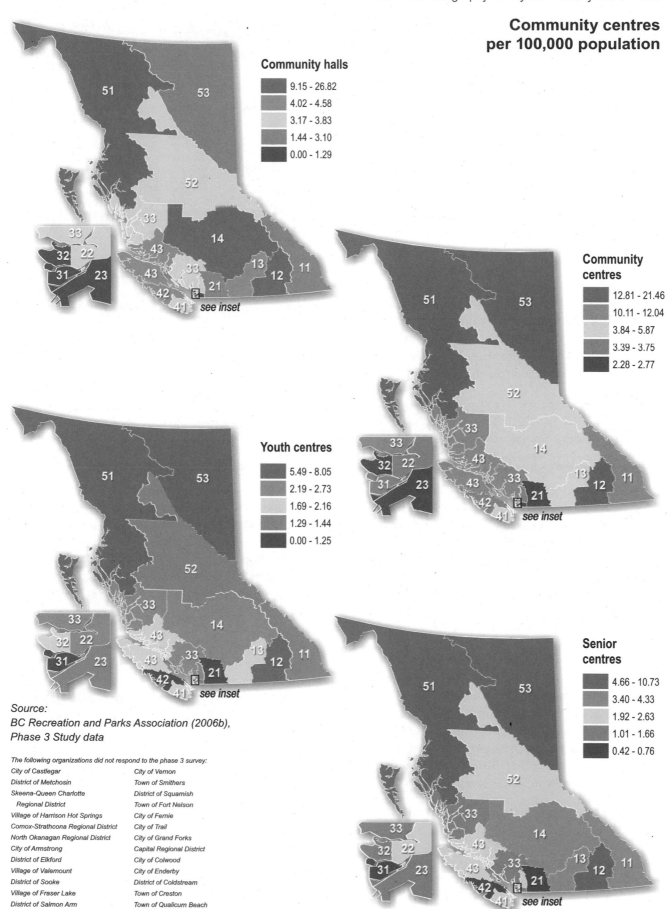

Community centres per 100,000 population

Community halls

	9.15 - 26.82
	4.02 - 4.58
	3.17 - 3.83
	1.44 - 3.10
	0.00 - 1.29

Community centres

	12.81 - 21.46
	10.11 - 12.04
	3.84 - 5.87
	3.39 - 3.75
	2.28 - 2.77

Youth centres

	5.49 - 8.05
	2.19 - 2.73
	1.69 - 2.16
	1.29 - 1.44
	0.00 - 1.25

Senior centres

	4.66 - 10.73
	3.40 - 4.33
	1.92 - 2.63
	1.01 - 1.66
	0.42 - 0.76

Source:
BC Recreation and Parks Association (2006b),
Phase 3 Study data

The following organizations did not respond to the phase 3 survey:

City of Castlegar	City of Vernon
District of Metchosin	Town of Smithers
Skeena-Queen Charlotte	District of Squamish
Regional District	Town of Fort Nelson
Village of Harrison Hot Springs	City of Fernie
Comox-Strathcona Regional District	City of Trail
North Okanagan Regional District	City of Grand Forks
City of Armstrong	Capital Regional District
District of Elkford	City of Colwood
Village of Valemount	City of Enderby
District of Sooke	District of Coldstream
Village of Fraser Lake	Town of Creston
District of Salmon Arm	Town of Qualicum Beach

Playing fields

A third key survey undertaken by the BC Recreation and Parks Association involved an inventory of the number of publicly owned or operated parks, natural areas, trails, and playing fields (BC Recreation and Parks Association, 2006a). Of the 185 local government organizations, 88% responded to the questionnaire. The data presented here again give rates of playing fields per 100,000 population. For those local government organizations responding, approximately 13,000 natural areas (112,000 hectares), 4,500 parks (65,000 hectares), 3,900 off-road trails (9,100 kms), and 3,600 playing fields were indentified. These are all major assets for health and wellness maintenance and improvement, and accessibility encourages use. (Due to space constraints, only a limited amount of this rich data base is presented here in map form, with a focus on playing fields.)

Health Service Delivery Area	Soccer pitches	Softball diamonds	Baseball diamonds	Football/ rugby fields
053 Northeast	51.22	55.88	40.36	6.21
031 Richmond	50.16	40.94	12.11	2.88
051 Northwest	43.51	36.71	9.52	1.36
022 Fraser North	42.67	37.34	21.87	3.20
033 North Shore/Coast Garibaldi	37.15	24.38	20.51	5.03
021 Fraser East	35.40	46.82	26.27	8.37
043 North Vancouver Island	33.53	53.18	15.03	17.34
023 Fraser South	30.33	19.54	11.73	1.88
013 Okanagan	28.25	27.09	16.64	2.71
052 Northern Interior	27.53	28.84	30.15	1.31
012 Kootenay Boundary	26.42	51.19	18.17	8.26
014 Thompson Cariboo Shuswap	22.51	39.65	14.68	3.92
011 East Kootenay	21.48	35.79	14.32	2.86
042 Central Vancouver Island	20.93	22.54	18.12	4.43
041 South Vancouver Island	18.12	14.56	18.44	1.94
032 Vancouver	12.81	12.47	10.79	2.02
999 Province	**29.37**	**28.05**	**17.25**	**3.56**

Soccer pitches

Nearly 1,200 soccer pitches were identified in the survey. Province-wide, there were 29.37 pitches per 100,000 population, varying from a high of over 50 per 100,000 in Northeast and in Richmond in the lower mainland to less than 20 per 100,000 in Vancouver and South Vancouver Island. There were no clear geographic trends, with both high and low rates in the urban southwest, while, with the exception of Northwest and Northeast, there were lower than average rates in much of the interior.

Softball diamonds

About 1,130 softball diamonds were identified, second only to soccer pitches in terms of numbers. Provincially, the rate was 28.05 per 100,000 population. Geographically, the highest rates were scattered around the province, with Northeast, North Vancouver Island, and Kootenay Boundary all having more than 50 pitches per 100,000 population. The lowest rates were found in the southwest part of the province, with Vancouver, South Vancouver Island, and Fraser South all having rates of less than 20 per 100,000 population.

Baseball diamonds

There were almost 700 baseball diamonds identified, for a provincial rate of 17.25 per 100,000 population. Northeast and Northern Interior had the highest rates,

both in excess of 30 per 100,000 population, while neighbouring Northwest, with less than 10 diamonds per 100,000 population, had the lowest rate. Low rates were also evident in parts of the lower mainland (Vancouver, Fraser South, and Richmond).

Football/rugby pitches

There were more than 140 football/rugby fields throughout the province (3.56 per 100,000 population). North Vancouver Island, with 17.34 fields per 100,000, had by far the highest rate, followed by Fraser East and Kootenay Boundary, both of which had less than half the rate of North Vancouver Island. The lowest rates were in the north of the province and in Fraser South in the lower mainland.

Provincially, soccer pitches and softball diamonds are much more common than any other sports fields. Of the four sets of sports fields presented here, Northeast is best served overall in terms of rates per capita. It should be noted, however, that this is one of the most rural of all HSDAs in the province. At the other extreme, Vancouver is not well-resourced with publicly owned and operated sports fields on a per capita basis.

Playing fields per 100,000 population

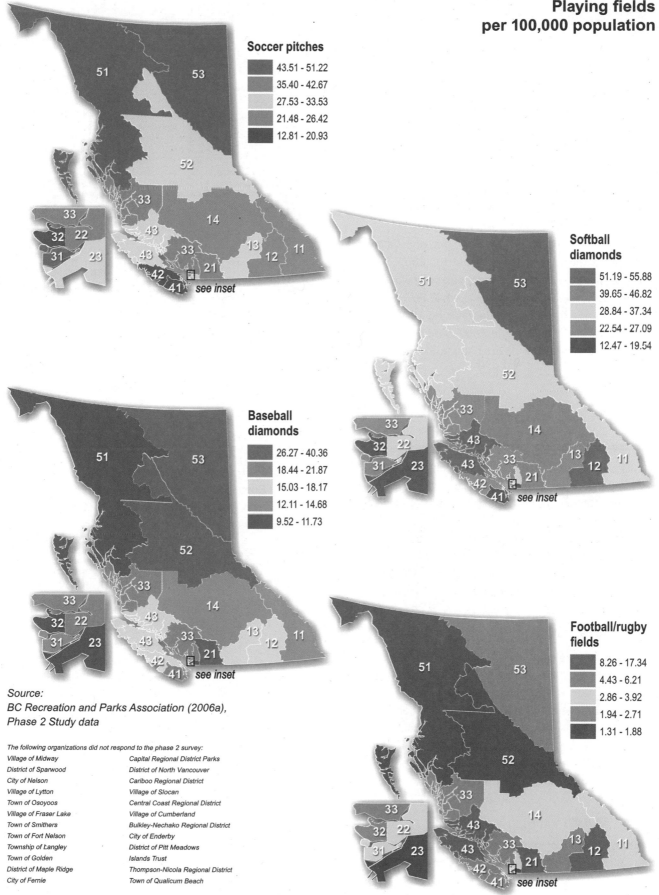

Soccer pitches

	43.51 - 51.22
	35.40 - 42.67
	27.53 - 33.53
	21.48 - 26.42
	12.81 - 20.93

Softball diamonds

	51.19 - 55.88
	39.65 - 46.82
	28.84 - 37.34
	22.54 - 27.09
	12.47 - 19.54

Baseball diamonds

	26.27 - 40.36
	18.44 - 21.87
	15.03 - 18.17
	12.11 - 14.68
	9.52 - 11.73

Football/rugby fields

	8.26 - 17.34
	4.43 - 6.21
	2.86 - 3.92
	1.94 - 2.71
	1.31 - 1.88

Source:
BC Recreation and Parks Association (2006a),
Phase 2 Study data

The following organizations did not respond to the phase 2 survey:

Village of Midway	Capital Regional District Parks
District of Sparwood	District of North Vancouver
City of Nelson	Cariboo Regional District
Village of Lytton	Village of Slocan
Town of Osoyoos	Central Coast Regional District
Village of Fraser Lake	Village of Cumberland
Town of Smithers	Bulkley-Nechako Regional District
Town of Fort Nelson	City of Enderby
Township of Langley	District of Pitt Meadows
Town of Golden	Islands Trust
District of Maple Ridge	Thompson-Nicola Regional District
City of Fernie	Town of Qualicum Beach

Playing fields

This second group of playing field assets are less numerous than those on the previous page, but nevertheless important from a physical activity perspective.

Running tracks

There were 95 running tracks in the province for an overall facility rate of 2.12 per 100,000 population. Tracks on a population rate basis were most numerous in Northwest (9.52 per 100,000 population) and North Vancouver Island (5.78 per 100,000). Rates were below average in the urban southwest of the province, except for Fraser North (3.56 per 100,000). Kootenay Boundary had no tracks recorded by the inventory, and South Vancouver Island had a rate of only 0.32 per 100,000 population.

Ultimate frisbee

This relatively new activity already had more fields per capita than more traditional sports such as field hockey or lacrosse. There were 1.84 per 100,000 population for the province as a whole. Fields for ultimate frisbee were most dominant in North Vancouver Island, with a rate of 10.40 per 100,000 population, and several lower mainland HSDAs also had rates above the provincial average. There were several HSDAs that recorded no fields for this sport from the municipalities responding to the questionnaire. These included South Vancouver Island, Richmond, Northeast, and Northern Interior.

Field hockey pitches

Provincially, there were 62 field hockey pitches, for a rate of 1.54 per 100,000 population. Rates were highest in North Shore/Coast Garibaldi and Kootenay Boundary, both with rates around 5 per 100,000 population or higher. The rates were lowest in the lower mainland and South Vancouver Island generally, although Northern Interior had none at all in those local governments responding to the questionnaire.

Lacrosse boxes

There was the same number of lacrosse boxes (62) as there were field hockey pitches, for a provincial rate of 1.54 per 100,000 population. Rates tended to be highest

Health Service Delivery Area	Running tracks	Ultimate frisbee	Field hockey pitches	Lacrosse boxes
051 Northwest	9.52	1.36	1.36	1.36
043 North Vancouver Island	5.78	10.40	1.16	2.31
052 Northern Interior	3.93	0.00	0.00	1.31
022 Fraser North	3.56	2.31	2.31	2.49
013 Okanagan	3.48	0.77	1.55	1.16
053 Northeast	3.10	0.00	3.10	0.00
014 Thompson Cariboo Shuswap	2.94	0.98	1.47	1.47
033 North Shore/Coast Garibaldi	1.93	1.55	5.80	1.93
021 Fraser East	1.90	0.76	0.38	0.38
042 Central Vancouver Island	1.61	2.01	1.21	2.82
011 East Kootenay	1.43	1.43	2.86	1.43
032 Vancouver	1.18	2.70	0.84	0.34
023 Fraser South	0.94	2.81	0.63	1.88
031 Richmond	0.58	0.00	2.31	1.73
041 South Vancouver Island	0.32	0.00	0.32	1.94
012 Kootenay Boundary	0.00	1.65	4.95	0.00
999 Province	**2.12**	**1.84**	**1.54**	**1.54**

in the lower mainland HSDAs (except Vancouver and Fraser East), as well as on Vancouver Island. Kootenay Boundary and Northeast had no lacrosse boxes in those local government organizations responding to the questionnaire.

There were major geographic variations in the sport field assets around the province. For this group of four sport field assets, North Vancouver Island was probably best served. Some caution is required in interpreting the rates, as only 88% of the local government organizations answered the questionnaire (see map on previous page).

Playing fields
per 100,000 population

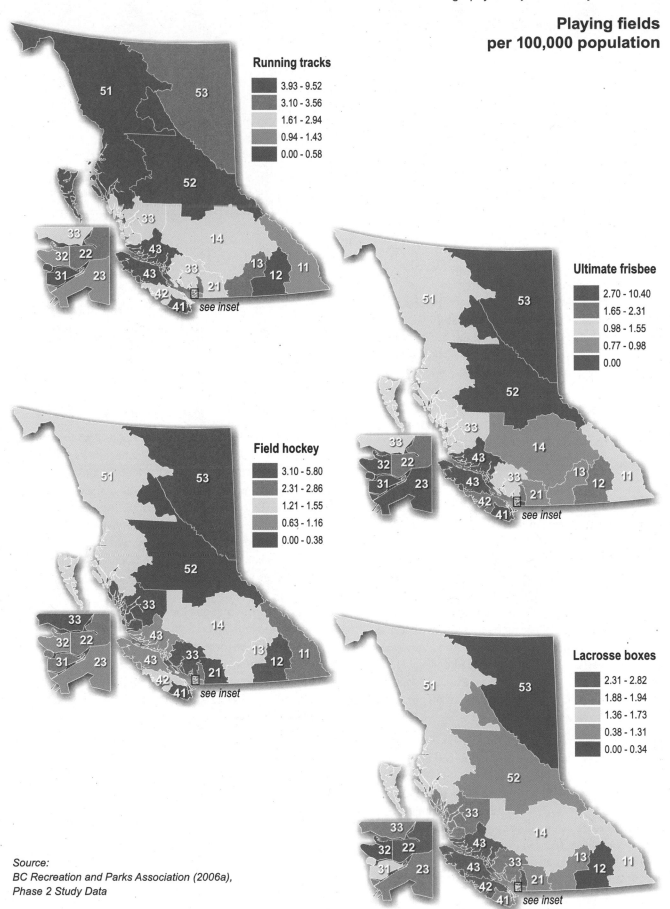

Running tracks

	3.93 - 9.52
	3.10 - 3.56
	1.61 - 2.94
	0.94 - 1.43
	0.00 - 0.58

Ultimate frisbee

	2.70 - 10.40
	1.65 - 2.31
	0.98 - 1.55
	0.77 - 0.98
	0.00

Field hockey

	3.10 - 5.80
	2.31 - 2.86
	1.21 - 1.55
	0.63 - 1.16
	0.00 - 0.38

Lacrosse boxes

	2.31 - 2.82
	1.88 - 1.94
	1.36 - 1.73
	0.38 - 1.31
	0.00 - 0.34

Source:
BC Recreation and Parks Association (2006a),
Phase 2 Study Data

Sports club membership

Sports BC has supplied participation rates in about 60 sports for which they provided funding support in 2005. The data are available geographically by eight distinct BC Games Zones that cover the province, and participation is also available by age group and by gender. It should be noted that participation by individuals can occur in more than one sporting activity. Also, sport membership rates are provided on the basis of club membership per 1,000 population between the ages of 4 and 74. Although not shown in the table, rates are included in the text for the following age groupings: 4 to 12 years (4 is an estimate of lower age limit for sport membership); 13 to 18 years; 19 to 34 years; and 35 to 74 years. The upper limit of 74 years may appear at first glance to be high for some of these sports, but increasingly there is a recognition that older adults participate in active, competitive sports, a trend that is forecast to increase over time (Turcotte and Schellenberg, 2007). Since there are only eight regions depicted, these maps are based on a high, medium, or low scale rather than a quintile scale.

Soccer

Overall, the membership rate of males up to age 74 in soccer was 33.31 per 1,000 population. Membership rates declined with age for the province as a whole, going from nearly 205 per 1,000 for those 4 to 12 years old to a rate of 1.59 per 1,000 for those aged 35 to 74. Geographically, the Thompson Okanagan and Vancouver Squamish zones had the highest rate overall, both over 37 per 1,000 population. Vancouver Squamish had consistently high rates for all age groups when compared to the provincial averages. Cariboo North East had the lowest at 20.88 per 1,000, and had relatively low rates for all age groups.

For females, the provincial membership rate of 23.69 per 1,000 was about 30% below the male rate. As with males, rates fell with age from 131.36 per 1,000 for those 4 to 12 years old to 0.14 per 1,000 for those aged 35 to 74. Only Vancouver Squamish had any registered players in the oldest age grouping. Thompson Okanagan and Fraser River Delta zones had the highest overall rates (both over 32 per 1,000), and Fraser Valley, at 18.26 per 1,000, had the lowest rate.

BC Games Zones	Soccer males	Soccer females	Golf males	Golf females
002 Thompson Okanagan	37.71	33.13	42.93	17.04
005 Vancouver Squamish	37.29	22.61	15.70	6.30
007 North West	36.91	27.10	23.50	8.33
004 Fraser River Delta	33.80	32.16	14.27	5.72
006 Vancouver Island Central Coast	32.55	20.86	32.38	10.87
003 Fraser Valley	31.86	18.26	11.37	3.86
001 Kootenays	27.44	20.49	60.79	25.23
008 Cariboo North East	20.88	22.81	29.14	10.92
999 Province	**33.31**	**23.69**	**23.29**	**8.72**

Golf

The membership rate for males was 23.39 per 1,000, with the highest rates in the 13 to 18 and 35 to 74 ages groups at 35.85 and 32.29 per 1,000 respectively. The lowest membership group was the 19- to 34-year-olds at 19.34 per 1,000, and there were no registered male golfers under the age of 12. Kootenays had the highest regional participation rate at 60.79 per 1,000, while Fraser Valley had the lowest rate at 11.37.

While the membership rates were not as high for women, there were age and regional similarities. Overall, the rate was 8.72 per 1,000, with the highest rate being the 35 to 74 age group at 15.16 per 1,000 and the lowest being the 19 to 34 age group at 3.66. As was the case for males, there were no registered female golfers under age 12. Geographically, Kootenays led the way with a participation rate of 25.23 per 1,000, and, similar to males, Fraser Valley was the lowest with 3.86.

For both soccer and golf there were quite high rates of club membership for both genders, but males were more likely to be involved than females. Unlike other sport membership, golf was well represented among the older age group. Thompson Okanagan had the highest membership rates for these sports combined, and Fraser Valley the lowest.

**Sports club membership
per 1,000 population**

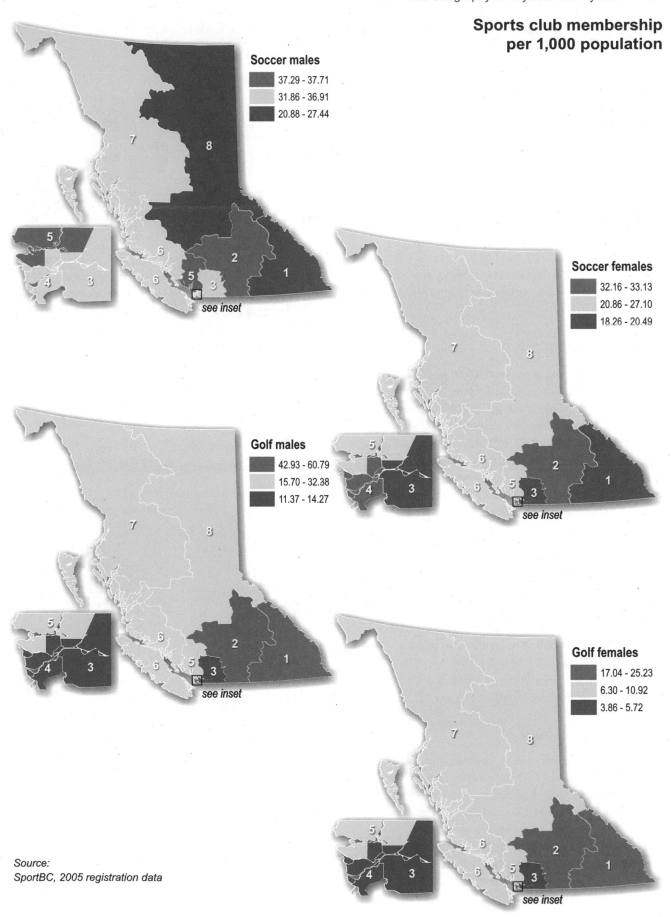

Soccer males

37.29 - 37.71
31.86 - 36.91
20.88 - 27.44

Soccer females

32.16 - 33.13
20.86 - 27.10
18.26 - 20.49

Golf males

42.93 - 60.79
15.70 - 32.38
11.37 - 14.27

Golf females

17.04 - 25.23
6.30 - 10.92
3.86 - 5.72

see inset

*Source:
SportBC, 2005 registration data*

Sports club membership

Baseball (males)

Only male membership rates are included here because significantly more males participated in baseball than females (the rate for males was 19.41 per 1,000, compared with only 1.48 for females). The highest rate was in the 4 to 12 age group at 147.31 per 1,000, while the 19 to 34 age group had a rate of 4.99. There were no members registered in the 35 to 74 age group. Kootenays boasted the highest rates at 29.03 per 1,000, but rates were reasonably distributed in other regions. The lowest membership region was North West at 7.23 per 1,000.

Softball (females)

The provincial female membership rate was 11.38 per 1,000 (compared to only 3.52 for males), with the highest rates being in the 4 to 12 age group at 62.09 per 1,000 and 13- to 19-year-olds at 59.25, and the lowest rate being those over 35 at 0.07 per 1,000. Geographically, females were active in softball relatively consistently across the province. Fraser Valley was most active for females with a rate of 15.63 per 1,000, and Vancouver Squamish was the least active at 6.46.

Hockey (males)

The overall membership rate for males in hockey was 18.11 per 1,000 (compared with only 2.88 for females), with the most active age group being the 4- to 12-year-olds at 111.51. The least active group was the over 35 group at 0.47 per 1,000. The most active regions were Cariboo North East at 35.73 and Kootenays at 31.17 per 1,000, in the interior of the province, while the least active region was Fraser Valley at 9.15 per 1,000.

Figure skating (females)

Figure skating was very much a female sport, with a membership of 7.15 per 1,000 females. By age, the 4- to 12-year-old group had the highest rate (76.73 per 1,000). Geographically, the sport was very prominent in the North West region with a rate over all age groups of 28.99 per 1,000 female population. Kootenays and Thompson Okanagan had rates in excess of 10 per 1,000. The lowest rate (3.53 per 1,000) was found in Fraser River Delta.

BC Games Zones	Baseball males	Softball females	Hockey males	Figure skating females
001 Kootenays	29.03	9.06	31.17	13.86
006 Vancouver Island Central Coast	23.52	13.21	18.43	6.29
004 Fraser River Delta	21.88	13.24	20.15	3.53
003 Fraser Valley	21.63	15.63	9.15	5.88
002 Thompson Okanagan	17.58	8.17	23.54	10.77
008 Cariboo North East	13.86	8.38	35.73	7.44
005 Vancouver Squamish	13.81	6.46	15.50	5.60
007 North West	7.23	9.16	30.52	28.99
999 Province	**19.41**	**11.38**	**18.11**	**7.15**

Membership in the clubs described in this section shows how males and females dominate different sports. Even for those presented here, males were much more likely to be involved in club membership than were females. Among these four sports, Kootenays had the highest overall membership rate, and Vancouver Squamish had the lowest.

Sports club membership per 1,000 population

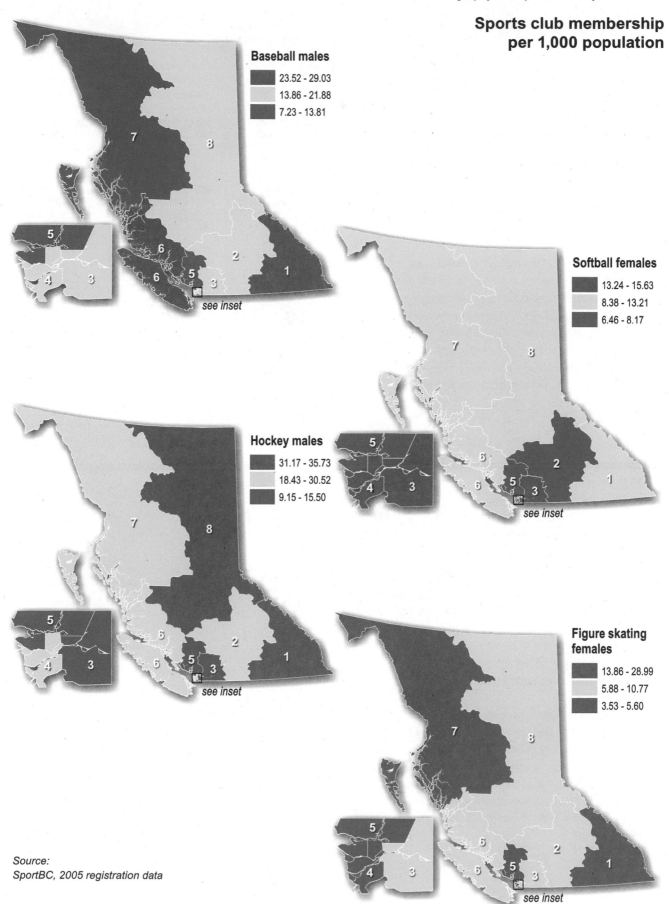

Baseball males

- 23.52 - 29.03
- 13.86 - 21.88
- 7.23 - 13.81

Softball females

- 13.24 - 15.63
- 8.38 - 13.21
- 6.46 - 8.17

Hockey males

- 31.17 - 35.73
- 18.43 - 30.52
- 9.15 - 15.50

Figure skating females

- 13.86 - 28.99
- 5.88 - 10.77
- 3.53 - 5.60

Source:
SportBC, 2005 registration data

Sports club membership

Athletics

The male membership for athletics (track and field) had a rate of 14.64 per 1,000, with the highest rate age group being 13- to 18-year-olds at 107.88 per 1,000 and the lowest being 19- to 34-year-olds at 0.47, closely followed by 35- to 74-year-olds at 0.91 per 1,000. Cariboo North East had the highest participation rates for males at 88.18 per 1,000, while Kootenays had the lowest at 0.28.

The athletics membership rate for females was slightly higher than that for males at 15.36 per 1,000, with the highest rate being for the 13 to 18 age group at 98.79. The age group with the lowest membership rate was 19- to 34-year-olds at 0.47 per 1,000, followed by 35- to 74-year-olds at 0.63. The most active region for females was Cariboo North East at 100.19 per 1,000, and Kootenays was the least active region at 0.25.

Curling

The membership rate for males in curling clubs was 7.77 per 1,000 provincially, with the most active group being the 35 to 74 age group at 12.15 per 1,000 and the least active being the 4- to 12-year-olds at 0.74. Kootenays had the most active membership rate at 23.30 per 1,000, while Vancouver Squamish was the least active at 3.07.

At 5.20 per 1,000, the overall membership rate for females was somewhat lower than that for males. As was the case for males, the 35 to 74 age group was most active for females at 8.11 per 1,000. The least active group was also the same for females as for males at 0.58 per 1,000 for the 4- to 12-year-olds. Again, Kootenays was most active (15.38 per 1,000), while Fraser River Delta was least active (2.72 per 1,000).

Both athletics and curling had some balance in club membership among the genders. Athletics had marginally more female members than males, but the opposite was true for curling. The latter had a larger membership among the older population than younger age groups. Among these two sports, Thompson Okanagan had the highest membership rate and Fraser Valley the lowest.

BC Games Zones		Athletics males	Athletics females	Curling males	Curling females
008	Cariboo North East	88.18	100.19	5.75	4.79
002	Thompson Okanagan	32.98	34.35	15.16	9.72
006	Vancouver Island Central Coast	17.01	17.37	10.31	6.54
005	Vancouver Squamish	9.38	9.61	3.07	3.23
004	Fraser River Delta	2.47	2.58	5.40	2.72
003	Fraser Valley	1.60	1.40	5.18	3.10
007	North West	0.33	1.05	11.01	9.38
001	Kootenays	0.28	0.25	23.30	15.38
999	**Province**	**14.64**	**15.36**	**7.77**	**5.20**

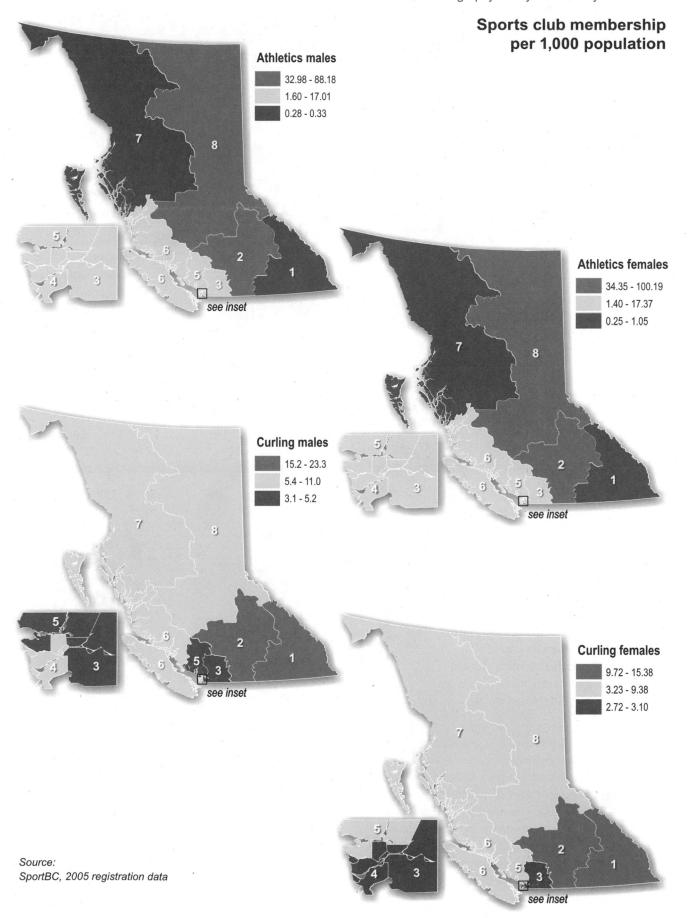

**Sports club membership
per 1,000 population**

Athletics males

32.98 - 88.18
1.60 - 17.01
0.28 - 0.33

see inset

Athletics females

34.35 - 100.19
1.40 - 17.37
0.25 - 1.05

see inset

Curling males

15.2 - 23.3
5.4 - 11.0
3.1 - 5.2

see inset

Curling females

9.72 - 15.38
3.23 - 9.38
2.72 - 3.10

see inset

*Source:
SportBC, 2005 registration data*

Provincial and national parks

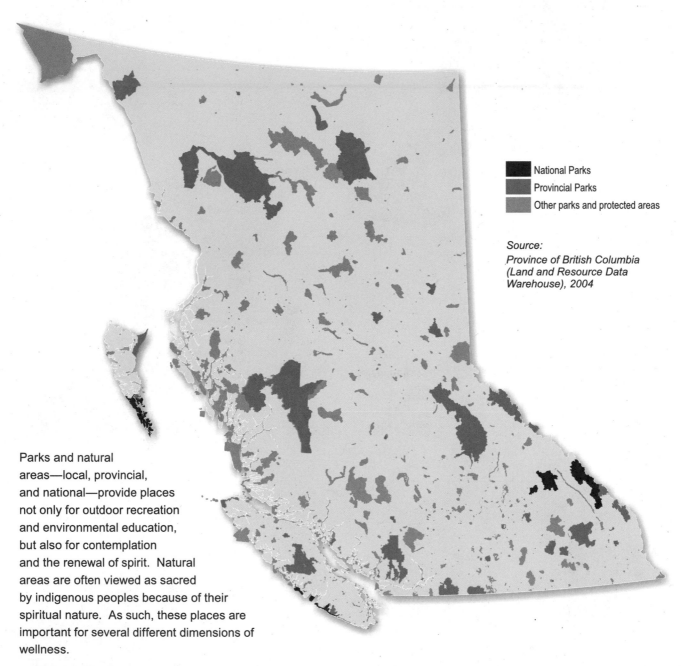

National Parks
Provincial Parks
Other parks and protected areas

Source:
Province of British Columbia
(Land and Resource Data
Warehouse), 2004

Parks and natural areas—local, provincial, and national—provide places not only for outdoor recreation and environmental education, but also for contemplation and the renewal of spirit. Natural areas are often viewed as sacred by indigenous peoples because of their spiritual nature. As such, these places are important for several different dimensions of wellness.

As of July 2006, BC had over 850 provincial parks and protected areas scattered around the province (see map, which shows the larger of these in light green). In total, they cover more than 13 million hectares, or nearly 14% of the total land mass of the province. Many are small and readily accessible to the urban population in the lower mainland and south and eastern Vancouver Island. However, the majority of the larger parks are less accessible, which is part of their spiritual and recreational attraction.

BC also has seven national parks (shown in dark green), some of which straddle the border with Alberta. These larger parks are less accessible than most provincial parks, but nevertheless provide spiritual and recreational wellness assets.

Summary

Increasing physical activity among the BC population is one of the key pillars of ActNow BC. This section of the Atlas has provided a diversity of wellness indicators related to this pillar which have been mapped in a variety of formats. Assets have included programs developed specifically to support ActNow BC initiatives by some of its key partners, such as 2010 Legacies Now, BC Recreation and Parks Association, and other partners from the BC Healthy Living Alliance. Other indicators are included from questions in the CCHS related to walking and physical activity. Still others look at the distribution of walking clubs and the use of public transit. There are several indicators related to activity assets that have been collected through questionnaire surveys, as well as data from SportsBC on sport club membership.

A key program, Action Schools! BC, is being used in every school district to get children more active. It has been adopted by more than 70% of all schools teaching kindergarten to Grade 7, as well as some with higher grades. There are still opportunities for greater adoption of the initiative by some school districts and by Aboriginal schools and independent schools. Active Communities is another key program to support ActNow BC, and in a very short time period, local government areas that are home to approximately 89% of the province's population have become Active Communities. There is still room for improvement, especially in the Northern Interior and other interior regions of the province.

BC respondents to the CCHS are more active in terms of leisure time pursuits and in daily living than their Canadian counterparts as a whole. However, even with this good news, only about 60% indicate that they are active enough to gain health benefits, and less than one-quarter of BC respondents walked for six or more hours a week in everyday chores or going to work/ school. The number of both teens and seniors who walk is low.

Walking clubs supported by the Heart and Stroke Foundation are scattered throughout the province, although many are located in the urban southwest corner. Further, public transit serves about 80% of the population, but it is only well used in the Greater Vancouver Regional District, and the Capital Regional District on Vancouver Island. People who use public transit rather than a car are more likely to walk and have healthier weights. There are very low rates of transit use in the north and interior parts of the province.

Publicly owned and/or operated recreational assets (pools, ice rinks, community activity centres) tend to be much more common outside of the urbanized lower mainland. The highest number on a per capita basis tend to be in the less densely populated rural areas of the interior in the southeast of the province. Because of low population densities in these regions, accessibility may be a barrier to use, while in the urban areas of the southwest part of the province private facilities may be more common.

Membership in sports organizations also varies substantially throughout the province, and also between genders and among different age groups. Generally, males have higher membership rates, but not always. Figure skating and athletics are higher for females. Most sport membership drops off with age, but not for golf and curling.

BC has a large number of provincial parks and protected areas, and while many are relatively remote, they can nevertheless provide spiritual assets for wellness when used.

Several of these indicators are novel, but most of them indicate that there are major geographical variations throughout the province in terms of wellness assets, whether they be physical assets or behavioural assets, and suggest that there is room for improvement.

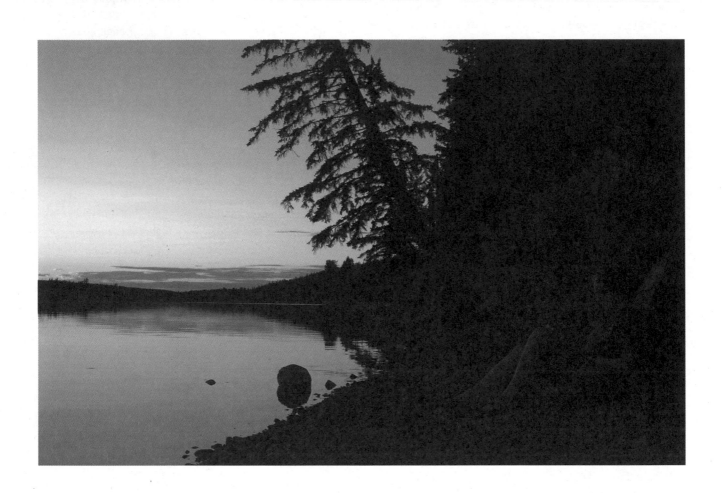

5.5 The Geography of Healthy Weight in BC

Healthy weight is an important wellness asset. A person's weight depends on nutrition and food security issues as well as physical activity, as discussed in the two previous sections of this Atlas.

There are many health problems and risks associated with being either underweight or overweight. Being underweight may be an indication of an underlying illness or an eating disorder. It may also cause osteoporosis and infertility. Being overweight or obese has several health risks, including Type 2 diabetes, hypertension, cardiovascular disease, some types of cancer, osteoarthritis, gallbladder disease, functional limitations, and impaired fertility, among others (Health Canada, 2003; Canadian Institute for Health Information, 2004, 2006a).

While there are several different measures utilized to assess healthy body weight, body mass index (BMI), which gives a value based on kilograms per metre squared (weight and height), is widely used internationally for assessing health risk. Any person with a BMI lower than 25 but higher than 18.5 is considered to have a "healthy body mass index" (Health Canada, 2003). Values lower than 18.5 are considered underweight, 25 to 29.9 is considered overweight, and those with a BMI in excess of 30 are considered obese.

In 1978-1979, the Canada Health Survey directly measured respondents' height and weight. After adjusting for age, this survey found that 50.8% of Canadians had a healthy measured BMI (i.e., BMI between 18.5 and 24.9). The CCHS conducted in 2004 (and also utilizing direct measures of height and weight) found that the age-adjusted rate of healthy BMI had decreased to 40.9%. The 2004 CCHS demonstrated clear gender differences, as 35% of males compared to 46.4% of females had healthy age-adjusted measured BMI. Healthy measured BMIs were highest for young adults (about 60%), but decreased steadily so that only about one-quarter of the population had healthy BMIs by age 75. After age 75, the healthy BMI rate increased somewhat (Tjepkema, 2006). Rates of healthy BMI have been decreasing in Canada since at least as far back as the early 1950s, with a more rapid rate of decline occurring over the past 15 years (Katzmarzyk, 2002).

Using the 2004 CCHS, Shields and Tjepkema (2006) investigated regional differences in healthy measured BMI. The province with the highest proportion of their population having a healthy BMI was Quebec (43.7%, followed closely by BC), and the province with the lowest proportion was Nowfoundland/Labrador (29%). Within all provinces, according to the Canadian Institute for Health Information (2006a), the rate of healthy BMI is higher in urban areas and lower in northern and remote rural regions. A recent 2006 telephone survey of 8,000 respondents in BC showed that, overall, 46% of respondents had a normal weight (BMI between 18.5 and 24.9), but the areas with the healthiest weights were in the lower mainland urban communities (Burnaby with 56%, Coquitlam with 57%, and Delta with 53% in the normal range for BMI) (Discovery Research, 2006).

While self-reports of height and weight are a less reliable basis for calculations of BMI than directly measured height and weight (there is a tendency to overestimate height and underestimate weight in self-reports; see Kendall, 2006), they can fairly reliably be used to estimate the regional, age, and gender variability in healthy BMI at a specific time.

Two questions were used from the CCHS to assess key weight and related wellness assets. The first question, *"Do you consider yourself overweight, underweight, or just about right?"* assessed individual's feelings about their own body weight. It is important in relation to the second question, which asked respondents (excluding pregnant women) their weight and height. Responses to this question were used to calculate the body mass index (BMI) for each respondent aged 18 years or older. For younger individuals, the 2003 McCreary Adolescent Health Survey data were used.

Weight is perceived to be just about right

Provincially, an average of 54.27% of respondents over the age of 12 felt that their weight was about right. (For Aboriginal respondents, the average was 53.28%). The top map opposite indicates a rough gradient, with the proportion of respondents feeling that their weight was just right being generally higher in the urban southwest and rural coastal regions compared to the interior and the north. For example, a low of 44.56% of respondents in the Northeast felt that their weight was just right compared to a high of 59.38% in Fraser North. As well, Vancouver and Fraser North had a significantly higher than average proportion of respondents who felt their weight was just right, while Central Vancouver Island, Northern Interior, Fraser East, and Northeast regions all had rates significantly lower than the provincial average.

The second two maps show the patterns for males and females separately. They illustrate that, in all regions (except Vancouver), a higher proportion of males than females were likely to feel that their weight was just right. These gender differences were statistically significant at the provincial level, and for 6 of the 16 regions (Fraser North, Fraser South, North Shore/Coast Garibaldi, East Kootenay, South Vancouver Island, and Thompson Cariboo Shuswap). The greatest gender difference was found in East Kootenay, where 60.23% of men compared with 46.24% of women felt their weight was about right. In general, the variation in responses to this question was greater across regions for females than for males.

As shown in the bottom two maps and the above table, on average, 72.43% of youths felt that their weight was about right, compared to 52.09% of 20- to 64-year-olds and 50.56% of seniors. Differences in the proportion of 12- to 19-year-olds who felt that their weight was just right were higher (and statistically significant) compared to 20- to 64-year-olds in all but three regions of the province. Geographically, Fraser East and Northeast had significantly lower values than the provincial average for males, while for females, Vancouver was significantly higher and Northern Interior was significantly lower than the provincial average.

When considering trends across regions of the province but within the two age groups 12 to 19 and 65 and over, there is very little variation in the proportion of respondents who felt that their weight was about right, although Kootenay Boundary was significantly higher than the average for teens. However, for 20- to 64-year-olds there were relatively large regional differences. For example, Northeast, Fraser East, and Northern Interior all had significantly low values for this age group, while Fraser North and Vancouver had significantly high values compared to the provincial average for this age group.

Health Service Delivery Area	All respondents (%)	Males (%)	Females (%)	Ages 12-19 (%)	Ages 20-64 (%)	Ages 65+ (%)
022 Fraser North	59.38	63.91†	54.97†	69.40	58.54	55.44
032 Vancouver	58.47	58.18	58.76	67.73	57.66	57.49
012 Kootenay Boundary	58.39	65.18	51.58	86.54‡	53.85	56.65
033 North Shore/Coast Garibaldi	57.87	64.09†	51.95†	81.94‡	56.42	47.38
043 North Vancouver Island	56.62	60.49	52.79	64.65	56.35	50.87
023 Fraser South	54.16	59.50†	48.93†	76.50‡	50.59	51.73
011 East Kootenay	53.32	60.23†	46.24†	83.62‡	49.05	47.38
013 Okanagan	53.22	56.10	50.50	69.68‡	50.02	53.95
041 South Vancouver Island	52.88	59.37†	47.02†	73.44‡	51.77	45.27
014 Thompson Cariboo Shuswap	52.39	58.26†	46.55†	68.87‡	50.21	48.71
031 Richmond	50.96	52.17	49.83	73.92‡	48.94	45.14
051 Northwest	48.71	54.31	42.65	72.49‡	44.65	41.89
042 Central Vancouver Island	48.58	50.86	46.38	72.41‡	46.13	42.20
052 Northern Interior	47.82	53.72	41.60	70.69‡	42.64	52.65
021 Fraser East	47.71	50.87	44.62	69.56‡	43.34	47.18
053 Northeast	44.56	46.50	42.48	66.52‡	40.20	42.42
999 Province	54.27	58.17†	50.48†	72.43‡	52.09	50.56

‡ Age group differs significantly from 20-64 group.
† Males differ significantly from females.

Weight is perceived to be just about right

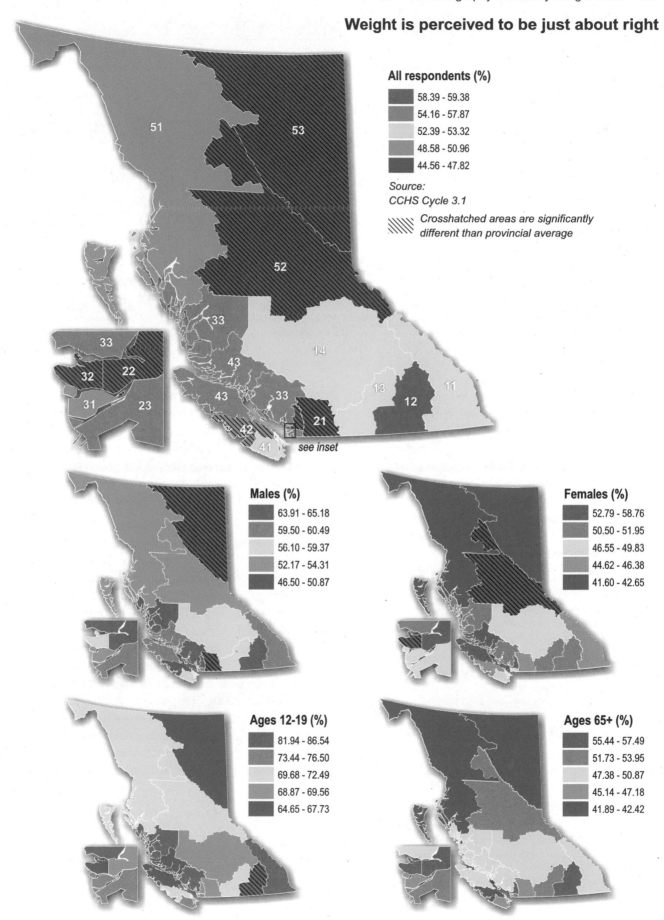

All respondents (%)

- 58.39 - 59.38
- 54.16 - 57.87
- 52.39 - 53.32
- 48.58 - 50.96
- 44.56 - 47.82

Source:
CCHS Cycle 3.1

Crosshatched areas are significantly different than provincial average

Males (%)

- 63.91 - 65.18
- 59.50 - 60.49
- 56.10 - 59.37
- 52.17 - 54.31
- 46.50 - 50.87

Females (%)

- 52.79 - 58.76
- 50.50 - 51.95
- 46.55 - 49.83
- 44.62 - 46.38
- 41.60 - 42.65

Ages 12-19 (%)

- 81.94 - 86.54
- 73.44 - 76.50
- 69.68 - 72.49
- 68.87 - 69.56
- 64.65 - 67.73

Ages 65+ (%)

- 55.44 - 57.49
- 51.73 - 53.95
- 47.38 - 50.87
- 45.14 - 47.18
- 41.89 - 42.42

Healthy body mass index based on self-reported height and weight

The following maps and tables are based on the CCHS except the map pertaining to youths aged 12 to 19. Because BMI calculations are complex for children and teens, the CCHS did not calculate a BMI for those under age 18. We substituted data from the 2003 McCreary Adolescent Health Survey for the map pertaining to the 12 to 19 age group (Grades 7 to 12) as it used a more accepted method for calculating BMI in young people (Cole, Bellizzi, Fliegal, and Dietz, 2000).

Health Service Delivery Area	All respondents (%)	Males (%)	Females (%)	Ages 12-19 (%)	Ages 20-64 (%)	Ages 65+ (%)
032 Vancouver	59.38	54.27†	64.51†	79.16‡	60.35	55.31
031 Richmond	56.09	50.20	61.64	77.99‡	55.60	52.49
033 North Shore/Coast Garibaldi	55.61	51.01	59.97	80.98‡	57.51	44.89‡
022 Fraser North	55.19	50.36	59.98	77.02‡	55.11	56.67
012 Kootenay Boundary	52.75	47.52	57.94	79.53‡	51.86	47.41
011 East Kootenay	48.45	43.49	53.62	78.40‡	50.10	37.77
023 Fraser South	48.36	39.57†	57.11†	F	48.28	45.75
013 Okanagan	47.50	38.69†	55.76†	80.66‡	47.68	44.56
043 North Vancouver Island	47.31	41.25	53.40	78.10‡	48.43	39.11
041 South Vancouver Island	47.01	46.02	47.91	78.96‡	46.67	46.13
042 Central Vancouver Island	44.32	37.59†	50.81†	76.76‡	45.10	35.70
052 Northern Interior	43.57	39.28	48.07	73.22‡	43.80	33.29E
014 Thompson Cariboo Shuswap	40.30	35.43	45.16	78.53‡	38.91	42.71
021 Fraser East	39.94	35.12	44.66	F	37.89	44.24
051 Northwest	39.86	39.70	40.05	80.72‡	38.53	33.55E
053 Northeast	36.62	33.40	40.17	F	35.72	35.41E
999 Province	**49.96**	**44.43†**	**55.39†**	**78.35‡**	**50.14**	**46.46‡**

‡ Age group differs significantly from 20-64 group
† Males differ significantly from females
E Interpret data with caution (16.77< coefficient of variation <33.3)
F Data not available

Based on self-reports of weight and height rather than direct measures, approximately half of all respondents in BC over the age of 18 had a healthy self-reported BMI. For Aboriginal respondents, however, only 41.74% had a self-reported healthy weight, although the difference was not statistically significant. When compared to the Canadian population as a whole, BC had a significantly higher percentage of respondents with a healthy BMI (49.96% compared to 46.18%). There is a gradient with the lowest proportion of respondents with healthy BMI generally in the northern and interior regions of the province and the highest proportion in the lower mainland. The range between the highest and lowest was more than 20 percentage points. Vancouver, Richmond, North Shore/Coast Garibaldi, and Fraser North (all over 55% with a healthy BMI) were significantly higher than the provincial average. Central Vancouver Island, Thompson Cariboo Shuswap, Fraser East, Northwest, and Northeast were all significantly lower.

For females, the proportion with healthy BMI is highest in Vancouver and Richmond and lowest in Fraser East and in the north and interior regions of the province. Geographically for males, Vancouver was significantly high and Thompson Cariboo Shuswap and Fraser East were significantly low when compared to the provincial average. For females, Vancouver was significantly high while South Vancouver Island, Thompson Cariboo Shuswap, Fraser East, Northwest, and Northeast were all significantly lower than the provincial average.

On average, 55.39% of females reported healthy BMIs compared to 44.43% of males. This difference was statistically significant. In all regions, a higher proportion of females reported healthy BMIs compared to males. These differences were statistically significant for 4 of the 16 regions (Vancouver, Fraser South, Okanagan, and Central Vancouver Island). The greatest difference was found in Fraser South, where 57.11% of women compared to 39.57% of men reported healthy BMIs.

For 12- to 19-year-olds, based on the 2003 McCreary Society survey, there was very little difference in the proportion of teens with healthy BMI across the regions, except for the Northern Interior, where only 73.22% of respondents had a healthy BMI. The difference from the provincial average (78.35%) for this age group was statistically significant. For the middle age cohort, the story is different. Among 20- to 64-year-olds, a high of 60.35% of respondents in Vancouver reported healthy BMIs compared to a low of 35.72% in the Northeast. Although the pattern of regional differences among seniors was similar to 20- to 64-year-olds, the magnitude of differences across regions was not as marked. Only Central Vancouver Island had a significantly different value (35.70%) from the average for seniors.

Healthy body mass index based on self-reported height and weight

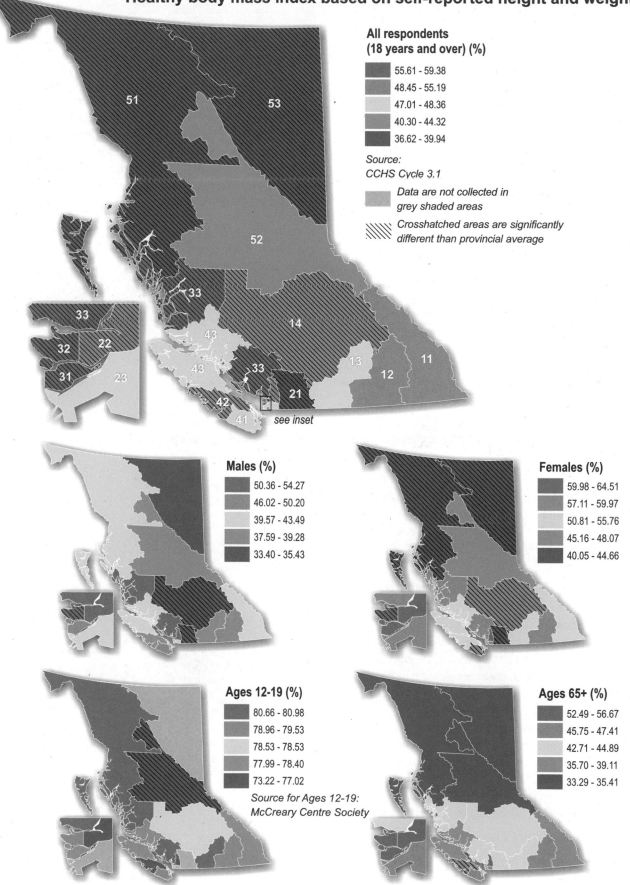

**All respondents
(18 years and over) (%)**

- 55.61 - 59.38
- 48.45 - 55.19
- 47.01 - 48.36
- 40.30 - 44.32
- 36.62 - 39.94

*Source:
CCHS Cycle 3.1*

*Data are not collected in
grey shaded areas*

*Crosshatched areas are significantly
different than provincial average*

Males (%)

- 50.36 - 54.27
- 46.02 - 50.20
- 39.57 - 43.49
- 37.59 - 39.28
- 33.40 - 35.43

Females (%)

- 59.98 - 64.51
- 57.11 - 59.97
- 50.81 - 55.76
- 45.16 - 48.07
- 40.05 - 44.66

Ages 12-19 (%)

- 80.66 - 80.98
- 78.96 - 79.53
- 78.53 - 78.53
- 77.99 - 78.40
- 73.22 - 77.02

*Source for Ages 12-19:
McCreary Centre Society*

Ages 65+ (%)

- 52.49 - 56.67
- 45.75 - 47.41
- 42.71 - 44.89
- 35.70 - 39.11
- 33.29 - 35.41

Summary

The proportion of the population that felt their weight was about right tended to be lower in rural than in urban regions. As well, three-quarters of youth felt their weight was about right compared to about half of those aged 20 and over. Across all but one region (Vancouver), a higher proportion of males felt their weight was about right compared to females. Finally, regional differences were quite marked for 20- to 64-year-olds but not for teens or seniors.

There was a rough urban/rural gradient for self-reported healthy BMI in BC, and a greater proportion in mainly urban regions had a healthy BMI. There was little regional variation in self-reported BMI among youth. The proportion of females reporting a healthy BMI in all regions of BC was, on average, about 10% greater than for males. These results, in conjunction with results from a recent study on rural health (Canadian Institute for Health Information, 2006), indicate that attention must be paid to the diets of populations living in the north and in rural and remote regions of BC.

According to BC's Select Standing Committee on Health (2006), obesity is a problem that we can no longer ignore. While this committee focused on childhood obesity, our maps indicate that obesity and being overweight may be a larger problem among older adults, particularly seniors. (Because a different data set was used for the youth analysis, extreme caution is required when interpreting differences between that age group and others.)

Committee members reporting on problems of childhood obesity have recommended that the broad framework brought to bear in developing this map also be utilized to develop a coherent policy response to problems of obesity in the province. In particular, the committee recommends an extremely broad policy thrust including: expanded data gathering and monitoring; improving food security through broad initiatives, such as improved promotion and marketing of BC vegetables and fruit, and through school-based programs aimed at increasing the availability of healthy foods in schools; a diabetes action plan; expanded ActNow BC initiatives; and improved promotion of breastfeeding and other early childhood initiatives (Select Standing Committee on Health, 2006).

More recently, Canada's House of Commons Standing Committee on Health (2007) has also expressed concern about the levels of childhood overweight and obesity:

26% of Canadians aged 2 to 17 years are overweight or obese, while for First Nations children, 55% on-reserve and 41% off-reserve are overweight or obese. The Committee has noted that many experts have predicted that "today's children will be the first generation for some time to have poorer health outcomes and a shorter life expectancy than their parents" (p. 1).

One of the key pillars of ActNow BC involves promoting healthy pregnancies, especially with respect to ensuring that mothers refrain from drinking alcohol during pregnancy.

Alcohol consumption during pregnancy acts as a toxic substance that can damage the brain and central nervous system cells in the developing fetus. The damage to the fetus is permanent, and children born with fetal alcohol spectrum disorder (FASD) have speech and vision impairment, learning problems, generally a poor memory, attention deficit disorder and hyperactivity, and overall poor conditions and prospects for healthy development into adulthood (Health Canada, 2001).

Fetal brain development occurs throughout pregnancy. Alcohol affects the ability of the brain to organize and communicate information. An important challenge for the individual with FASD is that emotions and consequences of decisions are often not well understood (Ministry of Health, 2005). Some children with FASD have no outward symptoms. Others have distinct physical facial features, such as shortened eye slits, flattened mid face, a flattened midline ridge between nose and lip, as well as a thin upper lip.

There does not appear to be any known safe amount of alcohol that can be consumed during pregnancy. The lifetime costs for those with FASD have been estimated in the order of $1.5 million. Individuals with FASD require a lot of nurturing, understanding, and community supports, as well as a stable home environment, and responsive school supports. Diagnosing this condition at birth is not always easy, and it may be several years before a diagnosis can be made.

The reader is cautioned that data with respect to FASD are very incomplete and, therefore, it is difficult to map it accurately for the whole province for the purposes of this Atlas. While sample responses were very small, the CCHS showed that approximately 84% of women aged 15 to 54 in BC answering the question about drinking during pregnancy indicated that they did not drink during their last pregnancy. However, only 79% of those aged 35 to 54 indicated that they did not drink during their last pregnancy.

Healthy pregnancy, healthy birth, and healthy mothers-to-be and new mothers are all important wellness indicators,

and there are a series of other key indicators that can be used to measure these components. There is much research to show the very important relationship of healthy beginnings for healthy child development and moving into healthy adulthood. Having a good start is an important asset for future wellness, and an important determinant of health and wellness.

A total of 11 maps are provided to measure healthy pregnancy, childbirth, and motherhood. The first two look at the rates of alcohol-free and smoking-free pregnancies. The following three show babies born without perinatal or maternal complications, and without congenital anomalies.

The next set of three maps looks at the percentage of mothers who have babies in the healthiest age period of their life for having children, those children with the healthiest birth weight, and those babies who are born at full term. These are all important wellness indicators.

The following two maps show babies born with the healthiest conditions, and infant survival rates.

Finally, a map showing the location of Pregnancy Outreach Programs is provided. These programs help pregnant women who are at risk of poor birthing outcomes. As such, they are an important community asset for women without established prenatal care.

There are some cautions and caveats with respect to the Vital Statistics data used for the majority of maps. With respect to perinatal and maternal complications, there is not always complete documentation on the Physician Notice of Birth record. Second, the data only cover births occurring in BC to BC mothers. Caution, therefore, is required in analysing the maps, as some complicated births to BC mothers take place in neighbouring Alberta, especially for those living in East Kootenay, and to a lesser extent in the Northeast.

Did not drink alcohol during last pregnancy

Health Canada has estimated that approximately 9 of every 1,000 infants are born with FASD annually (Ministry of Children and Family Development, 2006) as a result of alcohol consumption by expectant mothers. FASD is a national problem, but the rates in some First Nations and Inuit communities are much higher than the national average. These rates exist "within the context of the history of colonization and devaluation endured by First Nations and Inuit, which has resulted in a loss of culture" (Health Canada, 2001, p. 1). The prevalence of FASD in high-risk groups like Aboriginal peoples may be as high as 20% (Brynelsen, Conry, and Loock, 1998; Tait, 2003).

For BC as a whole, those women between the ages of 15 and 54 who answered negatively to the CCHS question about consuming alcohol during their last pregnancy represented 83.59% of respondents. A lower percentage of older women (aged 35-54) answered negatively (79.00%). Not all HSDAs can be mapped because of low numbers responding to the question. The range among HSDAs is more than 30 percentage points, indicating large variations between regions of the province for which data are available. Four HSDAs, Northwest, Thompson Cariboo Shuswap, Northern Interior, and Fraser East, all had alcohol-free pregnancies greater than 90%. The first two had significantly higher rates, statistically, than the provincial average. Okanagan in the interior, North Shore/Coast Garibaldi in the lower mainland, and South Vancouver Island all had values less than 80%.

Health Service Delivery Area	Females ages 15-54 (%)
051 Northwest	97.84
014 Thompson Cariboo Shuswap	95.06
052 Northern Interior	91.16
021 Fraser East	90.84
023 Fraser South	87.48
032 Vancouver	85.97
042 Central Vancouver Island	83.17
022 Fraser North	82.13
041 South Vancouver Island	76.17
033 North Shore/Coast Garibaldi	74.84
013 Okanagan	66.56
011 East Kootenay	F
012 Kootenay Boundary	F
031 Richmond	F
043 North Vancouver Island	F
053 Northeast	F
999 Province	**83.59**

F Data suppressed due to Statistics Canada sampling rules

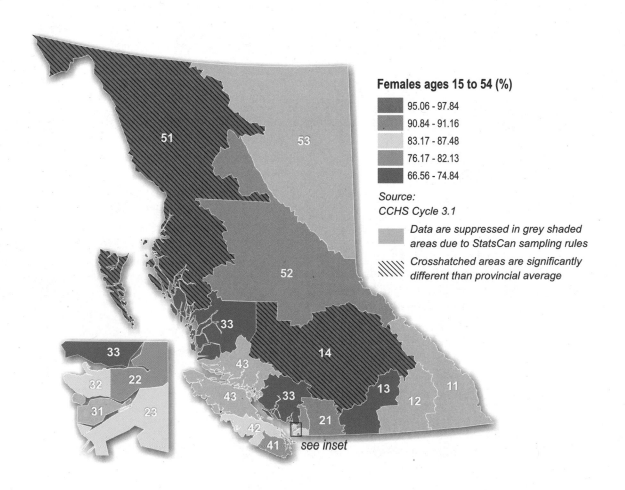

Females ages 15 to 54 (%)

- 95.06 - 97.84
- 90.84 - 91.16
- 83.17 - 87.48
- 76.17 - 82.13
- 66.56 - 74.84

Source:
CCHS Cycle 3.1

Data are suppressed in grey shaded areas due to StatsCan sampling rules

Crosshatched areas are significantly different than provincial average

Did not smoke during pregnancy

Tobacco smoke is one of the most important teratogens affecting pregnancy. In addition to concerns about birth defects, smoking is one of the main causes of low birth weight (<2,500 grams) by causing both pre-term delivery at less than 37 completed weeks of pregnancy, and intra-uterine growth restriction. Birth weight is an important indicator of wellness, and a healthy birth weight is a strong indicator for positive future development of the baby. A major focus of prenatal care in recent years has been smoking cessation among pregnant women.

Data from the BC Perinatal Database shows that, for the 4 year period 2000/01 to 2003/04, an average of 88.01% of women in BC did not smoke during their pregnancy. The range throughout the province, however, is quite high; 17 percentage points separate the highest (best) from the lowest HSDA, indicating large geographical variations in smoking rates during pregnancy.

In Vancouver, Richmond, North Shore/Coast Garibaldi, and Fraser North and Fraser South HSDAs, more than 90% of women did not smoke during their pregnancy. In the areas with the highest prevalence of smoking during pregnancy—Northeast, Thompson Cariboo Shuswap, and East Kootenay—less than 80% of women refrained from smoking during pregnancy.

Geographically, smoking during pregnancy increases eastward and northward as one moves away from the lower mainland HSDAs. Overall, the northern two-thirds of the province and East Kootenay region have the highest rates of smoking during pregnancy.

Health Service Delivery Area	Mothers did not smoke (%)
031 Richmond	95.74
032 Vancouver	95.37
033 North Shore/Coast Garibaldi	92.66
022 Fraser North	90.94
023 Fraser South	90.16
041 South Vancouver Island	85.03
021 Fraser East	84.96
012 Kootenay Boundary	83.99
013 Okanagan	83.78
042 Central Vancouver Island	81.78
051 Northwest	81.75
043 North Vancouver Island	81.35
052 Northern Interior	80.56
011 East Kootenay	79.57
014 Thompson Cariboo Shuswap	79.35
053 Northeast	78.51
999 Province	**88.01**

Mothers did not smoke (%)

- 92.66 - 95.74
- 85.03 - 90.94
- 81.78 - 84.96
- 80.56 - 81.75
- 78.51 - 79.57

Source:
BC Perinatal Database Registry

Births free of complications and anomalies

Data presented here are from the Vital Statistics Agency for the 5 calendar years 2001 to 2005, and include data only for babies born in BC to BC mothers. The cautions noted earlier need to be observed in viewing the patterns on the maps.

No maternal complications

For the 5 year period 2001 to 2005, on average less than 50% of all birthing mothers had a complication-free delivery. The range between the highest and lowest values for maternal complication-free births was 16 percentage points. The HSDAs in which mothers were most likely to remain healthy during pregnancy were Kootenay Boundary (58.44%), and Northeast, East Kootenay, Northern Interior, Fraser East, Okanagan, and Thompson Cariboo Shuswap, all with rates higher than 50%. This is a much different distribution than that reflecting complications between the fetus and neonate. Many lower mainland HSDAs had rates of complications higher than average, although the lowest rate of maternal complication-free birth was found in Central Vancouver Island (42.06%). Overall for the province, the number of pregnancies remaining free of complications, at 48.38%, leaves room for much improvement.

No perinatal complications

Perinatal complications affect the fetus after 20 weeks of pregnancy and/or the newborn up to 7 days of age. They affect one-third of BC babies. There was a range of 14 percentage points between HSDAs within the province, indicating substantial geographical variation in births with no perinatal complications. Similar to the areas in which women most often refrain from smoking, Richmond and Vancouver had the highest proportions of pregnancies free of perinatal complications at 70% or more. Fraser South and North Shore/Coast Garibaldi followed at 69.18% and 68.36% respectively, with Northeast at 67.70%. North and Central Vancouver Island had the lowest rate of pregnancies with healthy outcomes at 59.53% and 58.46% respectively.

No congenital anomalies

Congenital anomalies among the fetus/newborn generally occur in 2% to 5% of pregnancies. In BC during the 5 year period 2001 to 2005, the regions with

Health Service Delivery Area	No complications or anomalies maternal (%)	perinatal (%)	congenital (%)
012 Kootenay Boundary	58.44	65.86	94.39
053 Northeast	57.88	67.70	95.31
011 East Kootenay	53.46	61.72	94.61
052 Northern Interior	52.64	60.74	90.81
021 Fraser East	52.12	63.86	95.13
013 Okanagan	50.25	66.08	92.96
014 Thompson Cariboo Shuswap	50.22	61.37	92.26
041 South Vancouver Island	49.79	64.88	94.18
033 North Shore/Coast Garibaldi	49.11	68.36	93.07
051 Northwest	48.74	63.61	93.51
043 North Vancouver Island	46.80	59.53	93.97
023 Fraser South	46.69	69.18	94.23
031 Richmond	46.61	72.29	94.54
032 Vancouver	46.52	70.53	92.55
022 Fraser North	46.47	66.46	93.20
042 Central Vancouver Island	42.06	58.46	92.75
999 Province	**48.38**	**66.37**	**93.49**

rates less than 5% were Northeast and Fraser East. The lowest rates of pregnancies uncomplicated by congenital anomalies were in Northern Interior at 90.81%, followed by Thompson Cariboo Shuswap, Vancouver, Central Vancouver Island, and Okanagan, all being lower than 93%.

Births free of complications and anomalies

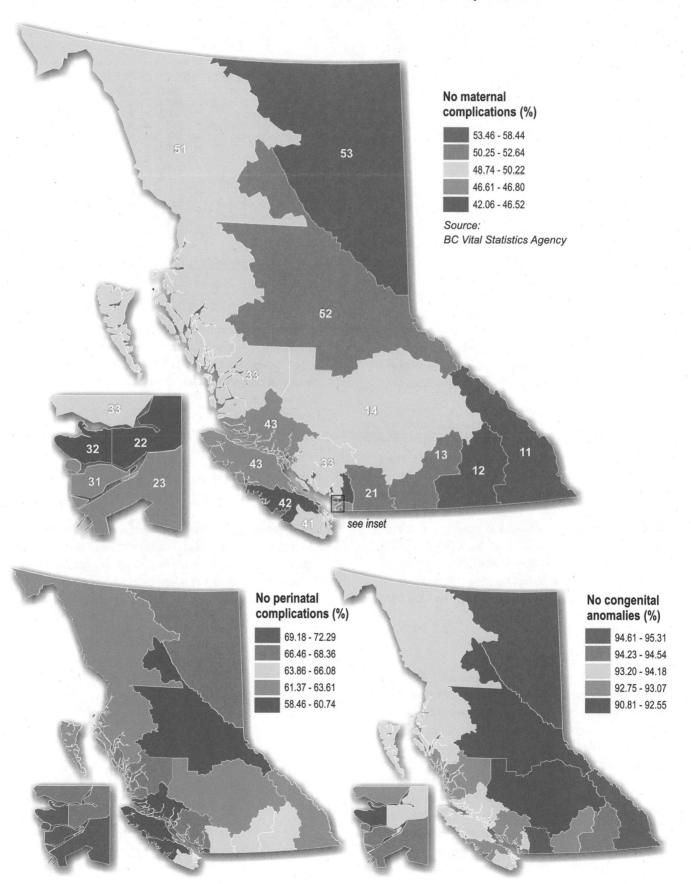

No maternal complications (%)

- 53.46 - 58.44
- 50.25 - 52.64
- 48.74 - 50.22
- 46.61 - 46.80
- 42.06 - 46.52

Source:
BC Vital Statistics Agency

No perinatal complications (%)

- 69.18 - 72.29
- 66.46 - 68.36
- 63.86 - 66.08
- 61.37 - 63.61
- 58.46 - 60.74

No congenital anomalies (%)

- 94.61 - 95.31
- 94.23 - 94.54
- 93.20 - 94.18
- 92.75 - 93.07
- 90.81 - 92.55

Healthiest pregnancies

The maps opposite provide three key indicators related to conditions for mother and child that improve the chances for the healthiest pregnancies and birth outcomes. These relate to the best age for pregnancy, baby's birthweight, and full gestational development of the baby.

Healthiest mother's age

Pregnancy complications such as prematurity and intrauterine growth restriction are more common among teen mothers. These complications and others, including pregnancy-related diabetes and hypertension, as well as hemorrhage, also occur more often in mothers aged 35 or older. During the last two decades, there has been a steady increase in the percentage of births occurring to women aged 34 or older, especially for women having their first baby, while live births to teenage mothers continue to fall. The net result, however, has been a reduction in the percentage of births to mothers in the healthiest age group (Vital Statistics Annual Report, 2005).

The percentage of births to mothers in the healthiest age group was 75.94%, but there was a 16 percentage point range in values among the HSDAs. Northeast, Fraser East, Northern Interior, and Thompson Cariboo Shuswap had the highest proportions of pregnancies occurring to mothers between 20 and 34 years of age (all over 80%). The lowest proportion of births to women in this age group was in North Shore/Coast Garibaldi at 66.32%, followed closely by Vancouver at 67.86%. Generally speaking, the percentage of healthiest age group pregnancies increased northward when moving from the lower mainland urban areas.

Healthy birthweight

The ideal weight for newborns is between 2,500 and 4,499 grams. Babies born too small for their gestational age (less than the 10th percentile) are vulnerable to hypoglycemia and other metabolic disorders. In addition to inadequate growth for a given gestational age, pre-term delivery is the major complication responsible for low birthweight. Premature birth is responsible for 75% of perinatal morbidity and mortality. Large babies are at risk for complications as well, but these are birth injuries related to a difficult delivery (e.g., facial palsy, and fractures of the clavicle).

Health Service Delivery Area	Mothers aged 20-34 years (%)	Birth weight 2500-4499g (%)	Full term live births (%)
053 Northeast	82.75	93.46	92.93
021 Fraser East	82.65	92.48	92.08
052 Northern Interior	81.25	91.54	90.93
014 Thompson Cariboo Shuswap	80.19	91.88	91.41
012 Kootenay Boundary	79.38	90.48	89.89
023 Fraser South	79.09	92.30	92.18
013 Okanagan	79.03	92.75	91.58
011 East Kootenay	78.47	94.12	92.92
042 Central Vancouver Island	78.01	91.90	91.24
051 Northwest	77.49	91.11	90.97
043 North Vancouver Island	76.38	91.54	90.72
041 South Vancouver Island	74.27	91.84	90.82
022 Fraser North	73.25	92.29	92.03
031 Richmond	70.70	92.93	92.88
032 Vancouver	67.86	92.67	91.50
033 North Shore/Coast Garibaldi	66.32	92.72	92.38
999 Province	**75.94**	**92.32**	**91.75**

The highest proportion of babies with an optimal birthweight was found in East Kootenay and Northeast at 94.12% and 93.46% respectively. The areas with the lowest proportion were Kootenay Boundary and Northwest, at 90.48% and 91.11%. The average for the province was 92.32%.

Full term live births

More than 9 out of every 10 babies were born at full term. The areas with the highest proportion of babies born at full term (37 to 41 weeks of pregnancy) were concentrated in the northeast, southeast (East Kootenay), and southwest (Richmond, North Shore/Coast Garibaldi, and Fraser North, South, and East). The lowest proportion of full term births were Kootenay Boundary at 89.89% and North and South Vancouver Island at 90.72% and 90.82%. Rates of full term birth across Canada range from 90 to 92%.

Healthiest pregnancies

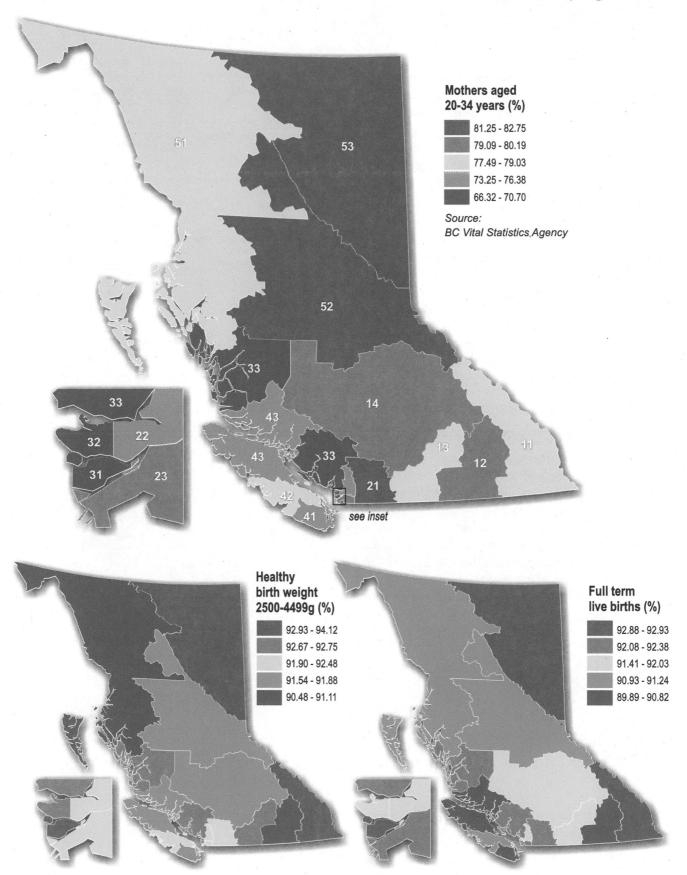

Mothers aged 20-34 years (%)

- 81.25 - 82.75
- 79.09 - 80.19
- 77.49 - 79.03
- 73.25 - 76.38
- 66.32 - 70.70

Source: BC Vital Statistics Agency

see inset

Healthy birth weight 2500-4499g (%)

- 92.93 - 94.12
- 92.67 - 92.75
- 91.90 - 92.48
- 91.54 - 91.88
- 90.48 - 91.11

Full term live births (%)

- 92.88 - 92.93
- 92.08 - 92.38
- 91.41 - 92.03
- 90.93 - 91.24
- 89.89 - 90.82

Healthiest babies

Data were collected for births with the following characteristics combined: no maternal or perinatal complications; no congenital anomalies; mother's age between 20 and 34 years old; birthweight between 2,500 and 4,499 grams; and full term. These are the characteristics associated with the healthiest babies overall, and therefore those babies with the potential for the healthiest start in life.

Provincially, less than half of babies were born with these combined characteristics (42.63%). The range from the highest percentage to the lowest was more than 13 percentage points, indicating much regional variation throughout the province. Overall, the highest proportion of healthiest babies was found in Kootenay Boundary, Northeast, and Vancouver and Richmond (all over 45%). The areas with the lowest proportions were found on Vancouver Island, with Central Vancouver Island at 34.39% and North Vancouver Island at 38.24%. Thompson Cariboo Shuswap was also below 40%.

Infant survival rate

Most babies survive their first year of life and go on to develop in a healthy manner. A very small minority does not survive for a variety of reasons, some of which are related to the conditions already described. No region of the province is immune to the tragic loss of a child in infancy but, overall, the rate of infant survival was uniformly high in BC for the 10 year period 1996 to 2005. The highest rates of survival were concentrated in East Kootenay, Northeast, and Fraser North and North Shore/ Coast Garibaldi. The lowest rates of survival were in North Vancouver Island, Kootenay Boundary, Northern Interior, and Northwest, all at 99.46% or lower.

Health Service Delivery Area	Healthiest babies (%)	Survival rate (%)
012 Kootenay Boundary	47.90	99.45
053 Northeast	47.54	99.65
032 Vancouver	45.65	99.59
031 Richmond	45.50	99.60
033 North Shore/Coast Garibaldi	44.71	99.65
013 Okanagan	43.83	99.59
041 South Vancouver Island	42.78	99.55
052 Northern Interior	42.73	99.46
011 East Kootenay	42.68	99.66
022 Fraser North	42.62	99.65
021 Fraser East	42.49	99.61
023 Fraser South	41.74	99.57
051 Northwest	40.93	99.45
014 Thompson Cariboo Shuswap	39.64	99.50
043 North Vancouver Island	38.24	99.42
042 Central Vancouver Island	34.39	99.52
999 Province	**42.63**	**99.58**

Healthiest babies

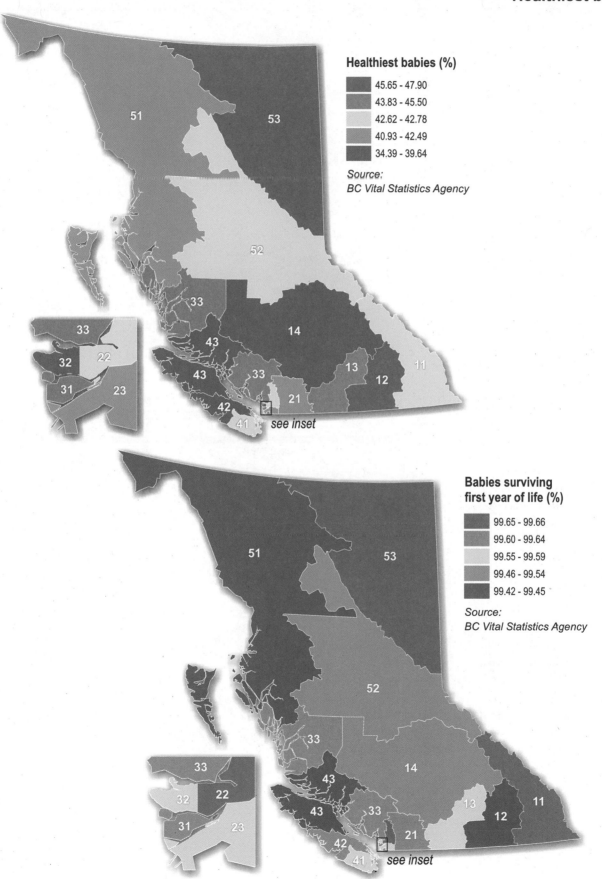

Healthiest babies (%)

- 45.65 - 47.90
- 43.83 - 45.50
- 42.62 - 42.78
- 40.93 - 42.49
- 34.39 - 39.64

Source:
BC Vital Statistics Agency

Babies surviving
first year of life (%)

- 99.65 - 99.66
- 99.60 - 99.64
- 99.55 - 99.59
- 99.46 - 99.54
- 99.42 - 99.45

Source:
BC Vital Statistics Agency

Pregnancy outreach programs

Located throughout the province, there is a series of centres providing specialized services supporting women to have healthy babies. Known as Pregnancy Outreach Programs, these centres have been created over the past two decades to reach out to women who do not have access to typical prenatal information and services. Many of these women are vulnerable to unhealthy pregnancies for several reasons, including substance abuse, spousal abuse, homelessness, and other conditions.

Pregnancy Outreach Programs are located in different types of centres for easy access. These include community centres, health centres, and native friendship centres. Women can access a variety of services at these centres, such as: nutrition and health counselling; food hampers, prenatal vitamins, and food vouchers; peer support groups; referrals to counselling services, life skills programs, parenting programs, and breastfeeding support; support to cut down or stop smoking and to reduce exposure to second-hand smoke; help to deal with an alcohol or drug issue; activities such as music therapy; and instruction on caring for and feeding a baby (Burglehaus, 2004).

In all, there are 46 Pregnancy Outreach Program centres scattered around the province to help improve the chances of healthy pregnancies and healthy beginnings.

1 Outreach Program
2 Outreach Programs

Source:
British Columbia Association of Pregnancy Outreach Programs, 2006

Summary

The previous maps indicate that there is a considerable amount of variation throughout the province for most wellness indicators related to healthy pregnancies and healthy beginnings. These variations are not always consistent geographically. For example, smoking in pregnancy is least prevalent in the urbanized lower mainland area of the province, and the central interior and northern areas have the highest prevalence. This pattern is similar to others discussed earlier in the smoke-free section of the Atlas. On the other hand, the percentage of births to mothers in the healthiest age group is highest in the north and interior parts of the province, and less so in the lower mainland. This pattern is also similar for maternal complications.

Perinatal complications are also least prevalent in the lower mainland area of the province, but high in the northern and central parts of Vancouver Island and in Northern Interior, while congenital anomalies are high in Vancouver and the interior part of the province.

Healthy birthweight and full term babies show somewhat similar geographical patterns to each other. The best results occur in Northeast, East Kootenay, and Richmond. The good results in the eastern parts of the province may be related to data collection issues as noted earlier.

The lowest percentage of healthy babies, based on the combined criteria used here, are found on Vancouver Island (Central and North Vancouver Island) and the interior part of the province (Thompson Cariboo Shuswap), while babies born with the healthiest indicators overall are in HSDAs scattered around the province in Vancouver, Northeast, and Kootenay Boundary.

While the overall infant survival rate in the province is uniformly high, the variations in other indicators suggest that there is clearly room for improvement in healthy beginnings for the province's infants.

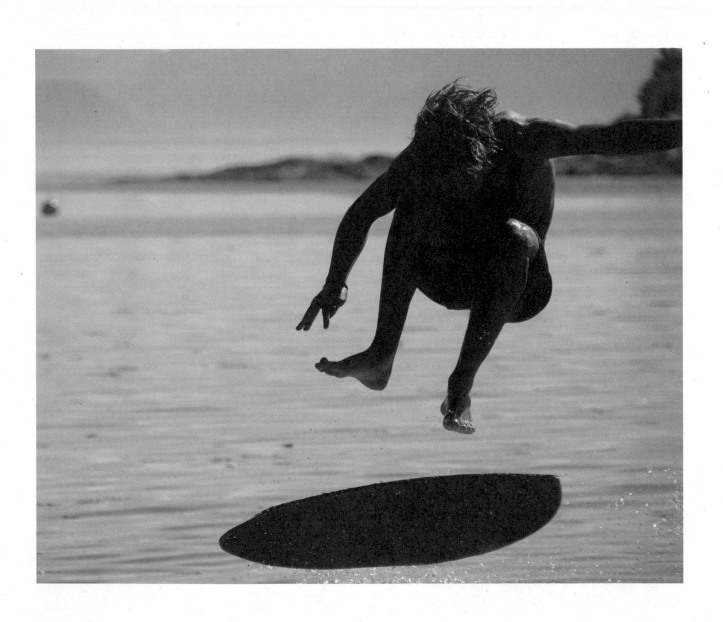

5.7 The Geography of Wellness Outcomes in BC

This section of the Atlas provides a series of health and wellness measures that logically follow as the outcomes from many of the indicators presented earlier in the Atlas. In fact, all of the sections so far build upon each other in some manner or form to result in these wellness outcomes.

There are 53 maps in total and 11 separate measures. All but one of the measures is derived from the CCHS. This is consistent with the personal and subjective nature of how wellness is defined. Each of the 11 measures (except for life expectancy at birth) is represented by five maps and a table and provides data for the total population, for males and females separately, and for teens and seniors, the model that has been used throughout the Atlas for CCHS-derived indicators. Again, the half-full or asset approach is followed rather than the half-empty or deficit approach.

The maps that follow are divided into several groupings. The first map looks at self-reported health, while the next two look at mental health reporting. One deals directly with mental health while the second provides information on the question about feeling sad, blue, or depressed for 2 or more weeks in the previous 12 months.

The next group of indicators deals with conditions that might restrict normal activity. These include lack of chronic conditions based on an amalgamation of responses to over 30 different questions in the CCHS. The next two deal with being injury-free over the previous 12 months, so that activities are not restricted. The following two indicators explore the level of being disability-free so that activities both inside and outside the home are not affected.

The Health Utilities Index is a combination of the results from several CCHS questions, and the higher the score, the healthier and more well the individual. This is followed by general satisfaction with life, an important wellness indicator and asset.

Finally, three maps are presented that show the life expectancy of BC residents for the total population, and separately for males and females.

Self-reported health is good to excellent

As noted earlier in the Atlas, individual perception of health is an important wellness asset. The CCHS asked the question *"In general would you say your health is...?"* In response, nearly 9 out of every 10 BC residents (88.14%) surveyed answered that they felt their health was good, very good, or excellent. For Aboriginal respondents, 85.66% felt their health was good to excellent, but this lower value was not statistically significantly different from the provincial average.

Health Service Delivery Area	All respondents (%)	Males (%)	Females (%)	Ages 12-19 (%)	Ages 20-64 (%)	Ages 65+ (%)
022 Fraser North	89.89	89.96	89.82	94.29	91.92	73.70‡
031 Richmond	89.80	93.21	86.61	95.96	93.46	66.49‡
043 North Vancouver Island	88.90	90.03	87.79	86.13	93.24	71.84‡
033 North Shore/Coast Garibaldi	88.75	89.83	87.73	92.90	89.90	80.53‡
021 Fraser East	88.53	90.97	86.15	92.30	91.56	71.56‡
014 Thompson Cariboo Shuswap	88.33	89.75	86.92	95.43	90.27	74.31‡
013 Okanagan	88.30	86.96	89.56	96.16	91.31	74.21‡
041 South Vancouver Island	88.07	87.19	88.86	95.89	89.51	78.09‡
023 Fraser South	88.02	89.74	86.33	97.12‡	89.15	72.49‡
032 Vancouver	87.21	90.08	84.41	94.30	89.28	71.54‡
042 Central Vancouver Island	86.89	86.87	86.92	90.51	89.63	75.52‡
012 Kootenay Boundary	86.88	87.62	86.14	96.45	88.03	75.81
053 Northeast	86.84	87.05	86.60	87.69	89.86	59.44‡
052 Northern Interior	86.55	81.59†	91.78†	94.74	87.57	67.55‡
011 East Kootenay	86.27	88.04	84.45	98.66‡	88.16	67.10‡
051 Northwest	86.17	87.08	85.19	98.30‡	86.36	65.55‡
999 Province	**88.14**	**89.00**	**87.32**	**94.54‡**	**90.17**	**73.48‡**

‡ Age group differs significantly from 20-64 group
† Males differ significantly from females

While the highest values in BC were recorded in Fraser North and Richmond (both nearly 90%), the lowest values were only marginally lower in the north and southeast of the province.

Provincially, males generally had higher levels of self-reported good to excellent health at 89%, compared to 87.32% for females; this difference was not significant. Males in most HSDAs reported higher good to excellent health than females, but they were not significantly different statistically. For Northern Interior, however, males (81.59%) were significantly lower than females (91.78%) in the HSDA (see above table), and significantly lower than the provincial average for males.

In terms of age, teens for the province overall were significantly more likely to perceive their health as good to excellent than the two older age groups, and Fraser South, East Kootenay, and Northwest teens were significantly higher than the older age cohorts in their HSDAs. Provincially, seniors as a group, at 73.48%, had lower values. In all but one HSDA, Central Vancouver Island, the percent of seniors reporting self-perceived health as good to excellent was significantly lower than younger age groups in their HSDAs.

Among teens, the highest values were recorded in the extreme northwest and southeast of the province. East Kootenay and Northwest both had values greater than 98%, and both were significantly statistically higher than the provincial average for their teen peers elsewhere in the province. The lowest value HSDAs were in the central and northern part of Vancouver Island and in the extreme northeast of the province.

For seniors, there was a large geographical variation in self-perceived health. North Shore/Coast Garibaldi, with 80.53% of its seniors indicating good to excellent health, was significantly higher statistically than the average for all seniors provincially. In contrast, Northeast had fewer than 6 out of every 10 seniors recording good to excellent health.

Self-reported health is good to excellent

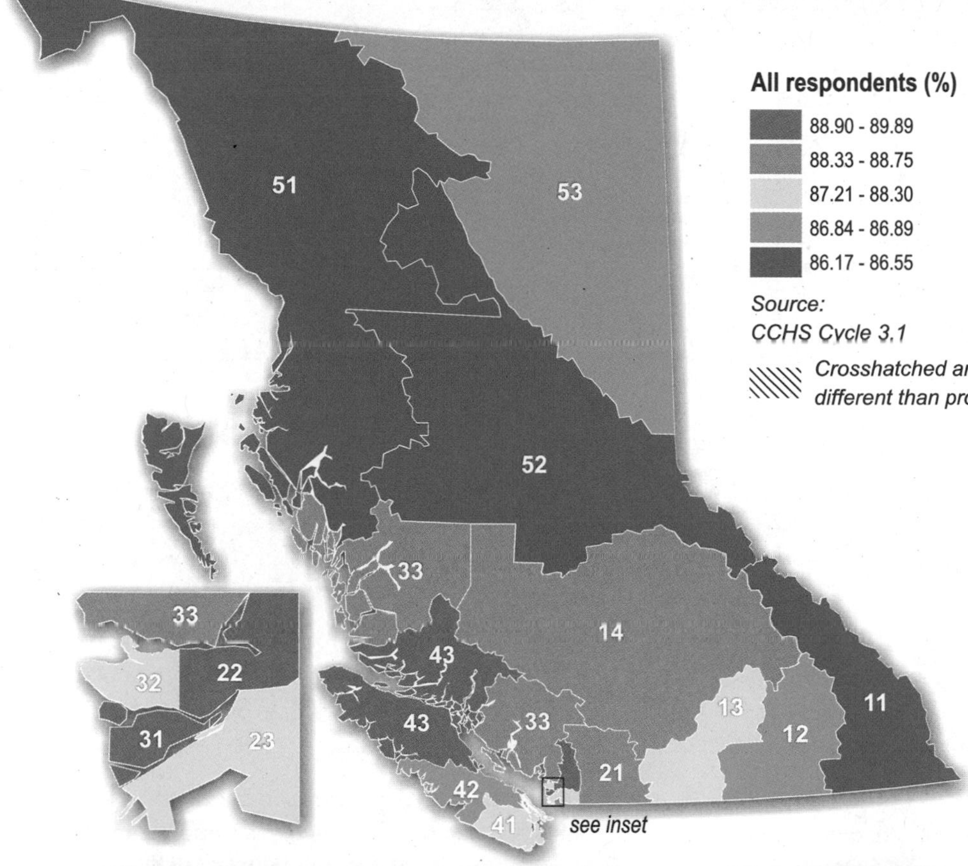

All respondents (%)

- 88.90 - 89.89
- 88.33 - 88.75
- 87.21 - 88.30
- 86.84 - 86.89
- 86.17 - 86.55

Source:
CCHS Cycle 3.1

Crosshatched areas are significantly different than provincial average

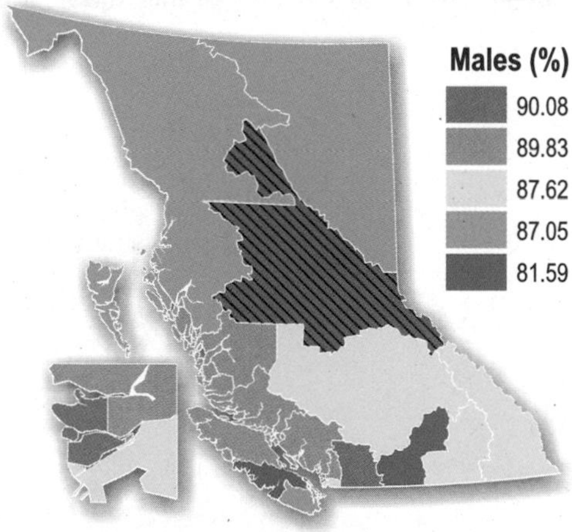

see inset

Males (%)

- 90.08 - 93.21
- 89.83 - 90.03
- 87.62 - 89.75
- 87.05 - 87.19
- 81.59 - 86.96

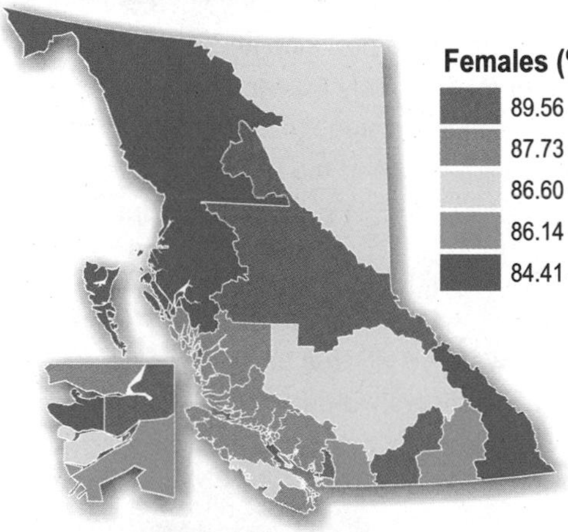

Females (%)

- 89.56 - 91.78
- 87.73 - 88.86
- 86.60 - 86.92
- 86.14 - 86.33
- 84.41 - 85.19

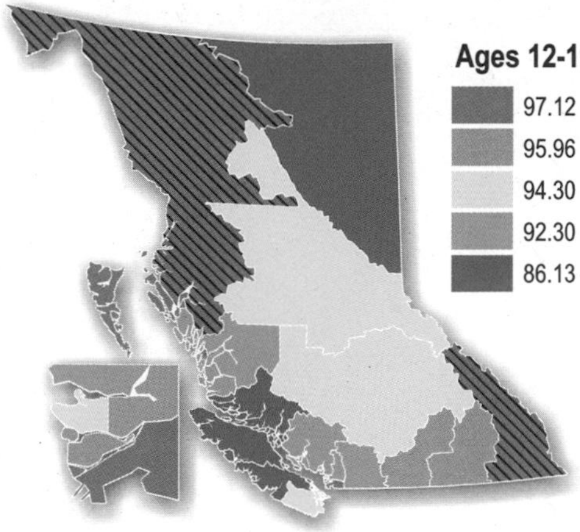

Ages 12-19 (%)

- 97.12 - 98.66
- 95.96 - 96.45
- 94.30 - 95.89
- 92.30 - 94.29
- 86.13 - 90.51

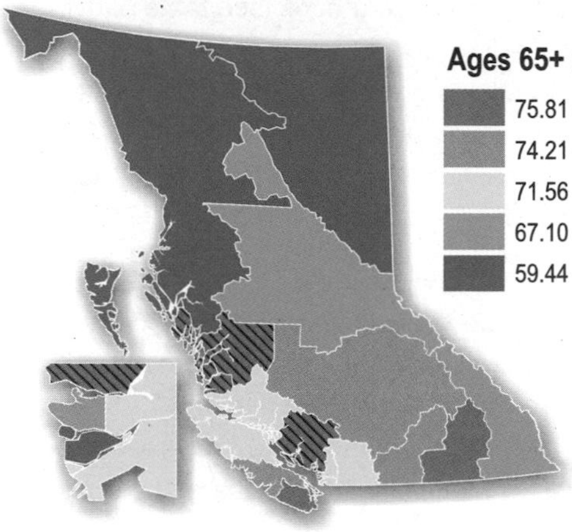

Ages 65+ (%)

- 75.81 - 80.53
- 74.21 - 75.52
- 71.56 - 73.70
- 67.10 - 71.54
- 59.44 - 66.49

Self-reported mental health is good to excellent

Feelings about mental health is also an important indicator of wellness among individuals. The CCHS asked respondents: *"In general, how would you say your mental health is...?"* and more than 9 out of every 10 (92.30%) respondents answered that it was good, very good, or excellent. Although the difference was small, the value for Canadians as a whole was significantly higher statistically at 93.22%, indicating that, overall, Canadians have a higher level of self-reported mental health than BC residents. For BC Aboriginal respondents, 89.82% felt their mental health was good to excellent. This response value was not statistically significantly different from the overall BC provincial value.

For all respondents, the geographical differences were small, although the lowest values occurred in the southwest of the province and the southern half of Vancouver Island. Only Fraser South respondents had significantly higher values than the provincial average. The difference between the highest and lowest value HSDAs was less than 4 percentage points.

Males as a group had marginally higher perceived mental health values than females, but not significantly so. There were no HSDAs for either males or females that were significantly different than the provincial averages by gender, indicating no real geographical variation through the province.

Among the three age groups (see table above), seniors were significantly less likely to perceive their mental health as good to excellent than were the other two age groups, but no individual HSDA had significantly lower values for seniors than other age groups.

For teens, there were some important geographical variations: 12- to 19-year-olds in the extreme corners of the province rated their mental health significantly better than their peers in the rest of BC. Northwest (98.69%) and East Kootenay (97.73%) teens both had significantly high values, statistically, when compared

to their provincial counterparts. The former also had significantly higher values than older age cohorts in the HSDA.

For the 20 to 64 age group, Fraser South in the lower mainland had significantly higher reported mental health than the provincial average for this age cohort.

Health Service Delivery Area	All respondents (%)	Males (%)	Females (%)	Ages 12-19 (%)	Ages 20-64 (%)	Ages 65+ (%)
023 Fraser South	94.47	95.43	93.53	94.12	95.34	89.96
011 East Kootenay	93.95	96.25	91.60	97.73	94.28	89.27
043 North Vancouver Island	93.62	94.81	92.44	86.93	95.26	92.06
033 North Shore/Coast Garibaldi	93.45	94.69	92.28	91.53	94.39	90.52
051 Northwest	93.42	93.40	93.44	98.69‡	93.88	81.52
013 Okanagan	92.83	92.34	93.30	93.80	93.55	90.02
022 Fraser North	92.39	93.28	91.53	90.34	93.44	87.93
031 Richmond	92.34	92.27	92.40	95.03	92.80	88.03
012 Kootenay Boundary	92.17	91.05	93.31	97.70	91.38	91.45
014 Thompson Cariboo Shuswap	92.15	94.21	90.10	96.27	92.77	86.19
053 Northeast	91.49	92.47	90.43	86.90	92.79	88.62
052 Northern Interior	91.45	89.96	93.02	88.65	92.76	85.93
021 Fraser East	91.30	91.57	91.03	90.82	91.91	88.99
041 South Vancouver Island	91.18	91.42	90.97	93.78	91.50	88.49
042 Central Vancouver Island	91.03	89.33	92.67	90.53	90.89	91.82
032 Vancouver	90.51	92.12	88.94	93.69	90.92	86.33
999 Province	**92.30**	**92.90**	**91.72**	**92.71**	**92.96**	**88.83‡**

‡ Age group differs significantly from 20-64 group

Self-reported mental health is good to excellent

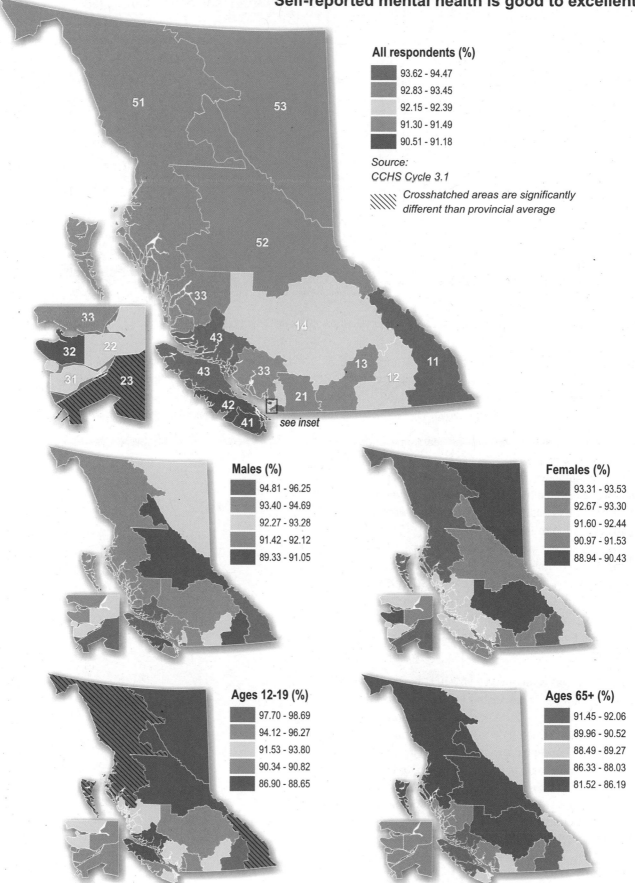

All respondents (%)

- 93.62 - 94.47
- 92.83 - 93.45
- 92.15 - 92.39
- 91.30 - 91.49
- 90.51 - 91.18

Source:
CCHS Cycle 3.1

Crosshatched areas are significantly different than provincial average

see inset

Males (%)

- 94.81 - 96.25
- 93.40 - 94.69
- 92.27 - 93.28
- 91.42 - 92.12
- 89.33 - 91.05

Females (%)

- 93.31 - 93.53
- 92.67 - 93.30
- 91.60 - 92.44
- 90.97 - 91.53
- 88.94 - 90.43

Ages 12-19 (%)

- 97.70 - 98.69
- 94.12 - 96.27
- 91.53 - 93.80
- 90.34 - 90.82
- 86.90 - 88.65

Ages 65+ (%)

- 91.45 - 92.06
- 89.96 - 90.52
- 88.49 - 89.27
- 86.33 - 88.03
- 81.52 - 86.19

Did not feel sad or blue for two or more weeks in the past year

Sometimes individuals, while not clinically depressed, can get "down in the dumps," thus interfering with their enjoyment of life and overall wellness. The CCHS asked the question: *"During the past 12 months was there ever a time when you felt sad, blue, or depressed for two weeks or more in a row?"* and 85.89% of respondents answered "never." It should be noted that the value is less than the value for the previous question on reported mental health.

Health Service Delivery Area	All respondents (%)	Males (%)	Females (%)	Ages 12-19 (%)	Ages 20-64 (%)	Ages 65+ (%)
051 Northwest	89.03	90.56	87.38	94.21	88.59	84.15
023 Fraser South	88.64	91.32	86.01	89.77	89.46	82.87
053 Northeast	88.06	89.09	86.94	87.79	87.89	89.98
013 Okanagan	87.79	90.33	85.40	86.25	87.85	88.49
012 Kootenay Boundary	87.69	87.76	87.62	95.81‡	86.12	88.20
022 Fraser North	87.27	89.86	84.75	84.50	87.61	87.70
031 Richmond	86.95	89.17	84.88	95.57‡	86.93	80.96
043 North Vancouver Island	86.02	91.96†	80.13†	85.96	85.70	87.52
011 East Kootenay	85.69	90.44	80.82	87.88	84.75	88.15
021 Fraser East	85.59	87.09	84.13	86.15	85.61	84.99
014 Thompson Cariboo Shuswap	85.33	90.50†	80.20†	87.04	85.65	82.58
041 South Vancouver Island	84.39	89.57†	79.72†	88.39	83.52	85.39
033 North Shore/Coast Garibaldi	83.90	88.92†	79.11†	84.03	84.05	83.13
032 Vancouver	83.70	84.92	82.51	90.87	82.97	83.51
052 Northern Interior	83.23	85.75	80.58	86.99	82.86	80.54
042 Central Vancouver Island	82.67	84.25	81.15	81.21	82.24	85.02
999 Province	**85.89**	**88.70†**	**83.17†**	**87.63**	**85.81**	**84.95**

‡ Age group differs significantly from 20-64 group
† Males differ significantly from females

For all respondents, the range in values between the highest and lowest value regions was small (less than 7 percentage points) and there was no significant geographical variation. The highest value was Northwest (89.03%) and the lowest was Central Vancouver Island (82.67%).

Geographically, there were no significant differences among males and females as separate groups. A look at the above table, however, shows that there was a significant difference between the genders based on the provincial average: males overall were significantly more likely to never feel sad, blue, or depressed for two weeks or more (88.70%) when compared to females (83.17%). The difference between the genders was consistent for each HSDA individually, and for North Vancouver Island, Thompson Cariboo Shuswap, South Vancouver Island, and North Shore/Coast Garibaldi these differences were significant statistically.

While there was a reduction with age in those never feeling sad, blue, or depressed for two or more weeks in a row in the previous 12 months, the differences were not significant. Among 12- to 19-year-olds, two HSDAs in different geographical regions were significantly less likely to feel sad, blue, or depressed for two or more weeks in a row than the teen average for the province: these were Richmond in the southwest and Kootenay Boundary in the south east. With values in excess of 95%, the teens in these two HSDAs also had significantly higher values statistically than the other age groups in their regions.

There were no significant differences among seniors geographically, although for the 20 to 64 age group, Fraser South in the southwest of the province had a significantly higher value than the same age cohort for the province as a whole.

Did not feel sad or blue for two or more weeks in the past year

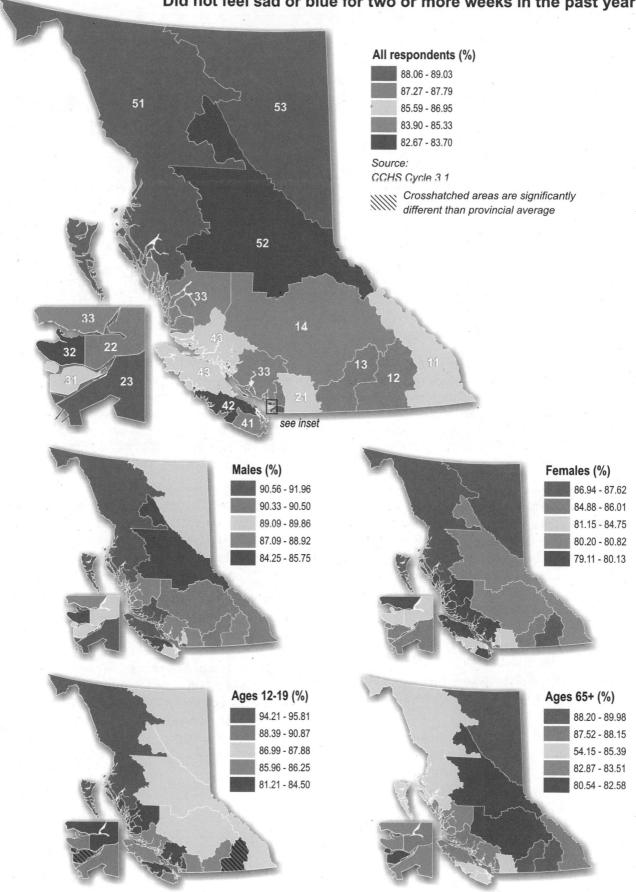

All respondents (%)

- 88.06 - 89.03
- 87.27 - 87.79
- 85.59 - 86.95
- 83.90 - 85.33
- 82.67 - 83.70

Source:
CCHS Cycle 3.1

Crosshatched areas are significantly different than provincial average

Males (%)

- 90.56 - 91.96
- 90.33 - 90.50
- 89.09 - 89.86
- 87.09 - 88.92
- 84.25 - 85.75

Females (%)

- 86.94 - 87.62
- 84.88 - 86.01
- 81.15 - 84.75
- 80.20 - 80.82
- 79.11 - 80.13

Ages 12-19 (%)

- 94.21 - 95.81
- 88.39 - 90.87
- 86.99 - 87.88
- 85.96 - 86.25
- 81.21 - 84.50

Ages 65+ (%)

- 88.20 - 89.98
- 87.52 - 88.15
- 54.15 - 85.39
- 82.87 - 83.51
- 80.54 - 82.58

No chronic conditions

As part of the CCHS, respondents were asked to answer "yes" or "no" to over 30 individual questions concerning different chronic conditions, including food allergies, asthma, arthritis/rheumatism, high blood pressure, chronic bronchitis, diabetes, heart disease, cancer, cataracts, and several mental disorders, to mention just a few. The results of those who answered "no" to all of the questions are referred to here as having no chronic conditions—an important wellness asset or indicator. For the provincial sample as a whole, only 3 out of every 10 answered negatively (31.39%) to all of the questions, indicating that most BC residents have some kind of chronic health-related problem. It should be noted that this is the same as the Canadian average. For BC Aboriginal respondents, only 25.03% had no chronic conditions, significantly lower than the BC population as a whole

Health Service Delivery Area	All respondents (%)	Males (%)	Females (%)	Ages 12-19 (%)	Ages 20-64 (%)	Ages 65+ (%)
031 Richmond	39.16	44.60	34.08	58.42‡	40.93	F
033 North Shore/Coast Garibaldi	37.41	43.29	31.80	52.38	40.24	F
032 Vancouver	37.05	42.13†	32.11†	54.98‡	39.54	F
021 Fraser East	34.16	38.07	30.35	47.82	35.94	F
051 Northwest	34.14	38.01	29.97	55.72	33.29	F
022 Fraser North	32.02	36.89†	27.28†	44.75	33.65	F
023 Fraser South	30.96	35.67†	26.35†	57.51‡	29.77	10.89E‡
052 Northern Interior	29.97	29.73	30.22	58.10‡	28.16	F
053 Northeast	29.73	29.82	29.64	53.62‡	27.47	F
014 Thompson Cariboo Shuswap	28.77	36.15†	21.43†	45.86	29.94	F
011 East Kootenay	28.38	34.10	22.52	51.96‡	27.30	F
042 Central Vancouver Island	26.41	31.84	21.19	48.35‡	27.79	F
013 Okanagan	26.29	28.71	24.02	45.28‡	29.20	F
041 South Vancouver Island	26.28	31.16†	21.87†	37.40	29.78	F
043 North Vancouver Island	24.14	27.72	20.60	F	23.18	F
012 Kootenay Boundary	22.22	28.37	16.04	F	21.44	F
999 Province	**31.39**	**36.00†**	**26.91†**	**50.24‡**	**32.77**	**10.10‡**

‡ Age group differs significantly from 20-64 group
† Males differ significantly from females
E Interpret data with caution (16.77< coefficient of variation <33.3)
F Data suppressed due to Statistics Canada sampling rules

For all respondents, there were clear geographical variations throughout the province. Most regions with values above the provincial average of 31.39% were located in the lower mainland. The one exception to this was Northwest. Richmond, North Shore/Coast Garibaldi, and Vancouver residents were significantly less likely, statistically, to have any chronic conditions (all more than 37% free from chronic conditions), while five HSDAs had values below 26.5% and all were significantly low compared to the provincial average. These were: North, Central, and South Vancouver Island, Okanagan, and Kootenay Boundary. The range in values between the highest and the lowest was 17 percentage points, reflecting the high level of regional variation throughout the province.

There was a significant difference between genders provincially. Males, with a value of 36%, were significantly more likely to be free of chronic conditions when compared to females (26.91%). With one exception (Northern Interior), this was consistent for every HSDA, and the difference was statistically significant for Vancouver, Fraser North, Fraser South, Thompson Cariboo Shuswap, and South Vancouver Island.

While the range from highest to lowest for males was about 16 percentage points, only one HSDA, Okanagan (28.71%), was significantly statistically lower than the average for males. For females, however, Richmond (34.08) and Vancouver (32.11) were significantly higher, and Kootenay Boundary (16.04%) significantly lower than the provincial average for females.

As expected, there was a very steep gradient by age, with the youth at 50.24% having a higher percentage being free of chronic conditions than 20- to 64-year-olds (32.77%), which in turn had a higher value than seniors (10.10%). These differences are statistically significant.

For teens, two HSDAs had too few data to be able to report the results (North Vancouver Island and Kootenay Boundary), but for the rest there was a 20 percentage point difference between the high of 58.42% for Richmond and the low of 37.40% for South Vancouver Island. The latter value was significantly lower statistically than the provincial average for youth. For seniors, only one HSDA had reportable findings indicating that there were very few seniors who did not have a chronic condition. The pattern for the 20 to 64 age group was very similar to that for the population as a whole.

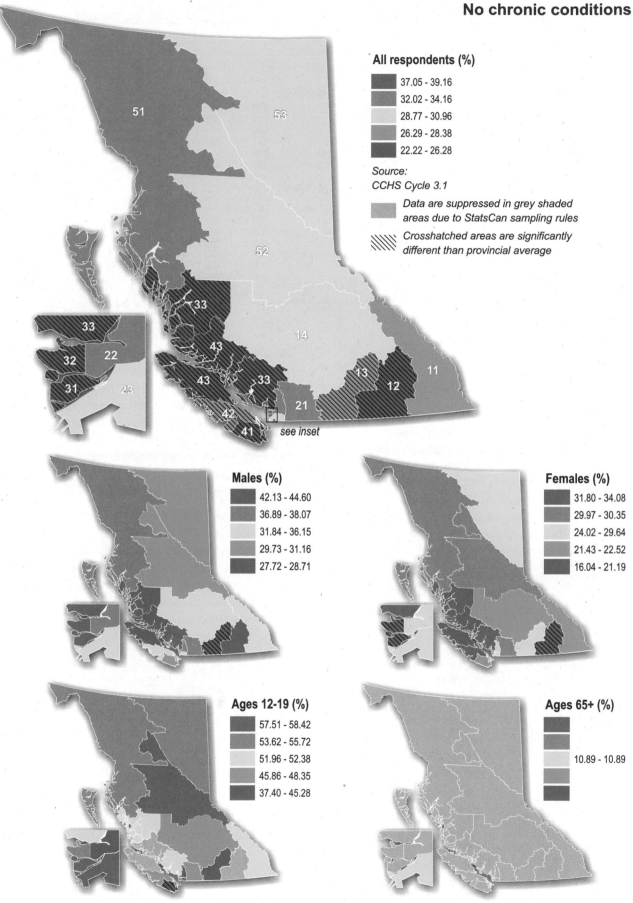

No chronic conditions

All respondents (%)
- 37.05 - 39.16
- 32.02 - 34.16
- 28.77 - 30.96
- 26.29 - 28.38
- 22.22 - 26.28

Source:
CCHS Cycle 3.1

Data are suppressed in grey shaded areas due to StatsCan sampling rules

Crosshatched areas are significantly different than provincial average

Males (%)
- 42.13 - 44.60
- 36.89 - 38.07
- 31.84 - 36.15
- 29.73 - 31.16
- 27.72 - 28.71

Females (%)
- 31.80 - 34.08
- 29.97 - 30.35
- 24.02 - 29.64
- 21.43 - 22.52
- 16.04 - 21.19

Ages 12-19 (%)
- 57.51 - 58.42
- 53.62 - 55.72
- 51.96 - 52.38
- 45.86 - 48.35
- 37.40 - 45.28

Ages 65+ (%)
- 10.89 - 10.89

Injury-free in the past year

The Atlas includes two questions from the CCHS related to injury-free status. Injuries can certainly detract from health and wellness, so being injury-free is a wellness asset. One question asked was: *"In the past 12 months did you have any injuries which were serious enough to limit your normal activities?"* and 82.23% of the respondents indicated that they had been free of injuries that might have curtailed activity during this period. While the difference is small, BC had a significantly lower level of injury-free status when compared to Canada as a whole (84.92%). For BC Aboriginal respondents, the value was 77.24%, which, while lower, was not significantly different from the provincial average.

For all respondents, there was a relatively small spread between the highest HSDA, Richmond at 86.90%, and the lowest, Northwest at 77.65%. Geographically there was no clear pattern, with relatively high percentages of injury-free individuals in both the lower mainland and extreme northeast, while Northwest, South Vancouver Island, and Okanagan had lower figures. Only Richmond had a value that was statistically significantly higher than the provincial average.

Females had higher levels of injury-free status than males, and for the province as a whole this difference was significant statistically. This difference was consistent for each HSDA, except North Vancouver Island and Northern Interior. The gender difference was only significant in three HSDAs: Central Vancouver Island, Fraser South, and Okanagan.

For males, there was no clear geographic pattern as no HSDA was statistically significantly different than the provincial average. For females, Richmond had a high of 90.04% and Northwest had a low of 77.74% of respondents who are injury-free. Both were significant statistically. The geographical patterns for both males and females were quite similar to that for the province as a whole.

There was a very clear and statistically significant gradient with age. Youth had lower injury-free status (71.01%), while seniors had the highest (88.12%).

Health Service Delivery Area	All respondents (%)	Males (%)	Females (%)	Ages 12-19 (%)	Ages 20-64 (%)	Ages 65+ (%)
031 Richmond	86.90	83.55	90.04	81.03	86.06	95.41‡
053 Northeast	86.90	83.79	90.24	80.35	88.19	87.74
032 Vancouver	84.50	81.24	87.67	79.70	84.80	85.67
021 Fraser East	84.46	84.10	84.82	74.74	86.01	86.46
012 Kootenay Boundary	83.31	80.77	85.86	77.67	81.52	94.16‡
043 North Vancouver Island	83.19	83.71	82.68	65.13	84.20	94.36‡
023 Fraser South	82.86	79.44†	86.21†	74.04	83.05	90.72‡
033 North Shore/Coast Garibaldi	82.85	79.63	85.92	62.42‡	85.91	83.41
022 Fraser North	82.64	79.87	85.33	70.97‡	83.09	90.41‡
042 Central Vancouver Island	81.43	76.41†	86.26†	67.31‡	81.83	88.73
052 Northern Interior	81.34	81.53	81.14	73.24	81.51	91.59
014 Thompson Cariboo Shuswap	79.37	75.21	83.51	62.20‡	81.66	83.10
011 East Kootenay	79.17	73.94	84.52	68.79	80.31	82.70
041 South Vancouver Island	78.76	76.07	81.19	66.20	78.83	85.72
013 Okanagan	78.21	72.36†	83.71†	65.76	77.16	88.62‡
051 Northwest	77.65	77.57	77.74	63.14	79.28	88.29
999 Province	**82.23**	**79.16†**	**85.22†**	**71.01‡**	**82.82**	**88.12‡**

‡ Age group differs significantly from 20-64 group
† Males differ significantly from females

For teens, every HSDA had a lower injury-free status than the older age groups, and North Shore/Coast Garibaldi, Fraser North, Central Vancouver Island, and Thompson Cariboo Shuswap were significantly lower than the 20- to 64-year-olds in the same HSDAs. For seniors, Richmond, Kootenay Boundary, North Vancouver Island, Fraser South and North, and Okanagan were all significantly higher statistically than the younger groups in their HSDAs.

While there was a large range between the highest and lowest HSDA for teens, there was no significant difference between any of these regions. This was also the case for the 20- to 64-year-olds. For seniors, however, several HSDAs were significantly higher statistically than the average for their age group: Richmond, North Vancouver Island, and Kootenay Boundary (all above 94% injury-free).

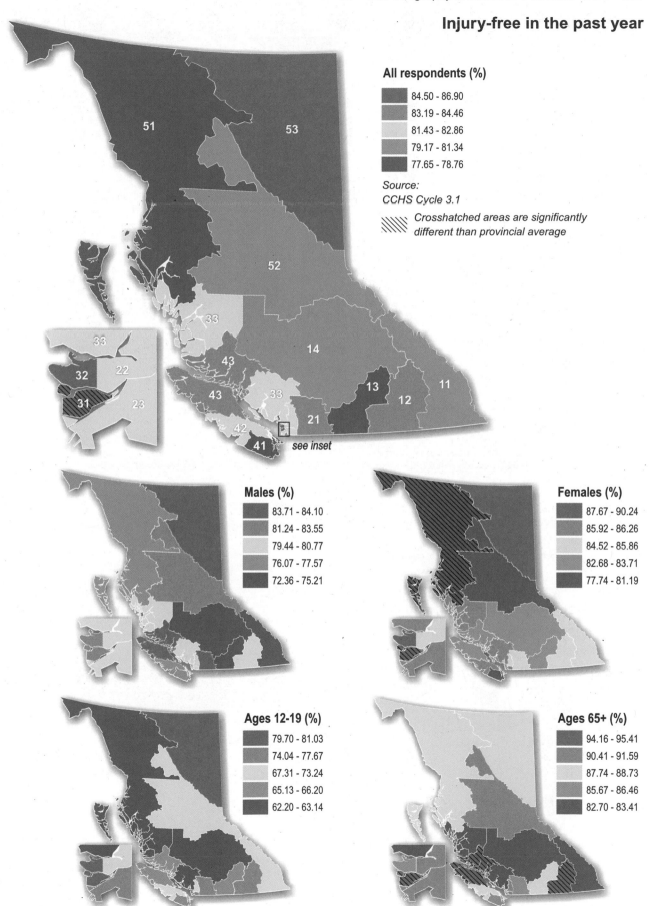

Injury-free in the past year

All respondents (%)

- 84.50 - 86.90
- 83.19 - 84.46
- 81.43 - 82.86
- 79.17 - 81.34
- 77.65 - 78.76

Source:
CCHS Cycle 3.1

Crosshatched areas are significantly different than provincial average

Males (%)

- 83.71 - 84.10
- 81.24 - 83.55
- 79.44 - 80.77
- 76.07 - 77.57
- 72.36 - 75.21

Females (%)

- 87.67 - 90.24
- 85.92 - 86.26
- 84.52 - 85.86
- 82.68 - 83.71
- 77.74 - 81.19

Ages 12-19 (%)

- 79.70 - 81.03
- 74.04 - 77.67
- 67.31 - 73.24
- 65.13 - 66.20
- 62.20 - 63.14

Ages 65+ (%)

- 94.16 - 95.41
- 90.41 - 91.59
- 87.74 - 88.73
- 85.67 - 86.46
- 82.70 - 83.41

No repetitive strain injury in the past year

Many tasks are repetitive in nature and can lead to repetitive strain injury. Similar in scope to the previous question, the CCHS canvassed this issue and asked: "*In the past 12 months, did you have any injuries due to repetitive strain which were serious enough to limit your normal activities?*" and more than 19 out of 20 respondents (95.35%) for the province answered negatively, indicating a high level of wellness on this indicator.

Geographically, there was very little variation among HSDAs throughout the province. Only North Shore/ Coast Garibaldi at 97.26% was significantly different from the provincial average for all respondents. The range from highest to lowest was a little more than 4 percentage points.

By gender there was little difference, but repetitive strain injury increased significantly with age. Seniors were much less likely to be free from repetitive strain injury than younger age groups. This difference was statistically significant. For most regions, seniors were significantly less likely to be free of the injury than their younger counterparts, a reversal in trend when compared to the results of the previous question. Only in Kootenay Boundary were seniors less likely to have this injury than the 20 to 64 age group.

Only three HSDAs recorded repetitive strain injury for youth, indicating that this condition is not one which affects teens and is very much related to the older age groups.

Health Service Delivery Area	All respondents (%)	Males (%)	Females (%)	Ages 12-19 (%)	Ages 20-64 (%)	Ages 65+ (%)
033 North Shore/Coast Garibaldi	97.26	97.10	97.41	100.0‡	98.34	90.34‡
031 Richmond	96.57	96.87	96.28	100.0‡	97.50	89.34‡
053 Northeast	96.30	95.72	96.92	100.0‡	97.02	83.52‡
032 Vancouver	96.10	96.38	95.83	98.96	96.68	91.21
041 South Vancouver Island	95.84	94.86	96.73	99.34	97.49	87.56‡
052 Northern Interior	95.43	94.31	96.60	100.0‡	96.55	80.82‡
043 North Vancouver Island	95.40	95.47	95.32	100.0‡	96.74	85.38‡
023 Fraser South	95.21	93.96	96.44	100.0‡	95.70	87.59‡
021 Fraser East	95.11	96.13	94.13	100.0‡	96.16	85.96‡
011 East Kootenay	95.09	95.42	94.76	100.0‡	96.70	83.58‡
013 Okanagan	95.01	94.94	95.08	99.11	96.78	87.05‡
042 Central Vancouver Island	94.75	92.94	96.49	100.0‡	96.24	86.57‡
014 Thompson Cariboo Shuswap	94.70	93.31	96.09	100.0‡	95.38	87.59
022 Fraser North	94.32	95.64	93.03	100.0‡	95.05	84.83‡
051 Northwest	94.07	94.01	94.14	100.0‡	93.84	86.40
012 Kootenay Boundary	92.95	89.65	96.25	100.0‡	91.59	93.33
999 Province	**95.35**	**95.07**	**95.63**	**99.77‡**	**96.26**	**87.56‡**

‡ Age group differs significantly from 20-64 group

No repetitive strain injury in the past year

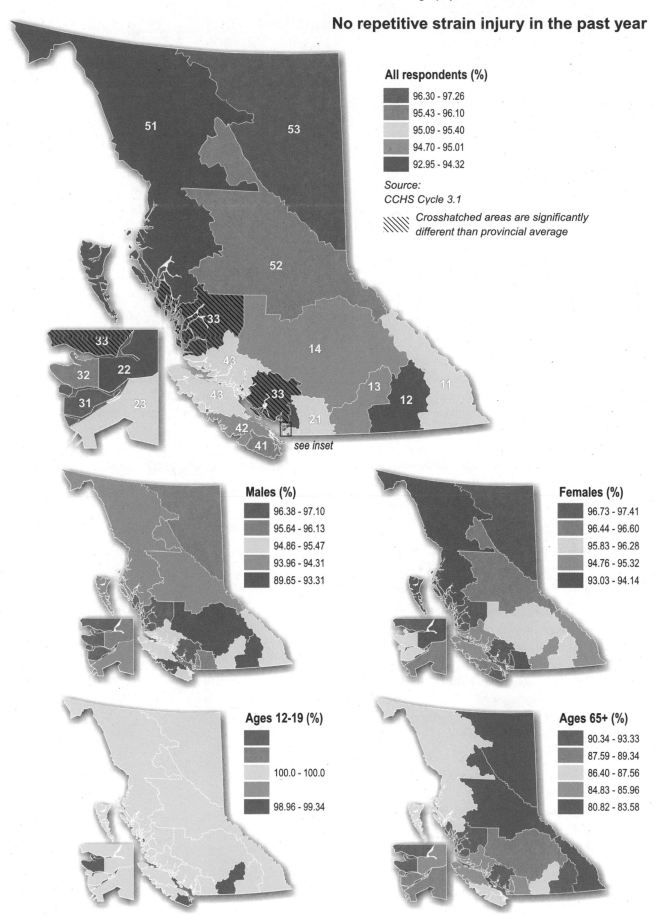

All respondents (%)

- 96.30 - 97.26
- 95.43 - 96.10
- 95.09 - 95.40
- 94.70 - 95.01
- 92.95 - 94.32

Source:
CCHS Cycle 3.1

Crosshatched areas are significantly different than provincial average

Males (%)

- 96.38 - 97.10
- 95.64 - 96.13
- 94.86 - 95.47
- 93.96 - 94.31
- 89.65 - 93.31

Females (%)

- 96.73 - 97.41
- 96.44 - 96.60
- 95.83 - 96.28
- 94.76 - 95.32
- 93.03 - 94.14

Ages 12-19 (%)

- 100.0 - 100.0
- 98.96 - 99.34

Ages 65+ (%)

- 90.34 - 93.33
- 87.59 - 89.34
- 86.40 - 87.56
- 84.83 - 85.96
- 80.82 - 83.58

No long-term physical, mental, or health condition that reduces activity at home

The CCHS asked a series of questions related to health and physical conditions that might interfere with an individual's ability to function well for certain activities. The first question was: *"Does a long-term physical condition or mental condition or health problem reduce the amount or kind of activity you can do at home (sometimes, often, never)?"* More than four in every five respondents (81.53%) answered negatively, indicating a relatively high ability to function because of no disabling conditions.

Health Service Delivery Area	All respondents (%)	Males (%)	Females (%)	Ages 12-19 (%)	Ages 20-64 (%)	Ages 65+ (%)
031　Richmond	88.00	91.59	84.64	93.78	89.70	75.10‡
032　Vancouver	87.28	89.56	85.06	93.78	88.96	74.12‡
033　North Shore/Coast Garibaldi	84.48	86.62	82.43	95.61‡	86.03	69.41‡
022　Fraser North	83.80	87.93†	79.78†	94.71‡	84.94	67.16‡
023　Fraser South	82.09	86.99†	77.28†	95.30‡	83.26	62.14‡
021　Fraser East	81.72	81.80	81.64	95.53‡	82.94	63.63‡
052　Northern Interior	80.46	81.45	79.41	95.09‡	80.11	62.19‡
051　Northwest	79.26	81.71	76.62	93.66‡	78.02	65.91
042　Central Vancouver Island	78.38	81.34	75.53	94.38‡	78.68	67.59‡
014　Thompson Cariboo Shuswap	78.14	83.11†	73.21†	92.26‡	80.07	58.60‡
043　North Vancouver Island	77.40	79.98	74.84	94.67‡	78.10	59.25‡
041　South Vancouver Island	76.91	77.83	76.09	91.13‡	77.96	64.78‡
013　Okanagan	76.35	77.22	75.54	91.18‡	78.57	60.85‡
053　Northeast	75.68	73.91	77.58	91.56	74.56	56.69
011　East Kootenay	74.77	77.38	72.09	85.05	75.62	62.18
012　Kootenay Boundary	74.73	74.61	74.85	90.97‡	74.51	64.38
999　Province	**81.53**	**84.18†**	**78.95†**	**93.73‡**	**82.84**	**65.73‡**

‡ Age group differs significantly from 20-64 group
† Males differ significantly from females

There were major geographical differences within BC. For all respondents, the lower mainland region had the best rates for being free of conditions that restrict activities in the home. Richmond and Vancouver both had significantly high rates statistically (both in excess of 87%), while five HSDAs had significantly low values when compared to the provincial average. These were South Vancouver Island, Okanagan, Northeast, East Kootenay, and Kootenay Boundary. With the exception of South Vancouver Island, they were all in the southeast or the extreme northeast of the province. Generally, lower values were recorded moving away from the urbanized lower mainland toward more rural areas.

Males were significantly more likely to answer the question negatively than females, indicating that they had fewer or less severe long-term conditions that hindered their activities around the home. This difference was consistent for all HSDAs (except Northeast), but only Thompson Cariboo Shuswap, Fraser South, and Fraser North were significantly different between genders at the HSDA level.

Generally, the geographical patterns were the same for the population as a whole as they were for males and females separately, but significant differences were much more dominant among males: Richmond and Vancouver were significantly high, and South Vancouver Island, Okanagan, Northeast, and Kootenay Boundary were significantly low. For females, only Vancouver at 85.06% was significantly different, statistically, from the provincial female average of 78.95%.

The restriction of activities increases with age for the province as a whole. At 93.73% for teens, 12 of the 16 HSDAs were significantly higher than the 20 to 64 age group, while 12 of the 16 areas were significantly lower for seniors than for 20- to 64-year-olds.

Geographically, there was no statistically significant variation for either teens or seniors, but for the 20 to 64 age group the geographical pattern was very similar to that of the population as a whole.

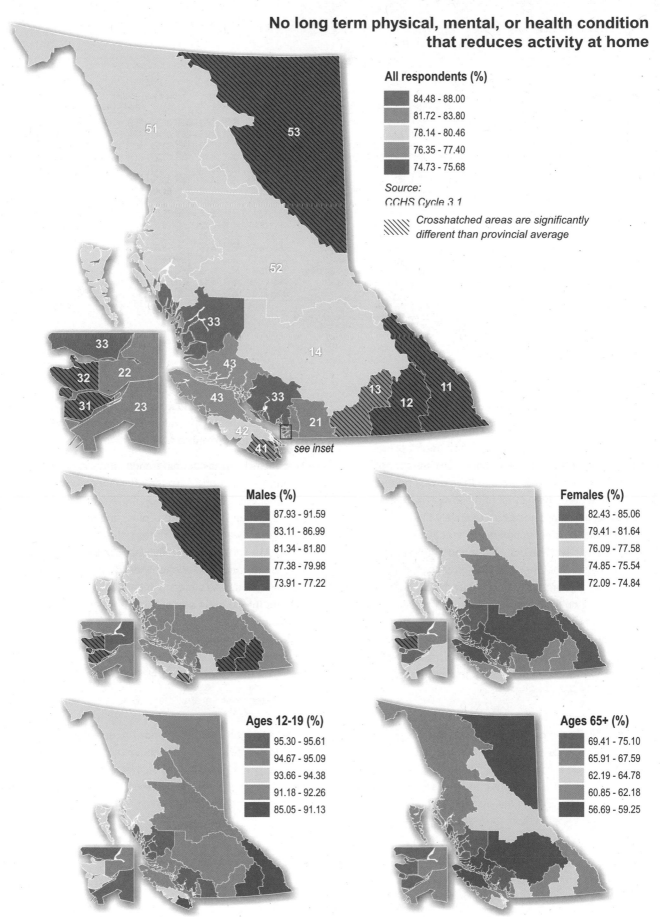

No long term physical, mental, or health condition that reduces activity at home

All respondents (%)

- 84.48 - 88.00
- 81.72 - 83.80
- 78.14 - 80.46
- 76.35 - 77.40
- 74.73 - 75.68

Source:
CCHS Cycle 3.1

Crosshatched areas are significantly different than provincial average

Males (%)

- 87.93 - 91.59
- 83.11 - 86.99
- 81.34 - 81.80
- 77.38 - 79.98
- 73.91 - 77.22

Females (%)

- 82.43 - 85.06
- 79.41 - 81.64
- 76.09 - 77.58
- 74.85 - 75.54
- 72.09 - 74.84

Ages 12-19 (%)

- 95.30 - 95.61
- 94.67 - 95.09
- 93.66 - 94.38
- 91.18 - 92.26
- 85.05 - 91.13

Ages 65+ (%)

- 69.41 - 75.10
- 65.91 - 67.59
- 62.19 - 64.78
- 60.85 - 62.18
- 56.69 - 59.25

No long-term physical, mental, or health condition that reduces activity outside the home

Various health- or disability-related conditions can interfere with individuals' abilities to undertake activities beyond the home environment. The CCHS canvassed this situation as follows: *"Does a long-term physical condition or mental condition or health problem reduce the amount or kind of activity you can do in other activities, for example, transportation or leisure?"* In BC, four out of every five respondents (80.69%) answered "never" to this question, indicating a relatively high level of disability-free living. Although the difference is small, the response was significantly lower than the Canada-wide response of 82.77% to this question, suggesting that BC residents have a higher level of restrictions on activities.

For all respondents, there were major geographical differences throughout the province and the range in values between the highest and lowest was nearly 16 percentage points. Most of the lower mainland or southwest of the province had relatively high values with respect to no reduction in other activities outside of the home. Two HSDAs, Richmond and Vancouver, were significantly higher than the provincial average. At the other extreme, East Kootenay, North Vancouver Island, and South Vancouver Island all had significantly lower than average values. Geographically, those with lower values tended to be more rural in nature, except South Vancouver Island, although the north region of the province was in the middle of the pack with respect to no reductions in activities.

By gender there was also a significant difference, statistically, for the province as a whole; males (82.69%) when compared to females (78.75%) were significantly less likely to be restricted by any of the above-noted conditions. By HSDA, all but one showed higher values for males (Fraser East is the exception), but only Fraser North showed a significant difference between genders.

Geographically, the patterns for males and females separately were very similar to that of the population as a whole. For males, Richmond and Fraser North, and South Vancouver Island and East Kootenay were high

Health Service Delivery Area	All respondents (%)	Males (%)	Females (%)	Ages 12-19 (%)	Ages 20-64 (%)	Ages 65+ (%)
031 Richmond	87.22	88.03	86.47	93.96	87.68	80.05
032 Vancouver	84.27	87.19	81.43	94.71‡	85.00	74.08‡
021 Fraser East	83.28	82.69	83.85	92.93	84.51	68.93‡
033 North Shore/Coast Garibaldi	82.82	83.76	81.93	93.85‡	83.75	70.68‡
022 Fraser North	82.60	86.85†	78.45†	93.84‡	84.44	61.39‡
023 Fraser South	82.35	84.64	80.10	95.58‡	82.78	66.55‡
051 Northwest	81.68	81.90	81.45	88.65	81.69	70.59
052 Northern Interior	79.05	80.44	77.58	91.48‡	78.57	64.87
013 Okanagan	77.40	78.84	76.05	89.31	79.84	62.88‡
053 Northeast	76.91	77.22	76.57	88.53	76.61	58.55
042 Central Vancouver Island	76.87	78.70	75.12	89.92‡	77.14	67.99
041 South Vancouver Island	76.67	76.85	76.50	92.52‡	77.32	65.06‡
012 Kootenay Boundary	76.66	77.35	75.97	86.29	77.60	66.36
014 Thompson Cariboo Shuswap	76.62	80.79	72.49	85.70	76.91	68.18
043 North Vancouver Island	73.15	75.12	71.20	86.45	72.46	64.70
011 East Kootenay	71.91	73.50	70.28	77.48	71.55	68.87
999 Province	**80.69**	**82.69†**	**78.75†**	**91.92‡**	**81.61**	**67.53‡**

‡ Age group differs significantly from 20-64 group
† Males differ significantly from females

and low, respectively, from a statistical significance perspective. For females, Richmond and Fraser East had significantly higher values than the average for females in the province.

There was a significant difference, statistically, among the age groups for the province as a whole. As expected, teens were much more restriction-free (91.92%) than 20- to 64-year-olds, and in turn, this latter group was much more restriction-free than seniors (67.53%). These differences were consistent not only for the province, but for each individual HSDA, and 7 of the 16 HSDAs were significantly higher for teens than for the 20 to 64 age cohort. For seniors, 7 HSDAs were significantly lower, statistically, than the 20 to 64 age group in their HSDA. They were Vancouver, Fraser East, North Shore/Coast Garibaldi, Fraser North, Fraser South, Okanagan, and South Vancouver Island.

Among the youth group, there was no significant difference geographically. For the 20 to 64 age group, however, significant differences occurred and the pattern was very similar for the population as a whole (see top map). For seniors, only Richmond, with a value of 80.05%, was significantly different from the provincial average for seniors of 67.53%.

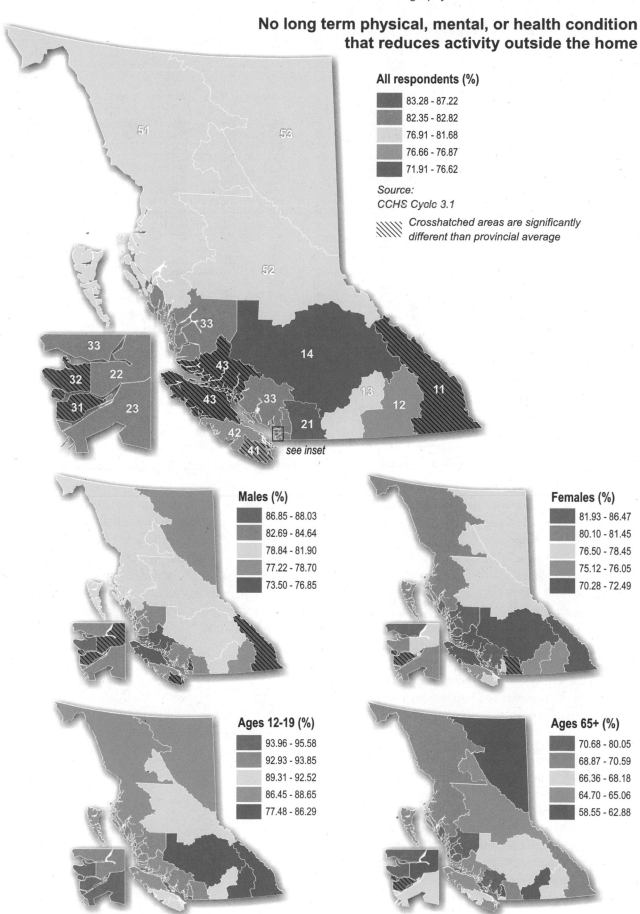

No long term physical, mental, or health condition that reduces activity outside the home

Good health utility index score

The Health Utility Index (HUI) is a multi-attribute health and wellness indicator and provides a single summary score for a variety of indicators (Horsman, Furlong, Feeney, and Torrance, 2003). Key attributes that go into the index include sensation (see, hear, speak), mobility, dexterity, emotion (happiness), cognition (learns and remembers), and pain status. A score of 0.8 or higher is considered to be very good or perfect health; scores below 0.8 are considered to indicate moderate or severe functional health problems. For BC respondents, 6.5% had index values below 0.50 and 12.6% had values between 0.5 and 0.79 (4.3% were not stated). The material presented here is based on mapping the percentage of the population by HSDA that scored at least 0.80 on the index.

The overall percentage for all respondents in the province scoring an index of at least 0.80 was 76.81% (or just over three out of every four respondents). For BC Aboriginal respondents, the percentage was a little higher (just above 78%), but not significantly so. The range from highest (North Shore/Coast Garibaldi, 80.70%) to lowest (North Vancouver Island, 71.16%) was nearly 9 percentage points, indicating a relatively small variation geographically. There was no clear pattern overall, although higher values prevailed in the extreme southwest of the province and South Vancouver Island. Only Central Vancouver Island, with a value of 71.75%, was statistically significantly different from the provincial average.

For males, higher values were evident in the southwest and lower values occurred in the eastern part of the province, although only North Vancouver Island was significantly lower than the provincial average for males; at 65.52% it was a clear outlier from the values for other HSDAs. For females, Northern Interior (81.48%) and Central Vancouver Island (66.98%) were statistically significantly higher and lower, respectively, than the provincial average for females. At the HSDA level, only Central Vancouver Island had a significantly higher

value for males than for females, although provincially, males had a higher percentage with the HUI at 0.80 or higher than females, but the difference was not significant statistically.

Geographically, there were no significant differences among the HSDAs for the 20 to 64 year and seniors age groups, but North Vancouver Island was statistically significantly lower than the provincial average for the youth group. While there was no significant difference provincially between the teen group and the middle age group, seniors had a significantly lower provincial value than the younger age groups. This pattern was evident for all but two (Richmond and Northwest) of the HSDAs (see above table).

Health Service Delivery Area	All respondents (%)	Males (%)	Females (%)	Ages 12-19 (%)	Ages 20-64 (%)	Ages 65+ (%)
033 North Shore/Coast Garibaldi	80.07	81.48	78.72	87.26	82.50	63.82‡
032 Vancouver	79.94	82.37	77.57	89.06	81.80	64.23‡
023 Fraser South	78.56	79.82	77.33	82.67	81.04	60.44‡
041 South Vancouver Island	77.86	78.26	77.50	80.05	81.47	62.89‡
022 Fraser North	77.63	77.92	77.34	83.89	80.07	57.26‡
031 Richmond	77.43	82.44	72.74	82.34	79.29	64.32
052 Northern Interior	77.18	73.09	81.48	78.18	79.25	60.81‡
014 Thompson Cariboo Shuswap	76.39	77.11	75.69	78.29	81.49	52.83‡
021 Fraser East	75.77	77.55	74.03	78.98	79.54	55.98‡
011 East Kootenay	74.07	73.70	74.45	78.54	76.68	58.30‡
012 Kootenay Boundary	73.55	73.27	73.83	83.59	76.83	53.87‡
051 Northwest	72.94	73.89	71.92	81.16	72.93	59.98
013 Okanagan	72.19	71.88	72.49	75.92	77.16	54.28‡
053 Northeast	71.91	73.46	70.24	75.45	73.90	48.50E‡
042 Central Vancouver Island	71.75	76.70†	66.98†	79.96	75.30	56.67‡
043 North Vancouver Island	71.16	65.52	76.74	60.66	76.43	56.60‡
999 Province	**76.81**	**77.85**	**75.80**	**81.00**	**79.81**	**59.17‡**

‡ Age group differs significantly from 20-64 group
† Males differ significantly from females
E Interpret data with caution (16.77< coefficient of variation <33.3)

Good health utility index score

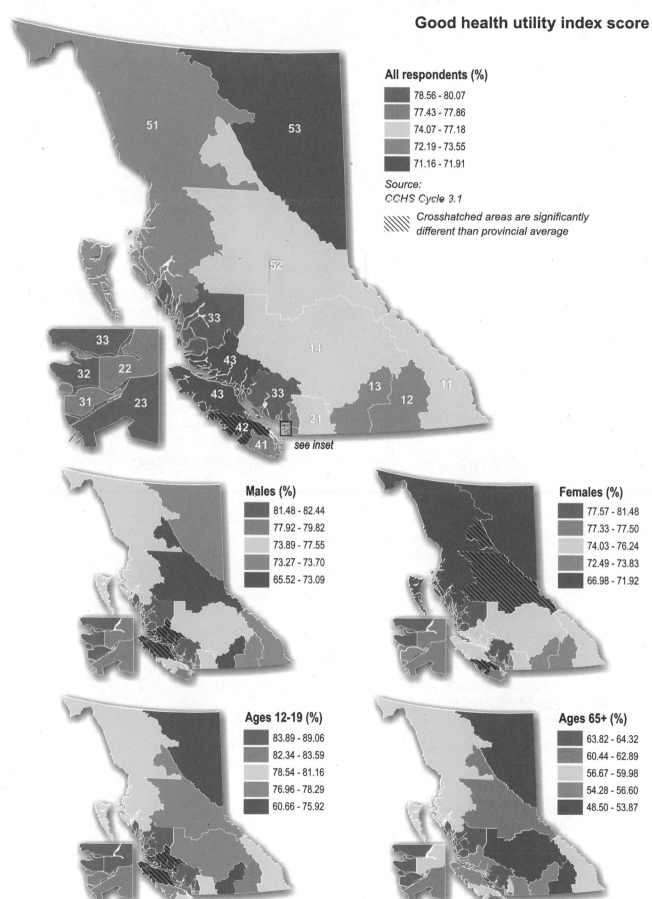

All respondents (%)

- 78.56 - 80.07
- 77.43 - 77.86
- 74.07 - 77.18
- 72.19 - 73.55
- 71.16 - 71.91

Source:
CCHS Cycle 3.1

Crosshatched areas are significantly different than provincial average

Males (%)

- 81.48 - 82.44
- 77.92 - 79.82
- 73.89 - 77.55
- 73.27 - 73.70
- 65.52 - 73.09

Females (%)

- 77.57 - 81.48
- 77.33 - 77.50
- 74.03 - 76.24
- 72.49 - 73.83
- 66.98 - 71.92

Ages 12-19 (%)

- 83.89 - 89.06
- 82.34 - 83.59
- 78.54 - 81.16
- 76.96 - 78.29
- 60.66 - 75.92

Ages 65+ (%)

- 63.82 - 64.32
- 60.44 - 62.89
- 56.67 - 59.98
- 54.28 - 56.60
- 48.50 - 53.87

Satisfied with life

Life satisfaction is an important measure of wellness. The CCHS asked the question: *"How satisfied are you with your life in general (very satisfied, satisfied, neither satisfied nor dissatisfied, dissatisfied, or very dissatisfied)?"* and 88.76% responded that they were very satisfied or satisfied. While the difference is small, the Canadian average at 89.78% was higher, and this difference was statistically significant. Of Aboriginal respondents in BC, 90.83% indicated they were satisfied or very satisfied with their life. This was not statistically significantly different from the provincial value for all respondents.

For the population as a whole, there were some interesting geographical differences, although the range in values was only 6 percentage points. The lowest values were recorded in the urbanized southwest of the province (South Vancouver Island, Vancouver, and Richmond), while the highest values were recorded in more rural areas, such as North Vancouver Island, Kootenay Boundary, and Thompson Cariboo Shuswap. The latter region, at 92.19%, was significantly higher than the provincial average of 88.76%.

There was no difference between the genders, and overall geographical patterns were quite similar to that for the population as a whole. Among males, Thompson Cariboo Shuswap (94.18%) was significantly higher for life satisfaction than the provincial male average. Females in Kootenay Boundary were significantly more satisfied with life than the provincial average for females.

Life satisfaction declined with age, but even seniors, although significantly lower than other age groups, had a high value for life satisfaction (85.33%).

There was little variation among teens, although Kootenay Boundary youth had a significantly high life satisfaction (97.36%) when compared to provincial teens as a whole (91.30%). The HSDA with the lowest value for teens was Fraser North (87.08%). For the 20 to 64 age cohort, Thompson Cariboo Shuswap was significantly higher than its peers. For the seniors group, the range between Northeast and North Vancouver Island was 22 percentage points. North Vancouver Island seniors were significantly more satisfied with life than their provincial peers.

Health Service Delivery Area	All respondents (%)	Males (%)	Females (%)	Ages 12-19 (%)	Ages 20-64 (%)	Ages 65+ (%)
014 Thompson Cariboo Shuswap	92.19	94.18	90.21	93.34	93.20	86.88
012 Kootenay Boundary	91.47	88.25	94.70	97.36	90.77	90.15
043 North Vancouver Island	91.12	90.62	91.61	94.97	89.78	93.78
052 Northern Interior	90.44	89.75	91.17	92.85	90.31	88.02
033 North Shore/Coast Garibaldi	90.08	92.34	87.92	94.62	90.24	86.10
022 Fraser North	89.64	90.79	88.52	87.08	90.51	86.68
021 Fraser East	88.96	90.23	87.72	90.38	89.38	85.77
013 Okanagan	88.83	88.04	89.58	90.71	89.22	86.54
042 Central Vancouver Island	88.75	86.60	90.81	91.70	88.17	88.87
051 Northwest	88.70	89.49	87.85	93.55	88.44	82.98
053 Northeast	88.67	88.00	89.39	91.34	90.12	71.45
023 Fraser South	88.60	88.66	88.54	90.90	88.87	84.76
011 East Kootenay	87.70	87.94	87.44	90.51	88.47	81.76
041 South Vancouver Island	87.46	88.07	86.90	90.00	87.81	84.66
031 Richmond	87.32	88.31	86.39	91.28	88.09	80.48
032 Vancouver	86.27	85.40	87.12	92.55	86.55	80.96
999 Province	**88.76**	**88.93**	**88.58**	**91.30**	**89.06**	**85.33‡**

‡ Age group differs significantly from 20-64 group

Satisfied with life

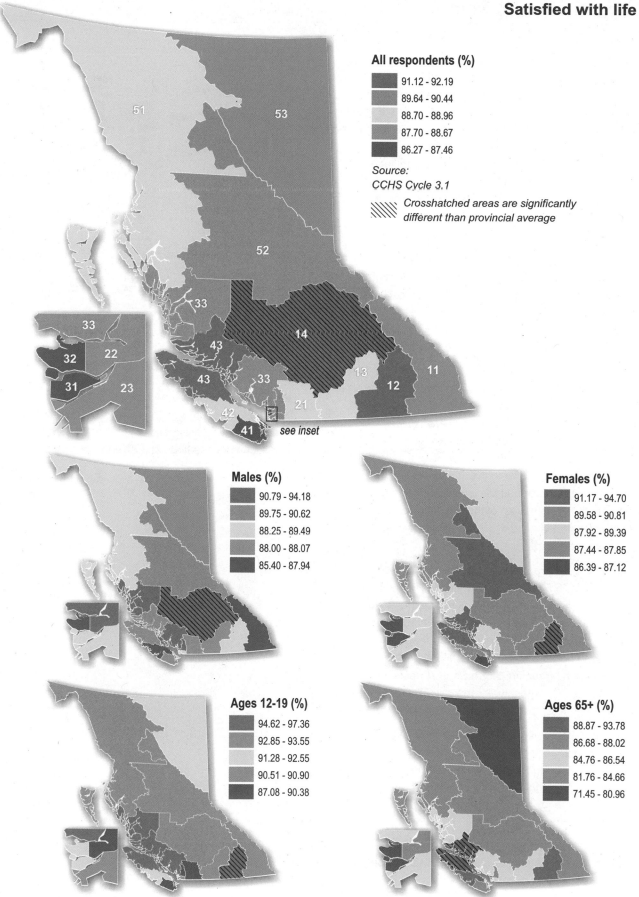

All respondents (%)

- 91.12 - 92.19
- 89.64 - 90.44
- 88.70 - 88.96
- 87.70 - 88.67
- 86.27 - 87.46

Source:
CCHS Cycle 3.1

Crosshatched areas are significantly different than provincial average

Males (%)

- 90.79 - 94.18
- 89.75 - 90.62
- 88.25 - 89.49
- 88.00 - 88.07
- 85.40 - 87.94

Females (%)

- 91.17 - 94.70
- 89.58 - 90.81
- 87.92 - 89.39
- 87.44 - 87.85
- 86.39 - 87.12

Ages 12-19 (%)

- 94.62 - 97.36
- 92.85 - 93.55
- 91.28 - 92.55
- 90.51 - 90.90
- 87.08 - 90.38

Ages 65+ (%)

- 88.87 - 93.78
- 86.68 - 88.02
- 84.76 - 86.54
- 81.76 - 84.66
- 71.45 - 80.96

Life expectancy at birth

A key health and wellness indicator is life expectancy at birth. This is an outcome of a combination of many of the assets and other indicators already mapped in this Atlas. It is an indicator that is recognized internationally as important for comparative purposes. Data were received from BC Statistics for the total population, and also for each gender. The three maps opposite provide the average life expectancy at birth for the 5 year period 2001 to 2005. More detailed data are provided in the table.

The top map opposite provides a picture of the variation in longevity rates for the total population. While there are five groupings, the table indicates that not each group is a perfect quintile. This is because several HSDAs had similar figures and we felt it best not to split them between two "quintiles," but rather to keep them together.

For BC, the average life expectancy at birth was 80.8 years for this 5 year period. This varied from a low of 78.4 years in Northern Interior to a high of 84.1 years in Richmond, a difference of 5.7 years. In terms of geographical patterns, there was a clear gradient moving east and north from the urbanized lower mainland and South Vancouver Island in the southwest corner of the province. The north had the lowest life expectancy rates, with the southeast of the province being in the middle for life expectancy, at the provincial overall rate or slightly below it.

For males, life expectancy was less than the provincial average, at 78.5 years. The range was 6 years between the best region, which was Richmond in the southwest at 82.3 years, compared with only 76.3 years for Thompson Cariboo Shuswap in the central interior of the province. Richmond had a 2.1 year greater life expectancy than the next highest region (North Shore/Coast Garibaldi at 80.2 years). Geographically, the overall pattern was very similar to that for the two sexes combined.

For females, the average life expectancy at 83.0 years for the 5 year period was 2.2 years greater than the provincial average. The range between Richmond, which was the highest life expectancy region at 85.6 years, and the lowest, which was Northern Interior at 80.6 years, was 5 years.

Each and every HSDA had a higher life expectancy for females than for males, and the geographical pattern was also similar to that for males.

Health Service Delivery Area	Both sexes	Age in years Males	Females
031 Richmond	84.1	82.3	85.6
033 North Shore/Coast Garibaldi	82.0	80.2	83.7
032 Vancouver	81.4	78.8	84.0
022 Fraser North	81.2	79.0	83.2
041 South Vancouver Island	81.1	78.9	83.0
011 East Kootenay	80.9	78.6	83.4
023 Fraser South	80.9	78.2	83.3
013 Okanagan	80.5	78.0	83.0
021 Fraser East	80.0	77.7	82.4
042 Central Vancouver Island	79.8	77.7	81.8
012 Kootenay Boundary	79.8	77.6	82.2
043 North Vancouver Island	79.6	77.3	82.0
053 Northeast	79.2	76.9	81.8
014 Thompson Cariboo Shuswap	78.8	76.3	81.5
051 Northwest	78.6	76.5	81.0
052 Northern Interior	78.4	76.5	80.6
999 Province	**80.8**	**78.5**	**83.0**

In summary, life expectancies were higher in the urban southwest corner of the province, lower in the southeast of the province, and lowest in the north. Provincially, the difference in life expectancy between the genders was 4.5 years, with Vancouver and Thompson Cariboo Shuswap having the greatest differential at 5.2 years, and Richmond the least at 3.3 years.

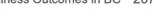
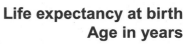

**Life expectancy at birth
Age in years**

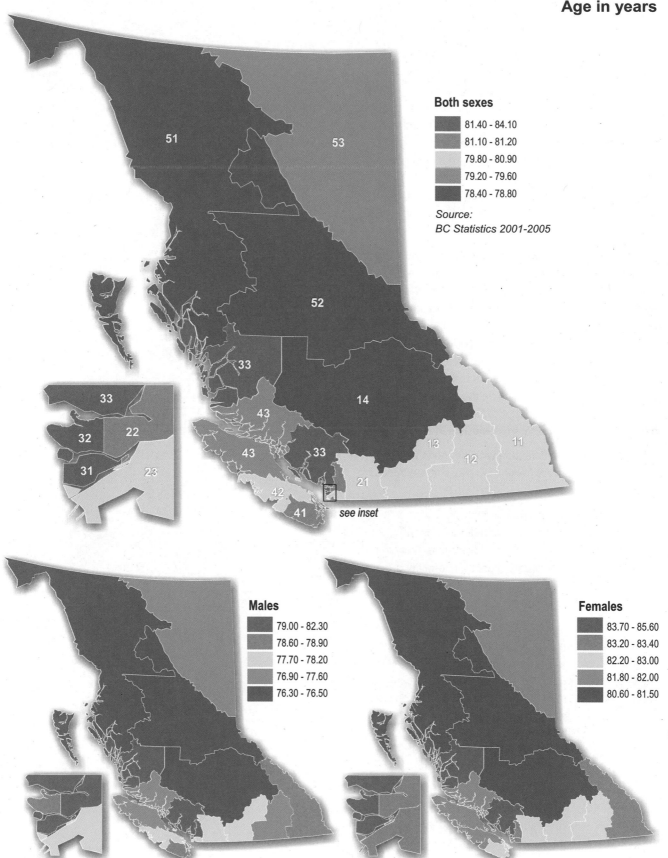

Both sexes

	81.40 - 84.10
	81.10 - 81.20
	79.80 - 80.90
	79.20 - 79.60
	78.40 - 78.80

*Source:
BC Statistics 2001-2005*

Males

	79.00 - 82.30
	78.60 - 78.90
	77.70 - 78.20
	76.90 - 77.60
	76.30 - 76.50

Females

	83.70 - 85.60
	83.20 - 83.40
	82.20 - 83.00
	81.80 - 82.00
	80.60 - 81.50

Summary

There were some major differences in wellness outcomes by geography, gender, and age. Not all of these differences were consistent; they varied depending on the indicator. For many indicators, such as perceived good to excellent health and mental health, not feeling sad or blue, being free of both injuries and repetitive strain injury and Health Utility Index, respondents generally showed high values. On the other hand, the majority of respondents had some type of chronic condition, some of which restricted activities both inside and outside the home.

Geographically, there was little variation for indicators with high overall values, but for the indicators with lower overall provincial values, regional variations were more evident. The large majority of respondents had some type of chronic condition, but those in the lower mainland fared better than those on Vancouver Island and the interior HSDAs of Kootenay Boundary and Okanagan. Similarly, with regard to conditions that interfered with activities both inside and outside the home, the lower mainland HSDAs were better off than many of those in parts of the interior and Vancouver Island.

When it comes to satisfaction with life, however, lower mainland HSDAs were lower than those in the interior of the province.

There were several differences based on gender. Males were less likely to feel sad or blue, or suffer from chronic conditions generally, and were less likely to have activities curtailed because of chronic conditions than females. Alternatively, females were more likely to be injury free than were males.

For all but two of the CCHS indicators, seniors did less well than the younger age groups. When it comes to not feeling sad or blue there was no significant difference between age groups, and seniors were significantly more likely to be injury free than their younger age cohorts. The youngest age group (12 to 19 years old) generally had significantly higher wellness values than both of the older age groups, except for injury-free status.

There was no significant difference between values for the provincial population as a whole and Aboriginal respondents for perceived health, mental health, satisfaction with life, injury free status, and the Health Utility Index. Aboriginal respondents, however, were significantly more likely to report chronic conditions.

Life expectancy showed clear geographical variations with higher values being prevalent in the lower mainland and South Vancouver Island HSDAs and lower values in the northern and interior HSDAs. These patterns were consistent when males and females were considered separately. For every HSDA, females had a higher life expectancy than did males.

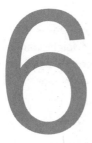

Benchmarking Wellness For British Columbia

This Atlas presents more than 120 different indicators related to wellness, some providing distinctions between gender and age, and over 270 maps showing how the values of these indicators vary within BC. One of the aims of the Atlas is to show how various aspects of wellness are distributed throughout the province.

While each map is accompanied by a brief description providing salient and significant points, the intention was always to let the "maps speak for themselves" in order to generate discussions about whether or not the geographical differences are important and, if so, what might or should be done to lessen the "inequities" in wellness between regions of the province. Understanding the reasons for the inequities is a job best left to those who live in communities within the administrative units that have been used for mapping purposes.

As noted at the beginning of the Atlas, the base geographical unit used for presenting the data is the Health Service Delivery Area (HSDA), of which there are 16 in the province. Examining the values of the various wellness indicators provides an opportunity to see which is the "best" HSDA for any particular indicator. Other regions that are below that value can set themselves a target of matching or even improving upon the "best" HSDA indicator value. Those areas with a lower value can also look to learn from those that have achieved the "best" result and examine why they are doing as well as they are: What are the characteristics that make a difference? Are there many Active Communities? Do they have more Action Schools? Do they have better local by-laws to encourage or discourage certain behaviours? Do they have public transit systems? Are their neighbourhoods safe and do they encourage walking? Are there accessible activity and recreation centres? Are sports clubs available? Are there

accessible stores selling fresh fruit and vegetables? These are just some of the questions that can be asked, but there are many more.

In order to give some examples of achievable wellness goals based on the information contained within this Atlas, this chapter provides some simple ways to determine the "best wellness" areas in the province based on different criteria.

For simplicity's sake, we focus only on one data set that is consistently available for all HSDAs. We examine the detailed responses to the questions that have been mapped from the Canadian Community Health Survey (CCHS) in 2005. There are several reasons for focusing on this data set. First, it is of high quality and provides coverage for the vast majority of the province, geographically. Some of the other data sets we have used have gaps because not all communities responded to community-based questionnaires. This affects, for example, some of the data collected for the BC Recreation and Parks Association. Also, the Vital Statistics data related to births cover only those events that occurred to BC mothers in BC. Key birth events in the eastern parts of the province may have occurred in Alberta hospitals, thus making us cautious about including those data in the construction of an overall wellness index. Second, approximately one-half of the maps and one-third of all the key wellness indicators contained in the Atlas are based on the CCHS. Third, wellness is subjective in nature, thus, using responses of individuals to survey questions captures, to some degree, this subjectivity. Fourth, the CCHS has wellness indicators from the major "pillars" of ActNow BC: smoke-free environments and behaviour; healthy nutrition; physical activity; healthy weight; and healthy pregnancy. While the CCHS collected data on alcohol consumption during pregnancy, the number of responses was too small for five HSDAs to provide complete provincial coverage for this indicator, and so it is not included in the group of maps in this chapter. The CCHS also provides data related to some key wellness determinants and wellness outcomes. The CCHS data are also collected across Canada so that provincial comparisons can be made if required.

What follows is a series of maps and tables that combine many of the indicators in a simple manner in order to identify the HSDAs that have the highest or "best" overall scores based on specific criteria. It also shows those that do less well, but our intent here is to highlight those that are the "best" based on the chosen indicators. The method used to develop these maps involves examining the responses to the CCHS questions and identifying those HSDAs having values that are statistically significantly higher or lower than the provincial average. Those that are significantly higher are given a "plus (+)" and those that are significantly lower are given a "minus (-)." The pluses and minuses are summed for each particular HSDA and then mapped based on the net score of pluses and minuses (negative numbers are taken away from positive numbers to give a net score). Although there are many different and sophisticated methods for combining indicators, our approach is simple, intuitive, and readily understandable by most individuals.

The first set of four maps presents information based on the set of indicators noted below for the age 12 and over population, the results of which are shown in the tables opposite.

Wellness determinants — Three indicators cover sense of belonging to community, emotional supports, and social supports.

Healthy outcomes — Eight indicators cover: mental health; free of chronic conditions; injury-free; repetitive strain injury-free; no restrictions to activities both inside and outside the home because of physical, mental, or other conditions; Health Utility Index (HUI); and satisfied with life. Two other variables in this group, perceived health and no sad or blue feeling, are not included because there were no HSDAs with either significantly high or low values and so there was no clear geographical variability in these indicators for the age 12 and over population as a whole.

Smoke-free environments and behaviour — Six indicators cover smoke-free public places, smoke-free work places, smoke-free vehicles, smoke-free homes, smoke-restricted homes, and non-smoking behaviour.

Healthy nutrition, physical activity, and weight — These three sets of indicators are dealt with as a single group because they are closely related from a wellness perspective. Six indicators cover fruit and vegetable consumption, availability of preferred foods, physical activity index, walking hours, satisfactory weight, and healthy BMI. Affordability of balanced meals was not included because there were no HSDAs with either significantly high or low values.

The second set of three maps provides a summary of 26 CCHS variables used in this Atlas together, based on the net results of totalling significantly high and significantly low (plus and minus) values by HSDA. Maps based on the table on page 212 are provided for the following groups:

• 20 to 64 middle age cohort for both sexes;

• 12 to 19 teen or youth age cohort for both sexes; and

• Age 65 and over seniors' cohort for both sexes.

This set of maps and tables enables us to identify an overall wellness value by HSDA based on the indicators included in the maps for the different sub-groups of the population based on age. The maps and supporting tables show which are the "best" or benchmark HSDAs based on differing age cohorts.

A final set of three maps, based on the table on page 213, provides the same information for age 12 and over, age 12 and over males, and age 12 and over females.

These maps and accompanying tables offer a variety of opportunities to identify those HSDAs that are the "best" or potential benchmarks in terms of wellness, and ones from which others may be able to learn if they wish to improve their own overall wellness. At the same time, they identify which HSDAs need most improvement and therefore provide an opportunity to target supports to enable them to improve certain wellness conditions.

Constructing benchmarks

Determinants of wellness

		Sense of belonging	Social supports	Emotional supports	Index
11	East Kootenay				0
12	Kootenay Boundary	+			+1
13	Okanagan		+		+1
14	Thompson Cariboo Shuswap	+			+1
21	Fraser East				0
22	Fraser North				0
23	Fraser South				0
31	Richmond		-	-	-2
32	Vancouver		-	-	-2
33	North Shore/Coast Garibaldi				0
41	South Vancouver Island				0
42	Central Vancouver Island				0
43	North Vancouver Island				0
51	Northwest	+			+1
52	Northern Interior				0
53	Northeast				0

Wellness outcomes

		Healthy	Mentally healthy	Not feeling sad or blue	No chronic conditions	Injury-free	No repetitive strain injury	No restricted activity outside	No restricted activity at home	Health Utilities Index	Satisfied with life	Index
11	East Kootenay							-	-			-2
12	Kootenay Boundary				-				-			-2
13	Okanagan				-				-			-2
14	Thompson Cariboo Shuswap										+	+1
21	Fraser East											0
22	Fraser North											0
23	Fraser South		+									+1
31	Richmond				+	+		+	+			+4
32	Vancouver				+			+	+			+3
33	North Shore/Coast Garibaldi				+		+					+2
41	South Vancouver Island				-				-			-3
42	Central Vancouver Island				-					-		-2
43	North Vancouver Island				-				-			-2
51	Northwest											0
52	Northern Interior											0
53	Northeast									-		-1

Smoke-free environments

		Smoke-free public	Smoke-free workplace	Smoke-free vehicles	Smoke-free home	Smoking restrictions in home	Currently non-smoker	Index
11	East Kootenay		-		-			-2
12	Kootenay Boundary							0
13	Okanagan							0
14	Thompson Cariboo Shuswap		-		-			-2
21	Fraser East	-	-					-2
22	Fraser North						+	+1
23	Fraser South	-						-1
31	Richmond		+	+			+	+3
32	Vancouver		+		+	-		+1
33	North Shore/Coast Garibaldi			+				+1
41	South Vancouver Island	+	+	+	+	+		+5
42	Central Vancouver Island		-					-1
43	North Vancouver Island						+	+1
51	Northwest							0
52	Northern Interior		-		-	-	-	-4
53	Northeast	-	-	-	-		-	-5

Healthy nutrition, physical activity, and weight

		Afford balanced meals	Always had preferred food	Fruits and vegetables	Physical Activity Index	Hours walking	Weight about right	Self-estimated BMI	Index
11	East Kootenay			+	+	+			+3
12	Kootenay Boundary					+			+1
13	Okanagan					-			-1
14	Thompson Cariboo Shuswap							-	-1
21	Fraser East					-	-	-	-3
22	Fraser North						+	+	+2
23	Fraser South					-			-1
31	Richmond					-		+	0
32	Vancouver		-			-	+	+	0
33	North Shore/Coast Garibaldi				+			+	+2
41	South Vancouver Island			+	+	+			+3
42	Central Vancouver Island			+		+	-	-	0
43	North Vancouver Island					-			-1
51	Northwest							-	-1
52	Northern Interior			-				-	-2
53	Northeast					-	-	-	-3

Overall wellness by age group: 26 CCHS indicators

Ages 12-19

#	Region	Sense of belonging	Social supports	Emotional supports	Smoke-free public	Smoke-free workplace	Smoke-free vehicles	Smoke-free home	Smoking restrictions in home	Currently non-smoker	Afford balanced meals	Always had preferred food	Fruits and vegetables	Physical Activity Index	Hours walking	Weight about right	Self-estimated BMI	Healthy	Mentally healthy	Not feeling sad or blue	No chronic conditions	Injury-free	No repetitive strain injury	No restricted activity outside	No restricted activity at home	Health Utilities Index	Satisfied with life	Index
11	East Kootenay													+	+			+	+									+4
12	Kootenay Boundary												+			+				+							+	+4
13	Okanagan																											0
14	Thompson Cariboo Shuswap																											0
21	Fraser East	+																										+1
22	Fraser North																											0
23	Fraser South																											0
31	Richmond						+	+												+								+3
32	Vancouver																											0
33	North Shore/Coast Garibaldi																											0
41	South Vancouver Island								+													-						0
42	Central Vancouver Island																											0
43	North Vancouver Island																											0
51	Northwest					+												+	+									+3
52	Northern Interior												-				-											-2
53	Northeast					-																						-1

Ages 20-64

#	Region	Sense of belonging	Social supports	Emotional supports	Smoke-free public	Smoke-free workplace	Smoke-free vehicles	Smoke-free home	Smoking restrictions in home	Currently non-smoker	Afford balanced meals	Always had preferred food	Fruits and vegetables	Physical Activity Index	Hours walking	Weight about right	Self-estimated BMI	Healthy	Mentally healthy	Not feeling sad or blue	No chronic conditions	Injury-free	No repetitive strain injury	No restricted activity outside	No restricted activity at home	Health Utilities Index	Satisfied with life	Index
11	East Kootenay					-								+	+	+								-	-			0
12	Kootenay Boundary															-									-			-2
13	Okanagan		+																									+1
14	Thompson Cariboo Shuswap	+				-											-										+	0
21	Fraser East					-									-	-	-											-4
22	Fraser North							+								+												+2
23	Fraser South				-											-						+	+					0
31	Richmond		-	-		+	+		+							-				+				+	+			+3
32	Vancouver		-	-		+	+	-								-	+	+		+				+	+			+3
33	North Shore/Coast Garibaldi						+							+			+			+			+					+5
41	South Vancouver Island					+	+	+	+					+	+	+								-	-			+5
42	Central Vancouver Island					-								+		+												+1
43	North Vancouver Island						-	+						+								-						0
51	Northwest	+			+												-											+1
52	Northern Interior		+			-		-	-								-											-3
53	Northeast					-		-	-	-	+			-		-	-											-6

Ages 65+

#	Region	Sense of belonging	Social supports	Emotional supports	Smoke-free public	Smoke-free workplace	Smoke-free vehicles	Smoke-free home	Smoking restrictions in home	Currently non-smoker	Afford balanced meals	Always had preferred food	Fruits and vegetables	Physical Activity Index	Hours walking	Weight about right	Self-estimated BMI	Healthy	Mentally healthy	Not feeling sad or blue	No chronic conditions	Injury-free	No repetitive strain injury	No restricted activity outside	No restricted activity at home	Health Utilities Index	Satisfied with life	Index
11	East Kootenay															+												+1
12	Kootenay Boundary	+																						+				+2
13	Okanagan											+																+1
14	Thompson Cariboo Shuswap																											0
21	Fraser East											+			-													0
22	Fraser North																											0
23	Fraser South																											0
31	Richmond																					+		+				+2
32	Vancouver		-	-											-													-3
33	North Shore/Coast Garibaldi						+				+							+										+3
41	South Vancouver Island					+										+												+2
42	Central Vancouver Island																-											-1
43	North Vancouver Island			+																		+					+	+3
51	Northwest						+																					+1
52	Northern Interior					-					-	-	-			-												-5
53	Northeast					-						-				-												-3

Overall wellness for ages 12 and over

Both Sexes

	Region	Sense of belonging	Social supports	Emotional supports	Smoke-free public	Smoke-free workplace	Smoke-free vehicles	Smoke-free home	Smoking restrictions in home	Currently non-smoker	Afford balanced meals	Always had preferred food	Fruits and vegetables	Physical Activity Index	Hours walking	Weight about right	Self-estimated BMI	Healthy	Mentally healthy	Not feeling sad or blue	No chronic conditions	Injury-free	No repetitive strain injury	No restricted activity outside	No restricted activity at home	Health Utilities Index	Satisfied with life	Index
11	East Kootenay					-		-					+	+	+									-	-			-1
12	Kootenay Boundary	+														+					-				-			0
13	Okanagan		+													-					-				-			-2
14	Thompson Cariboo Shuswap	+				-		-									-										+	-1
21	Fraser East					-	-									-	-	-										-5
22	Fraser North									+						+	+											+3
23	Fraser South				-											-			+									-1
31	Richmond		-	-		+	+			+						-		+			+	+		+	+			+5
32	Vancouver		-	-		+		+	-		-					-	+	+						+		+	+	+2
33	North Shore/Coast Garibaldi						+							+			+				+		+					+5
41	South Vancouver Island				+	+	+	+	+				+	+	+									-	-	-		+5
42	Central Vancouver Island					-							+			+	-	-			-						-	-3
43	North Vancouver Island							+								-					-				-			-2
51	Northwest	+															-											0
52	Northern Interior					-		-	-	-			-			-												-6
53	Northeast					-	-	-	-	-						-	-										-	-9

Males

	Region	Sense of belonging	Social supports	Emotional supports	Smoke-free public	Smoke-free workplace	Smoke-free vehicles	Smoke-free home	Smoking restrictions in home	Currently non-smoker	Afford balanced meals	Always had preferred food	Fruits and vegetables	Physical Activity Index	Hours walking	Weight about right	Self-estimated BMI	Healthy	Mentally healthy	Not feeling sad or blue	No chronic conditions	Injury-free	No repetitive strain injury	No restricted activity outside	No restricted activity at home	Health Utilities Index	Satisfied with life	Index
11	East Kootenay					-							+	+	+									-				+1
12	Kootenay Boundary																								-		-	-1
13	Okanagan																				-				-			-2
14	Thompson Cariboo Shuswap					-											-										+	-1
21	Fraser East															-	-	-										-3
22	Fraser North																							+				+1
23	Fraser South																											0
31	Richmond		-			+																		+	+			+2
32	Vancouver		-	-		+		+	-								+							+				+1
33	North Shore/Coast Garibaldi						+																					+1
41	South Vancouver Island				+		+	+								+	+							-	-			+3
42	Central Vancouver Island					-											+											0
43	North Vancouver Island							+																			-	0
51	Northwest	+																										+1
52	Northern Interior					-													-									-2
53	Northeast					-	-	-	-	-						-	-										-	-8

Females

	Region	Sense of belonging	Social supports	Emotional supports	Smoke-free public	Smoke-free workplace	Smoke-free vehicles	Smoke-free home	Smoking restrictions in home	Currently non-smoker	Afford balanced meals	Always had preferred food	Fruits and vegetables	Physical Activity Index	Hours walking	Weight about right	Self-estimated BMI	Healthy	Mentally healthy	Not feeling sad or blue	No chronic conditions	Injury-free	No repetitive strain injury	No restricted activity outside	No restricted activity at home	Health Utilities Index	Satisfied with life	Index
11	East Kootenay	-														+												0
12	Kootenay Boundary															+					-						+	+1
13	Okanagan																											0
14	Thompson Cariboo Shuswap	+															-											0
21	Fraser East							+									-							+				+1
22	Fraser North	-																										-1
23	Fraser South																											0
31	Richmond		-	-			+		+							-					+	+				+		+2
32	Vancouver		-	-		+			-							-	+	+						+			+	+1
33	North Shore/Coast Garibaldi																											0
41	South Vancouver Island						+						+	+	+	-												+3
42	Central Vancouver Island					+		+								+											-	+2
43	North Vancouver Island							+								+												+2
51	Northwest																-							-				-2
52	Northern Interior		+	+						-						-											+	+1
53	Northeast					-	-	-									-											-4

Determinants and outcomes of wellness

We have combined these two clusters as they provide some of the key indicators that help determine overall wellness and show wellness outcomes.

Determinants of wellness index

Looking at the summary map and tables for this group of three variables (sense of belonging, social supports, and emotional supports), it is clear that for most HSDAs there was little difference among them. Of the 16 regional HSDAs, 10 had an overall score of zero (0), indicating that they were not significantly different in a statistical sense from provincial average values for any of these indicators.

A second group consists of four HSDAs that did have a statistically significantly higher value than for the province as a whole for one of the three indicators and are shown with a positive value (score of +1). All four of the HSDAs were in the interior or northern parts of the province, which are more rural in nature and whose populations are spread out among smaller communities. A higher than average sense of belonging was evident in Kootenay Boundary, Thompson Cariboo Shuswap, and Northwest, while stronger social supports emerged in the Okanagan.

The third group consists of two urban HSDAs, Vancouver and Richmond in the southwest, which both had significantly lower values for emotional and social support (score of -2).

Health Service Delivery Area	Determinants
012 Kootenay Boundary	+1
013 Okanagan	+1
014 Thompson Cariboo Shuswap	+1
051 Northwest	+1
011 East Kootenay	0
021 Fraser East	0
022 Fraser North	0
023 Fraser South	0
033 North Shore/Coast Garibaldi	0
041 South Vancouver Island	0
042 Central Vancouver Island	0
043 North Vancouver Island	0
052 Northern Interior	0
053 Northeast	0
031 Richmond	-2
032 Vancouver	-2

Wellness outcomes index

This summary map shows greater variation than for determinants, which is expected, given that there are twice as many indicators in this cluster of variables (perceived health, mental health, feeling sad or blue, no chronic conditions, injury-free, no repetitive strain injury, no restrictions of activity inside or outside the home, Health Utilities Index, and satisfied with life). Three major groups of HSDAs emerged. Five HSDAs had positive numbers overall. With one exception (Thompson Cariboo Shuswap in the central interior of the province), all were located in the urban lower mainland. Richmond had significant positive values for 4 of the 10 indicators (score +4), while Vancouver (score +3) and North Shore/Coast Garibaldi (score +2) also scored relatively well.

There were seven HSDAs with overall negative values. These were clustered on Vancouver Island and in the northeast, southeast, and southern interior parts of the province. All other regions (score of 0) were the same as average provincial values for these indicators.

Health Service Delivery Area	Outcomes
031 Richmond	+4
032 Vancouver	+3
033 North Shore/Coast Garibaldi	+2
014 Thompson Cariboo Shuswap	+1
023 Fraser South	+1
021 Fraser East	0
022 Fraser North	0
051 Northwest	0
052 Northern Interior	0
053 Northeast	-1
042 Central Vancouver Island	-2
011 East Kootenay	-2
012 Kootenay Boundary	-2
013 Okanagan	-2
043 North Vancouver Island	-2
041 South Vancouver Island	-3

What is this telling us?

There was relatively little differentiation between regions in the province related to determinants indicators. What emerges is that the urban southwest of the province, especially Vancouver and Richmond, had significantly high percentages of respondents who were not well-connected within their communities. On the other hand, in more rural areas there was a strong attachment to community. From a benchmarking perspective, no HSDA dominates. From an outcome perspective, it was the lower mainland HSDAs that were prominent. Although Richmond rated low on the determinants scale, ironically, it was the benchmark (best) HSDA for outcomes.

Determinants and outcomes of wellness

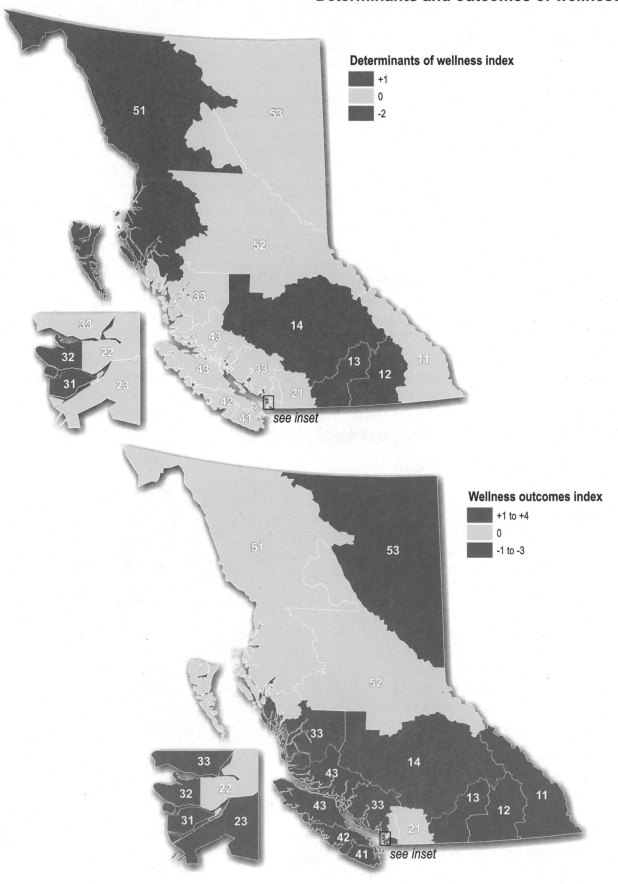

Determinants of wellness index

- +1
- 0
- -2

Wellness outcomes index

- +1 to +4
- 0
- -1 to -3

Smoke-free index

As noted earlier, the effect of smoking on health and wellness, particularly as it affects chronic disease, is still very high in BC despite the province having the lowest smoking rate in the country. The map of combined smoke-free behaviours and environments shows some major geographical variations and points to at least one HSDA that could be considered a leader based on this cluster of six indicators (smoke-free public places, smoke-free workplaces, smoke-free vehicles, smoke-free homes, smoking restrictions in home, and non-smoking behaviour).

There was a large range in scores among the regions, with a general southwest to northeast gradient based on positive to negative scores. The highest net positive scores occurred in the southwest of the province, particularly South Vancouver Island (score of +5), Richmond (score of +3), and Fraser North, Vancouver, and North Shore/Coast Garibaldi (all with scores of +1). North Vancouver Island was an outlier in terms of its positive score outside of the lower island and lower mainland. Vancouver was also unusual in that it scored significantly high for two indicators but significantly low on another for a net score of +1.

At the other extreme, northern and interior communities were more likely to have negative scores among this cluster of indicators. Northeast (score of -5) and Northern Interior (-4) had significantly poorer smoke-free environments than the province as a whole. Thompson Cariboo Shuswap in the central interior, East Kootenay in the southeast, and Fraser East (all with scores of -2) scored poorly among this group of indicators. Other negative scores occurred for Fraser South in the lower mainland and Central Vancouver Island (both with scores of -1).

Health Service Delivery Area	Smoke-free index
041 South Vancouver Island	+5
031 Richmond	+3
022 Fraser North	+1
032 Vancouver	+1
033 North Shore/Coast Garibaldi	+1
043 North Vancouver Island	+1
012 Kootenay Boundary	0
013 Okanagan	0
051 Northwest	0
023 Fraser South	-1
042 Central Vancouver Island	-1
011 East Kootenay	-2
014 Thompson Cariboo Shuswap	-2
021 Fraser East	-2
052 Northern Interior	-4
053 Northeast	-5

What is this telling us?

South Vancouver Island was clearly the benchmark HSDA, scoring significantly higher than the provincial average on five of the six indicators included in this analysis. A consideration of some of the other indicators related to smoke-free environments shows that South Vancouver Island also has very strong municipal by-laws related to no smoking and has had restrictions in place for well over a decade. Victoria, within the HSDA, had its first municipal no smoking by-law as early as 1984 and, as the seat of provincial administration, the introduction of a smoke-free workplace for provincial offices in 1990 also likely helped in promoting the need for smoke-free environments.

Richmond, with significantly positive scores for half of the indicators, is also worth considering as a benchmark. It too has a strong municipal no smoking by-law, thus setting an example for the region.

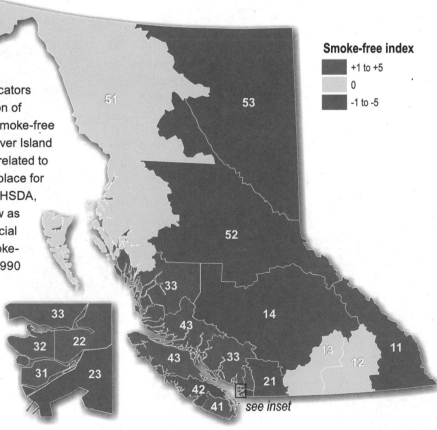

Smoke-free index
- +1 to +5
- 0
- -1 to -5

see inset

Nutrition, activity, and weight index

Three separate but related groups of indicators are provided. They deal with indicators for nutrition (afford balanced meals, availability of preferred food, fruit and vegetable consumption), physical activity (Physical Activity Index, hours walking), and healthy weights (satisfied with weight, BMI). The scores ranged from +3 to –3. The southwest and southeast regions of the province both had net positive scores.

South Vancouver Island in the southwest and East Kootenay in the southeast had leading scores of +3. Both had significantly higher values for fruit and vegetable consumption, Physical Activity Index, and walking 6 or more hours a week. Other HSDAs with net positive scores were found in the lower mainland and the southeast. Fraser North was significantly high for the two weight indicators. Vancouver also rated high on these two indicators, but these were negated by significantly low values for two other indicators.

Much of the northern half of the province was significantly lower than the provincial average on several indicators, as was part of the interior, North Vancouver Island, and Fraser South in the lower mainland. Northeast (score -3), Northern Interior (score -2), and Fraser East (score -3) had the poorest net scores.

Along with Vancouver, two other HSDAs, Richmond and Central Vancouver Island, had net scores of zero (0), as positive attributes were cancelled out by negative ones within the cluster of six indicators.

Health Service Delivery Area	Nutrition, activity, and weight index
011 East Kootenay	+3
041 South Vancouver Island	+3
022 Fraser North	+2
033 North Shore/Coast Garibaldi	+2
012 Kootenay Boundary	+1
031 Richmond	0
032 Vancouver	0
042 Central Vancouver Island	0
013 Okanagan	-1
014 Thompson Cariboo Shuswap	-1
023 Fraser South	-1
043 North Vancouver Island	-1
051 Northwest	-1
052 Northern Interior	-2
021 Fraser East	-3
053 Northeast	-3

What is this telling us?

There are three benchmark HSDAs worth considering based on this cluster of indicators. South Vancouver Island, as a largely urban region, scored well for nutrition and physical activity, as did East Kootenay, a rural region. Both were neutral on the weight indicators, but Fraser North scored significantly higher than the provincial average for the two healthy weight indicators.

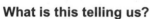

Nutrition, activity, and weight index

- +1 to +3
- 0
- -1 to -3

see inset

Overall wellness index by age group: 26 CCHS indicators

The three maps and table have combined 26 of the CCHS indicators contained within the Atlas and provide an overall wellness index score based on these indicators. Indicators are given equal weight. Scores can range from +26 to -26. The highest potential positive score (+26) would be achieved if one HSDA had a statistically significantly higher value than the provincial averages for each of the 26 indicators. Likewise, there is a lowest possible score (-26). The three age groups used here are the ones used throughout the Atlas: 20- to 64-year-olds; 12- to 19-year-olds; and, 65 and older. It is possible to identify which HSDAs can be viewed as the benchmark for the three age groups individually.

Health Service Delivery Area	Ages 20-64	Ages 12-19	Ages 65+
033 North Shore/Coast Garibaldi	+5	0	+3
041 South Vancouver Island	+5	0	+2
032 Vancouver	+3	0	-3
031 Richmond	+3	+3	+2
022 Fraser North	+2	0	0
042 Central Vancouver Island	+1	0	-1
013 Okanagan	+1	0	+1
051 Northwest	+1	+3	+1
011 East Kootenay	0	+4	+1
023 Fraser South	0	0	0
043 North Vancouver Island	0	-1	+3
014 Thompson Cariboo Shuswap	0	0	0
012 Kootenay Boundary	-2	+4	+2
052 Northern Interior	-3	-2	-5
021 Fraser East	-4	+1	0
053 Northeast	-6	-1	-3

20 to 64 age group index

The range from highest to lowest went from +5 to -6. Eight HSDAs had positive scores and four had negative scores. The remainder had a net score of zero. The higher positive scores were clustered in the urban southwest and southern part of Vancouver Island, while negative scores were more prominent in the north and interior.

North Shore/Coast Garibaldi and South Vancouver Island had the highest scores (+5) and, from a benchmarking perspective, they were the best overall HSDAs in this age category. While the former had five significantly high indicators and no significantly low indicators, South Vancouver Island had seven positive indicators offset by two negative ones (both related to restricted activities because of chronic conditions). Richmond and Vancouver (both with scores of +3) had a higher number of positive variables, but scores were reduced because of offsetting negative score variables.

12 to 19 age group index

This group ranged from +4 to -2. Half of the HSDAs (8) had net values of zero (0). Geographically, the southeast part of the province had the best values, with youth in both East Kootenay and Kootenay Boundary having scores of +4. Neither had any significantly negative score indicators, and these would be the benchmark HSDAs for youth. Richmond, Northwest, and Fraser East were positive overall. Only Northern Interior, North Vancouver Island, and Northeast had negative scores.

65 and over age group index

The seniors group had a range of eight points between HSDAs. North Shore/Coast Garibaldi and North Vancouver Island were the benchmarks (both with scores of +3). Neither HSDA had any significantly negative values for the 26 indicators. There was no clear overall geographic pattern for seniors, although two northern regions had negative scores (Northern Interior with -5 and Northeast with -3). Vancouver in the lower mainland (-3) and Central Vancouver Island (-1) were also negative.

What is this telling us?

For the middle age cohort, 20 to 64 years, there were two HSDAs, both urban, that can be considered benchmarks. These were South Vancouver Island and North Shore/Coast Garibaldi. Both rated highly overall, although South Vancouver Island had several indicators that were significantly negative, offsetting other positive scores. For youth (12 to 19 age group), the two HSDAs in the rural southeast of the province, East Kootenay and Kootenay Boundary, rated highest and can be considered benchmark regions. For the urban areas, Richmond might also be considered a benchmark. North Vancouver Island for rural communities can be considered the benchmark for seniors (65 years and over), while North Shore/Coast Garibaldi might be best for urban regions.

Overall wellness index by age group: 26 CCHS indicators

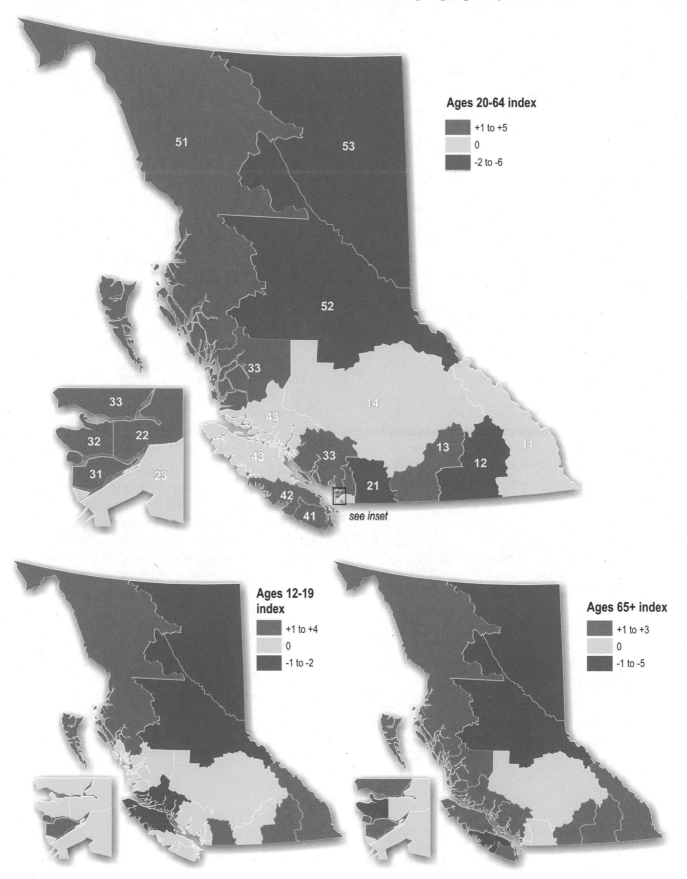

Ages 20-64 index

- +1 to +5
- 0
- -2 to -6

Ages 12-19 index

- +1 to +4
- 0
- -1 to -2

Ages 65+ index

- +1 to +3
- 0
- -1 to -5

see inset

Overall wellness index for ages 12 and over

The three maps and table presented here provide scores for the total CCHS sample, and individually for males and females. The scores are developed in the same way as for the previous three maps. Positive and negative indicators are offset against each other to give an overall wellness score.

Provincial population, 12 and over index

The range between the highest and lowest scoring HSDAs was 14. The highest, and therefore the benchmarks for the total sample group, were South Vancouver Island, North Shore/Coast Garibaldi, and Richmond, all with a net positive score of +5. In achieving these scores, North Shore/Coast Garibaldi had no negative value indicators, while South Vancouver Island and Richmond both had a total of eight statistically significantly high value indicators offset by three statistically significantly low values. For South Vancouver Island, these low values were related to chronic conditions and conditions that interfered with normal activities both inside and outside the home. For Richmond, the negative values related to emotional and social supports and hours walking. At the other end of the spectrum, Northern Interior (-6), Northeast (-9), and Fraser East (-5) had negative scores overall, and none of the three had any significantly positive value indicators.

Males index

There was a range of 11 points for males. Southern Vancouver Island with a score of +3 was the benchmark HSDA. Richmond (score of +2) and Vancouver, Northwest, East Kootenay, and North Shore/Coast Garibaldi (all with scores of +1) were also positive. Close to half of the HSDAs had overall net negative scores. Northeast was particularly notable for its high negative score (-8).

As the benchmark HSDA for males, South Vancouver Island had a total of five significantly positive indicators offset by two significantly low value indicators (both related to conditions that restrict activities inside and outside the home).

Females index

The range was only 7 points for females, indicating relatively more equity in wellness than for males among the regions. Only three HSDAs had net negative scores

Health Service Delivery Area	All respondents	Males	Female
041 South Vancouver Island	+5	+3	+3
031 Richmond	+5	+2	+2
033 North Shore/Coast Garibaldi	+5	+1	0
022 Fraser North	+3	+1	-1
032 Vancouver	+2	+1	+1
051 Northwest	0	+1	-2
012 Kootenay Boundary	0	-1	+1
011 East Kootenay	-1	+1	0
023 Fraser South	-1	0	0
014 Thompson Cariboo Shuswap	-1	-1	0
042 Central Vancouver Island	-2	0	+2
043 North Vancouver Island	-2	0	+2
013 Okanagan	-2	-2	0
021 Fraser East	-5	-3	+1
052 Northern Interior	-6	-2	+1
053 Northeast	-9	-8	-4

(Northeast, -4; Northwest, -2; and Fraser North, -1). South Vancouver Island had the highest positive score (+3), followed by Central and North Vancouver Island and Richmond (all with scores of +2). Vancouver (+1) had the highest number of statistically significantly positive indicators (5), but these were offset by negative indicators (4).

What is this telling us?

For all age groups combined (ages 12 and over), South Vancouver Island, Richmond, and North Shore/Coast Garibaldi were the "best" HSDAs and can be considered as the overall benchmarks for wellness in the province. South Vancouver Island and Richmond, though, both had a couple of significant negative factors that need to be taken into account. For both males and females individually, South Vancouver Island was also the benchmark HSDA.

Overall wellness index for ages 12 and over

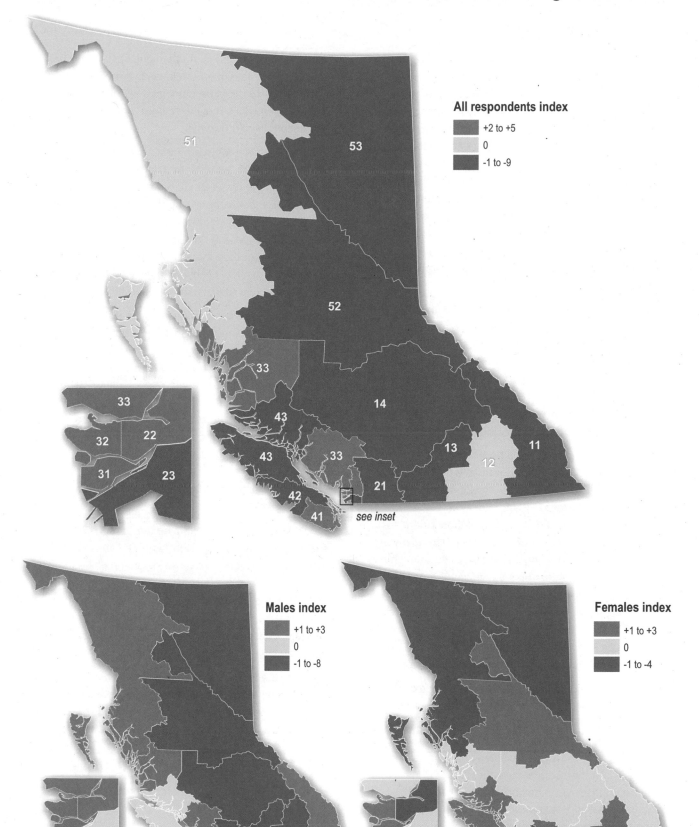

All respondents index
- +2 to +5
- 0
- -1 to -9

Males index
- +1 to +3
- 0
- -1 to -8

Females index
- +1 to +3
- 0
- -1 to -4

see inset

A Final Word

We hope that the data, tables, and maps produced in this Atlas will give users enough information to ask themselves: Why do we get so much regional variation in wellness-related indicators? Is this variation something that should be addressed? If so, what can be done, and which areas rate highly enough that we might want to learn from them? As noted earlier, the maps should, to a large degree, "speak for themselves." The text just points out some of their key features. It should be emphasized, however, that the maps are static and give a pattern at one point in time, in most cases 2005, the year that ActNow BC was initiated. Updates can be provided over time as new information becomes available.

For many of the indicators we have used in this Atlas, wellness decreased as distance from the urban lower mainland part of the province and South Vancouver Island increased. This is a very dominant pattern throughout the Atlas. It confirms other studies that have noted the difference in health and wellness between urban and rural regions, not only in BC, but elsewhere in Canada.

The examples used to develop benchmarks are just that—examples. Users can develop their own group or clusters of indicators in order to develop benchmarks that might be important to them. For example, some indicators could be given more weight than others so that, say, "non-smoking behaviour" has twice as much importance as "frequenting public places that are smoke free." Nutrition indicators may be weighted more highly than activity-related indicators. Groups of indicators and weights might be developed through a community process, through the use of technical groups, or through focus groups. Analyses and comparisons can be made in numerous ways, depending on community priorities.

Other wellness indicators can be added. For example, many of the non-CCHS indicators could be included by giving a positive value for those HSDAs that are in the highest quintile, and a negative value for those in the lowest quintile. Negative values could be ignored altogether. Further, communities or HSDAs can compare themselves to neighbouring HSDAs or to those in the same Health Authority. For example, South Vancouver Island could become the benchmark for the Vancouver Island Health Authority, or Richmond for the Vancouver Coastal Health Authority. Individuals

specifically interested in youth might want to convert the school district data to HSDA level data so that indicators from the CCHS might be combined with school district data, or even with survey data from the McCreary Adolescent Health Surveys.

The main points to note are, first, that the possibilities are immense and, second, that different geographical areas within the province can learn from each other in terms of what has been accomplished on different wellness indicators. How did the "best" become the "best"? Our approach has been to use clusters of indicators rather than focusing on just a very limited number of factors. This helps to achieve, we believe, an overall picture of wellness in a particular area.

In conclusion, we see this Atlas as the start, not the finish, of understanding geographical variations in wellness throughout the province. We have taken available data that can be updated over time, and combined indicators to develop benchmark HSDAs. These are HSDAs that have achieved the "best" statistically significant results somewhere in the province. There will undoubtedly be better results at a smaller community level. There will be geographical "highs" and "lows" within all of the HSDAs because they cover a large geographical area and/or have a large population.

A next step might be to examine the "best" HSDAs and see what they are doing "right" to obtain the results that they have achieved. Are there key communities within them that make the difference? A good understanding of the processes and conditions that help to create the "best" results can then be used, to some degree, by others to do the same. Processes can be adapted to the local conditions within any HSDA.

We hope that this Atlas will contribute to the discussion of why some regions are more "well" than others and what might be done about it, and how ActNow BC can help focus and target its resources and those of its numerous partners to achieve overall improvements in the health and wellness of people in British Columbia.

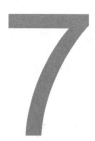

References

ActNowBC (2006). *Measuring our success: Baseline document*. Victoria: ActNowBC.

Adams, T., Bezner, J., and Steinhardt, M. (1997). The conceptualization and measurement of perceived wellness: Integrating balance across and within dimensions. *American Journal of Health Promotion*, 11, 208-218.

Adams, T.B. (2003). The power of perceptions: Measuring wellness in a globally acceptable, philosophically consistent way. Wellness Management. *www.hedir.org*.

Anderson, G.S, Snodgrass, J., and Elliott, B. (2007). Determining physical activity patterns of suburban British Columbia residents. *Canadian Journal of Public Health*, 98(1), 70-73.

Annas, J. (1993). *The morality of happiness*. Oxford: Oxford University Press.

Anspaugh, D., Hamrick, M., and Rosato, F. (2004). *Wellness: Concepts and applications*, 6th ed. Boston: McGraw Hill.

Ardell, D.B. (2005). What is wellness? *Ardell Wellness Report*, 69(Winter), 1.

Arnup, K. (1994). *Education for motherhood: Advice for mothers in twentieth-century Canada*. Toronto: University of Toronto Press.

Atlas of Canada (2004). People and society. Quality of life. *http://atlas.nrcan.gc.ca/site/english/maps/peopleandsociety#QOL*.

Barrett, P.H. (1980). *Metaphysics, materialism, and the evolution of mind. Early writings of Charles Darwin*. Chicago: University of Chicago Press.

Banks, R. (1980). Health and the spiritual dimension: Relationships and implications for professional preparation programs. *Journal of School Health*, 50, 195-202.

Barr, S. (2004). *British Columbia Nutrition Survey: Report on physical activity and body weight*. Victoria: Ministry of Health Services.

Bellows, A.C., and Hamm, M.W. (2003). International origins of community food security policies and practices in the US. *Critical Public Health*, 13(2), 107-123.

Berghaus, H.K.W. (1845). *Physikalischer Atlas*, 2 vols. Gotha.

Berkman, L., and Kawachi, I. (Eds.) (2000). *Social epidemiology*. Oxford, NY: Oxford University Press.

Blot, W.J., Harrington, J.M., Toledo, A., Hoover, R., Heath, C.W. Jr., and Fraumeni, J.F. Jr. (1978). Lung cancer after employment in shipyards during World War II. *New England Journal of Medicine*, 299, 620-624.

Blot, W.J., Davies, J.E., Brown, L.M, Nordwall, C.W., Buiatti, E., Ng, A., and Fraumeni. J.F. Jr. (1982). Occupation and the high risk of lung cancer in Northeast Florida. *Cancer*, 50, 364-371.

Blot, W.J., Morris, L.E., Stroube, R., Tagnon, I., and Fraumeni, J.F. Jr. (1980). Lung and laryngeal cancers in relation to shipyard employment in coastal Virginia. *Journal of the National Cancer Institute*, 65, 571-575.

Bouchard, C., Shephard, R.J., and Stephens, T. (1994). *Physical activity, fitness and health*. Champaign, IL: Human Kinetics.

Boulos, M.N.K. (2004). Towards evidence-based, GIS-driven national spatial health information infrastructure and surveillance services in the United Kingdom. *International Journal of Health Geographics*, 3, 1.

Breastfeeding Committee for Canada (BCC) (2003). *The Ten Steps and Practice Outcome Indicators for Baby-Friendly™ Hospitals*. Toronto: BCC.

Bridge, J., and Turpin, B. (2004). *The cost of smoking in British Columbia and the economics of tobacco control*. Ottawa: Health Canada.

BC Select Standing Committee on Health (2004). *The path to health and wellness: Making British Columbians healthier by 2010: Select Standing Committee on Health first report*. Victoria, BC: Legislative Assembly, Select Standing Committee on Health.

BC Select Standing Committee on Health (2006). *A strategy for combating childhood obesity and physical inactivity in British Columbia*. Victoria, BC: Legislative Assembly, Select Standing Committee on Health.

BC Healthy Living Alliance (2005a). *The winning legacy: A plan for improving the health of British Columbians by 2010*. Vancouver: Author.

BC Healthy Living Alliance (2005b). *Risk factor Interventions: An overview of their effectiveness*. Vancouver: Author.

BC Recreation and Parks Association (2004). *Phase One – Inventory. British Columbia community recreation facilities assessment study*. Prepared by Hughes Condon Marler for BCRPA, Burnaby.

BC Recreation and Parks Association (2006a). *Phase 2 – Inventory. Parks and natural areas comparative study*. Prepared by Hughes Condon Marler for BCRPA, Burnaby.

BC Recreation and Parks Association (2006b). *Phase 3 – Inventory. Community centres, youth centres, senior centres and community halls*. Prepared by Hughes Condon Marler for BCRPA, Burnaby.

BC Stats (2003). Special feature: BC immigrant population. Victoria: Ministry of Management Services. *www.bcstats.gov.bc.ca/data/dd/details.asp*. Accessed December, 2006.

BC Stats (2004). Socio-economic profiles: Health Service Delivery Areas. Victoria: Ministry of Labour and Consumer Services. *www.bcstats.gov.bc.ca/data/sep/hsda/hs_main.asp*. Accessed December, 2006.

BC Stats (2004a). 2001 census facts: BC Aboriginal identity population. August. Victoria: Ministry of Management Services. *www.bcstats.gov.bc.ca/data/cen01/facts/cff0108.PDF*. Accessed December, 2006.

BC Stats (2004b). 2001 census fast facts: BC Aboriginal identity population. Band membership, status, on/off reserve. August. Victoria: Ministry of Management Services. *www.bcstats.gov.bc.ca/data/cen01/facts/cff0109.PDF*. Accessed December, 2006.

BC Stats (2007). Social Statistics. *www.bcstats.gov.bc.ca/data/lss/social.asp*. Accessed July, 2007.

Broemeling, A-M., Watson, D., and Black, C. (2005). *Chronic conditions and co-morbidity among residents of British Columbia*. Vancouver: UBC Centre for Health Services and Policy.

Brynelsen, D., Conry, J., and Loock, C. (1998). *Community action guide: Working together for the prevention of fetal alcohol syndrome*. BC FAS Resource Society. Victoria, BC: Ministry for Children and Families.

Bullen, N., Moon, G., and Jones, K. (1996). Defining localities for health planning: A GIS approach. *Social Science Medicine*, 42(6), 801-816.

Burglehaus, M. (2004). Pregnancy outreach programs. *Visions Journal*, 2(4), 47.

Burr, K.F., McKee, B., Foster, L.T., and Nault, F. (1995). Interprovincial data requirements for local indicators: The British Columbia experience. *Health Reports*, 7(2), 17-24.

Campbell, D.E. (2006). What is education's impact on civic and social engagement? In R. Desjardins and T. Schuller (Eds.), *Proceedings of the Copenhagen Symposium: Measuring the effects of education on health and civic engagement* (pp. 25-108). Paris: Organisation for Economic Co-operation and Development.

Canada Mortgage and Housing Corporation (CMHC). (1996). *Quality of life indicators: A pilot test of the community-oriented model of lived environment*. Ottawa: Canada Mortgage and Housing Corporation.

Canadian Council on Learning (2006). Composite learning index. *www.experiencedesignernetwork.com/archives/000708.html*. Accessed February 15, 2007.

Canadian Council on Learning (2007). State of learning in Canada: No time for complacency. *www.ccl-cca.ca/CCL/Reports/StateofLearning?Language=EN*. Accessed March 10, 2007.

Canadian Institute for Advanced Research (1991). *The determinants of health* (CIAR Publication No. 5). Toronto: Author.

Canadian Institute for Health Information (2004). *Improving the health of Canadians*. Ottawa: Canadian Population Health Initiative.

Canadian Institute for Health Information (2005). *Improving the health of young Canadians*. Ottawa: Canadian Population Health Initiative.

Canadian Institute for Health Information (2005a). *Developing a healthy communities index: A collection of papers.* Ottawa: Author.

Canadian Institute for Health Information (2005b). Select Highlights on Public Views about the Social Determinants of Health. *http://secure.cihi.ca/cihiweb/products/CPHI_Public_Views_FINAL_e.pdf.* Accessed March, 2007.

Canadian Institute for Health Information (2006). *How healthy are rural Canadians? An assessment of their health status and health determinants.* Ottawa: Author.

Canadian Institute for Health Information (2006a). *Improving the health of Canadians: Promoting healthy weights.* Ottawa: Canadian Population Health Initiative.

Canadian Institute for Health Information (2006b). *Improving the health of Canadians: An introduction to health in urban places.* Ottawa: Canadian Population Health Initiative.

Canadian Public Health Association (2004). ParticipACTION: The mouse that roared. A marketing and health communications success story. *Canadian Journal of Public Health,* 95(2).

Centre for Health Services and Policy Research (nd). Mapping Health and Health Care in British Columbia. Vancouver: Centre for Health Services and Policy Research, University of British Columbia. *www.chspr.ubc.ca/cgi-bin/pub.* Accessed February, 2007.

Clark, C.C. (1996). *Wellness practitioner: Concepts, research, and strategies.* New York: Springer Publishing Co.

Cole, T.J., Bellizzi, M.C., Fliegal, K.M., and Dietz, W.H. (2000). Establishing a standard definition for child overweight and obesity worldwide: International survey. *British Medical Journal,* 320, 1-6.

Cooper, K.H. (1968). *Aerobics.* New York: Bantam

Cooper, K.H. (1970). Guidelines in the management of the exercising patient. *Journal of the American Medical Association,* 211(10), 1663-1667.

Cooper, K.H. (1975). An aerobics conditioning program for the Fort Worth, Texas, School District. *Research Quarterly,* 46(3), 345-50.

Cooper, K.H. (1977). *The aerobics way.* New York: Evans.

Cowley, P., and Easton, S. (2006). *Report card on Aboriginal education in British Columbia. Studies in Education Policy.* Vancouver: The Fraser Institute.

Crose, R., Nicholas, D.R., Gobble, D.C., and Frank, B. (1992). Gender and wellness: A multidimensional systems model for counseling. *Journal of Counseling and Development,* 77, 149-156.

Cutter, S.L., (1985). *Rating places: A geographer's view on quality of life.* Washington, DC: Association of American Geographers.

Danderfer, K., Wright, M., and Foster, L.T. (2006). *Towards improving well-being of children from deprived backgrounds.* Paper presented at the World Forum 2006: Future directions in child welfare. Vancouver, November, 22.

Danderfer, R.J., and Foster, L.T. (Eds.) (1993). *Selected vital statistics and health status indicators: One hundred and twenty-first annual report 1992.* Victoria, BC: Crown Publications Inc.

Danderfer, R.J., and Cronin, R.E. (Eds.) (1994). *Selected vital statistics and health status indicators: One hundred and twenty-second annual report 1993.* Victoria, BC: Crown Publications Inc.

Danderfer, R.J., and Cronin, R.F. (Eds.). (1995). Selected vital statistics and health status indicators: one hundred and twenty-third annual report 1994. Victoria, British Columbia: Crown Publications Inc

DeNeve, K.M., and Cooper, H. (1998). The happy personality: A meta-analysis of 137 personality traits and subjective well-being. *Psychological Bulletin,* 124, 197-229.

Depken, D. (1994). Wellness through the lens of gender: A paradigm shift. *Wellness Perspectives: Research, Theory, and Practice,* 70, 54-69.

Desjardins, R., and Schuller, T. (2006). Introduction: Understanding the social outcomes of learning. In R. Desjardins and T. Schuller (Eds). Proceedings of the Copenhagen Symposium: Measuring the effects of education on health and civic engagement. Organisation for Economic Co-operation and Development.

Devesa, S.S., Grauman, D.J., Blot, W.J., Pennello, G.A., Hoover, R.N., and Fraumeni, J.F. Jr. (1999). *Atlas of Cancer Mortality in the United States: 1950-1994* NIH Publication No. 99-4564. Washington: National Cancer Institute.

Diener, E., Eunkook, M., Suh, M., Lucas, E., and Smith, H.L. (1999). Subjective well-being: Three decades of progress. *Psychological Bulletin: American Psychological Association,* 125(20), 273-302.

Diez-Roux, A.V. (1998). Bringing context back into epidemiology: Variables and fallacies in multilevel analysis. *American Journal of Public Health,* 88, 216-222.

Discovery Research (2006). *International Physical Activity Questionnaire (IPAQ) Telephone survey: BC results*. Burnaby, BC: British Columbia Recreation and Parks Association.

Donatelle, R., Snow, C., and Wilcox, A. (1999). *Wellness: Choices for health and fitness* (2nd edition). Belmont, CA: Wadsworth Publishing Company.

Dunn, H.L. (1977). *High-level wellness*. Thorofare, NJ: Charles B. Slack.

Dunn, J.R., and Hayes, M.V. (2000) Social inequality, population health and housing: A study of two Vancouver neighbourhoods. *Social Science and Medicine*, 51, 563-587.

Durlak, J. (2000). Health promotion as a strategy in primary prevention. In D. Cicchetti, J. Rappaport, I. Sandler, and R. Weissberg (Eds.), *The promotion of wellness in children and adolescents* (pp. 221–241). Washington, DC: Child Welfare League Association Press.

Egbert, E. (1980). Concept of wellness. *Journal of Psychiatric Nursing and Mental Health Services*, 18(1), 9-12.

Ekos Research Associates Inc. (2004). *Stakeholder and public consultations on the Canadian index of well-being: Executive Summary*. Canadian Index of Wellbeing Project. Toronto: Atkinson Charitable Foundation.

Elliott, S., and Foster, L. (1995). Mind-body-place: A geography of Aboriginal health in British Columbia. In P. Stephenson, S. Elliott, L.T. Foster, and J. Harris (Eds.), *A persistent spirit: Towards understanding Aboriginal health in British Columbia* (pp. 94-127). Victoria, BC: Canadian Western Geographical Series, Vol. 31.

Evans, G.W., Saegert, S., and Harris, R. (2001). Residential density and psychological health among children in low-income families. *Environment and Behavior*, 33, 165-180.

Federation of Canadian Municipalities (FCM) (2001). *FCM Quality of Life Report 2001*. Ottawa: Federation of Canadian Municipalities.

Food and Agricultural Organization (1996). Report of the World Food Summit (WFS). Rome: Food and Agricultural Organization.

Food Security Standing Committee (2004). *Making the connection: Food security and public health*. Vancouver: Community Nutritionists' Council of BC.

Forster-Coull, L. (2004). *British Columbia Nutrition Survey: Report on energy and nutrition intakes*. Victoria, BC: Ministry of Health Services.

Foster, H.D. (1987). Landform and natural hazard. In C.N. Forward (Ed.), *British Columbia: Its resources and people* (pp. 43-63). Victoria, BC: Canadian Western Geographical Series, Vol. 22.

Foster, L.T. (2005). Youth in BC: Selected demographic, health and well-being trends and patterns over the last century. In R.S. Tonkin and L.T. Foster (Eds.), *The youth of British Columbia: Their past and their future* (pp. 15-37). Victoria, BC: Canadian Western Geographical Series, Vol. 39.

Foster, L.T., Burr, K., and Mohamed, J. (1992). *Identifying healthy communities in British Columbia*. Tenth Annual Pacific Health Forum. October 12, Vancouver.

Foster, L.T., Burr, K., and Mohamed, J. (1994). *Screening for health-care benchmarks in British Columbia: The use of Vital Statistics data*. Victoria, BC: Ministry of Health and Ministry Responsible for Seniors, Division of Vital Statistics.

Foster, L.T., and Edgell, M.C.R. (1992). *The geography of death: Mortality atlas of British Columbia* (pp. 63-165). Victoria, BC: Canadian Western Geographical Series, Vol. 26.

Foster, L.T., Kierans, W.J., and Macdonald, J. (2002). Chapter 4. Sudden infant death syndrome: A literature review and a summary of BC trends. In M.V. Hayes and L.T. Foster (Eds.), *Too small to see, too big to ignore: Child health and well being in British Columbia* (pp. 51-74). Victoria, BC: Canadian Western Geographical Series, Vol. 35.

Foster, L.T., Macdonald, J., Tuk, T.A., Uh, S.H., and Talbot, D. (1996). Native health in British Columbia: A vital statistics perspective. In P.H. Stephenson, S.J. Elliott, L.T. Foster, and J. Harris. (Eds), *A persistent spirit: Towards understanding Aboriginal health in British Columbia* (pp. 41-93). Victoria, BC: Canadian Western Geographical Series, Vol. 31.

Foster, L.T., and Wharf, B. (2007). *People, politics and child welfare in British Columbia*. Vancouver: University of British Columbia Press.

Foster, L.T., and Wright, M. (2002). Patterns and trends in children in the care of the Province of British Columbia: Ecological, policy and cultural perspectives. In M.V. Hayes and L.T. Foster (Eds.), *Too small to see, too big to ignore: Child health and well-being in British Columbia* (pp. 103-140). Victoria, BC: Canadian Western Geographical Series, Vol. 35.

Governor General of Canada (1999). *Building a higher quality of life for all Canadians: Speech from the Throne to Open the Second Session of the Thirty-sixth Parliament of Canada*. 12 October 1999. Canada. Governor General.

Greenberg, J.S. (1985). Health and wellness: A conceptual differentiation. *Journal of School Health*, 55, 403-406.

Gregory, I., Dorling, D., and Southall, H. (2001). A century of inequality in England and Wales using standardised geographical units. *Area*, 33(3), 297-311.

Hales, D. (2005). *An invitation to health*, 11th ed. "An Invitation to Health for the Twenty-First Century." Belmont, CA: Thomson & Wadsworth.

Hancock, T., Labonte, R., and Edwards, R. (1999). *Indicators that count! Measuring population health at the community level. Issues in health promotion.* HP-10-0207. Toronto: University of Toronto.

Harrington, R., and Loffredo, D.A. (2001). The relationship between life satisfaction, self consciousness, and the Myers-Briggs type inventory dimensions. *Journal of Psychology*, 135(4), 439-450.

Harrower, M., Keller, P., and Hocking, D. (1997). Cartography on the internet: Thoughts and a preliminary user survey. *Cartographic Perspectives*, 27(Winter), 27-37.

Hatch, R.L., Burg, M.A., Naberhaus, D.S., and Hellmich, L.K. (1998). The Spiritual involvement and beliefs scale: Development and testing of a new instrument. *Journal of Family Practice*, 46(6), 476-484.

Hayes, M.V., Foster, L.T., and Foster, H.D. (1994). *The determinants of population health: A critical assessment.* Victoria, BC: Canadian Western Geographical Series, Vol. 29.

Hayes, M.V., Ross, I.E., Gasher, M., Gutstien, D., Dunn, J.R., and Hackett, R.A. (2007). Telling stories: News media, health literacy and public policy in Canada. *Social Science and Medicine*, 64, 1842-1852.

Health Canada (2001). *It takes a community: Framework for the First Nations and Inuit Fetal Alcohol Syndrome and Fetal Alcohol Effects Initiative.* A resource manual for community-based prevention of fetal alcohol syndrome and fetal alcohol effects. Ottawa: Author.

Health Canada (2003). *Canadian guidelines for body weight classification in adults.* Catalogue No. H49-179. Ottawa: Health Canada.

Helburn, N. (1982). Geography and the quality of life. *Annals of the Association of American Geographers*, 72, 445-456.

Helliwell, J.F. (2005). *Well-being, social capital and public policy: What's new?* Cambridge, MA: National Bureau of Economic Research.

Hertzman, C., McLean, S.A., Kohen, D.E., Dunn, J., and Evans, T. (2002). *Early development in Vancouver: Report of the Community Asset Mapping Project (CAMP).* Vancouver: Human Early Learning Partnership, University of British Columbia; and Ottawa: Canadian Institute for Health Information.

Hettler, B. (1980). Wellness promotion on a university campus. Family and Community Health. *Journal of Health Promotion and Maintenance*, 3, 77-95.

Hettler, B. (1984). Wellness: Encouraging a lifetime pursuit of excellence. *Health Values: Achieving High Level Wellness*, 8, 13-17.

Hocking, D., and Keller, P. (1992). A user perspective on atlas content and design. *Cartographic Journal*, 29(December), 109-117.

Hocking, D., and Keller, P. (1993). Alternative atlas distribution formats: A user perspective. *Cartography and Geographic Information Systems*, 20(3), 157-166.

Hoge, D.R. (1972). A validated intrinsic religious motivation scale. *Journal for the Scientific Study of Religion*, 11, 369-376.

Hollander, M., Foster, L.T., Curtis, G., and Galloway, A. (1992). Factors related to the adoption of municipal bylaws to restrict smoking. In M.V. Hayes, L.T. Foster, and H.D. Foster (Eds), *Community, environment and health: Geographic perspectives* (pp. 343-370). Victoria, BC: Canadian Western Geographical Series, Vol. 27.

Horne, G. (2004). *British Columbia's heartland at the dawn of the 21st century.* BC Statistics. Victoria, BC: Ministry of Management Services.

Horsman, J., Furlong, W., Feeney, D., and Torrance, G. (2003). The Health Utilities Index (HUI): Concepts, measurement properties and applications. Health and Quality of Life Outcomes 2003, 1:54. *www.hqlo.com/content/1/1/54.* Accessed April, 2007.

House of Commons Standing Committee on Health (2007). *Healthy weights for healthy kids.* Report of the Standing Committee on Health. Seventh Report March. 39th Parliament, 1st Session. Ottawa.

Human Early Learning Partnership (HELP) (2005). Mapping Overview. Vancouver: HELP, University of British Columbia. *www.chspr.ubc.ca/Research/primarycaremapping/.* Accessed November 1, 2006.

Ingersoll, R.E. (1994). Spirituality, religion, and counseling: Dimensions and relationships. *Counseling and Values*, 38, 98-111.

Institute for Clinical Evaluative Sciences (ICES) (2007). Atlases that can be found at *www.ices.on.ca/webpage.cfm?site_id=1&org_id=67*. Accessed March, 2007. Toronto: ICES.

Jensen, L.A., and Alien, M.N. (1994). A synthesis of qualitative research on wellness-illness. *Qualitative Health Research*, 4(4), 349-369.

Johnston, R.J. (1982). On the nature of human geography. *Transactions of the Institute of British Geographers*, 7, 123-125.

Jonas, S. (2005). The wellness process for healthy living: A mental tool for facilitating progress through the stages of change. *American Medical Athletic Association Journal*, 8(2), 5-7.

Kasser, T., and Ryan, R.M. (1993). The dark side of the American dream: Correlates of financial success as a central life aspiration. *Journal of Personality and Social Psychology*, 65, 410-422.

Kasser, T., and Ryan, R.M. (1996). Further examining the American dream: Differential correlates of intrinsic and extrinsic goals. *Personality and Social Psychology Bulletin*, 22, 280-287.

Katzmarzyk, P. (2002). The Canadian obesity epidemic: An historical perspective. *Obesity Research*, 10(7), 666-674.

Katzmarzyk, P.T., Gledhill, N., and Shephard, R.J. (2000). The economic burden of physical inactivity in Canada. *Canadian Medical Association Journal*, 163 (11), 1435-1440.

Kawachi, I., and Berkman, L.F. (Eds). (2003). *Neighborhoods and health*. Oxford, NY: Oxford University Press.

Keller, P. (1995a). Visualizing digital atlas information products and the user perspective. *Cartographic Perspectives*, 20(Winter), 21-28.

Keller, P. (1995b), Letting the user talk: New insights into cartographic products. *Geomatica*, 49(1), 31-37.

Keller, P., Hocking, D., and Wood, C.J. (1995). Planning the next generation of regional atlases: Input from educators. *Journal of Geography*, March/April, 403-409.

Kelly, J.G. (2000). Wellness as an ecological enterprise. In D. Cicchetti, J. Rappaport, I. Sandier, and R.P. Weissberg (Eds.), *Promotion of wellness in children and adolescents* (pp. 101-131). Washington, DC: CWLA Press.

Kendall, P.R.W. (2001). Health status of children and youth in care in British Columbia: What do the mortality data show? A report from the Provincial Health Officer. Victoria, BC: Ministry of Health and Ministry Responsible for Seniors. *www.health.gov.bc.ca/library/publications/year/2001//cyicreportfinal.pdf*. Accessed April, 2007.

Kendall, P.R.W. (2002). The health and well-being of Aboriginal people in British Columbia. Provincial Health Officer's Annual Report, 2001. Victoria, BC: Ministry of Health. *www.health.gov.bc.ca/pho/pdf/phoannual2001pres.pdf*. Accessed April, 2007.

Kendall, P.R.W. (2003). An ounce of prevention: A public health rationale for the school as a setting for health promotion. A report of the Provincial Health Officer. Victoria, BC: Ministry of Health Planning. *www.health.gov.bc.ca/pho/pdf/o_prevention.pdf*. Accessed April, 2007.

Kendall, P.R.W. (2006). Food, health and well-being in British Columbia. Provincial Health Officer's annual report, 2005. Victoria, BC: Ministry of Health. *www.health.gov.bc.ca/pho/pdf/phoannual2005.pdf*. Accessed April, 2007.

Kendall, P.R.W. (2007). The health and well-being of the Aboriginal population in British Columbia: Interim update. February. Victoria, BC: Ministry of Health. *www.healthservices.gov.bc.ca/pho/pdf/Interim_report_Final.pdf*. Accessed April, 2007.

Kendall, P.R.W., and Morley, J. (2006). Health and well-being of children in care in British Columbia: Report 1 on health services utilization and mortality. Joint special report. Victoria, BC: Office of the Provincial Health Office. *www.healthservices.gov.bc.ca/pho/pdf/cyo/Introduction.pdf*. Accessed April, 2007.

Kendall, P.R.W., and Turpel-Lafond, M.E. (2007). Health and well-being of children in care in British Columbia: Educational experience and outcomes. Joint special report. Provincial Health Officer and Representative for Children and Youth. Victoria, BC: Office of the Provincial Health Officer. *www.health.gov.bc.ca/pho/pdf/joint_special_report.pdf*. Accessed April, 2007.

Kershaw, P., Irwin, L., Trafford, K., Hertzman, C., Schaub, P., Forer, B., Foster, L.T., Wiens, M., Hertzman, E., Guhn, M., Schroeder, J., and Goelman, H. (2005). *The British Columbia atlas of child development*. Victoria, BC: Canadian Western Geographical Series, Vol. 40.

Khan, O., and Skinner, R. (2003). *Geographic information systems and health applications*. Hershey, PA: Idea Group Publishing.

Kierans, W.J., Collison, M.A., Foster, L.T., and Uh, S.H. (1993). *Charting birth outcome in British Columbia: Determinants of optimal health and ultimate risk*. Victoria, BC: British Columbia Vital Statistics Agency.

Kierans, W.J., Kramer, M.S., Wilkins, R., Liston, R., Foster, L., Uh, S.H., and Mohamed, J. (2004). *Charting birth outcome in British Columbia: Determinants of optimal health and ultimate risk. An expansion and update.* Victoria, BC: British Columbia Vital Statistics Agency.

Kierans, W.J., Kendall, P.R.W., Foster, L.T., Liston, R.M., and Tuk, T. (2006). New birth weight and gestational age charts for the British Columbia population. *BC Medical Journal,* 48(1), 28-32.

Kierans, W.J., Kendall, P.R.W., Foster, L.T., Liston, R.M., and Tuk, T. (2007). New birth body length and head circumference charts for the British Columbia population. *BC Medical Journal,* 49(2), 72-77.

Kierans, W.J., Verhulst, L.A., Mohamed, J., and Foster, L.T. (in press). Neonatal mortality risk related to birth weight and gestational age in British Columbia. *Journal of Obstetrics and Gynaecology Canada,* 29(7), 568-574.

Koch, T. (2004). The map as intent: Variations on the theme of John Snow. *Cartographica,* 39(4), 1-14.

Koenig, H., Parkerson, G.R., and Meador, K.G. (1997). Religion index for psychiatric research. *American Journal of Psychiatry,* 153(6), 885-856.

Kuo, F.E. (2001). Coping with poverty impacts of environment and attention in the inner city. *Environment and Behavior,* 33, 5-34.

Lafferty, J. (1979). A credo for wellness. *Health Education,* 10, 10-11.

Lalonde, M. (1974) *The Lalonde Report: A New Perspective on the Health of Canadians.* Ottawa: Ministry of Supplies and Services.

Larson, J.S. (1999). The conceptualization of health. *Medical Care Research and Review,* 56(2), 123-136.

Leafgren, F. (1990). Being a man can be hazardous to your health: Life-styles issues. In D. Moore and F. Leafgren (Eds.), *Problem solving strategies and interventions for men in conflict* (pp. 265-311). Alexandria: American Association for Counseling and Development.

Lorion, R.P. (2000). Theoretical and evaluation issues in the promotion of wellness and the protection of "well enough." In D. Cicchetti, J. Rappaport, I. Sandier, and R.P. Weissberg (Eds.), *Promotion of wellness in children and adolescents* (pp. 1-27). Washington DC: CWLA Press.

Macintyre, S., Ellaway, A., and Cummins, S. (2002). Place effects on health: How can we conceptualize, operationalise and measure them? *Social Science and Medicine,* 55, 125-139.

MacMurchy, H. (1927). *The Canadian mother's book.* Ottawa: Department of Health.

McBride, M. (2005). *School smoking policy. A discussion paper.* Prepared for the British Columbia Ministry of Health, Victoria.

McCreary Centre Society (2004). *Healthy youth development: Highlights from the 2003 Adolescent Health Survey III.* Vancouver: McCreary Centre Society.

McCreary Centre Society (2006). *Promoting healthy bodies: Physical activity, weight, and tobacco use among BC youth.* Vancouver: McCreary Centre Society.

McLintock, B. (2004). *Smoke-free: How one city successfully banned smoking in all indoor public places.* Vancouver: Granville Island Publishing.

MacDonald, D.A. (2000). Spirituality: Description, measurement, and relation to the Five Factor model of personality. *Journal of Personality,* 68(1), 153-197.

McGrail, K., and Schaub, P. (2002). The British Columbia Health Atlas. 1st Edition. Vancouver: Centre for Health Services and Policy Research, University of British Columbia. *www.chspr.ubc.ca/node/191.* Accessed November, 2005.

McGrail, K., Schaub, P., and Black, C. (2004). The British Columbia Health Atlas. 2nd Edition. Vancouver: Centre for Health Services and Policy Research, University of British Columbia. *www.chspr.ubc.ca/healthatlas/2004.* Accessed March, 2007.

McKay, M. (2004). Action Schools! BC: Phase 1 (pilot) evaluation report and recommendations. A report to the Ministry of Health Services. November. *www.actionschoolsbc.ca.* Accessed December, 2006.

McNally, E., Hendricks, S., and Horowitz, I. (1985). A look at breastfeeding trends in Canada (1963-1982). *Canadian Journal of Public Health,* 76(2), 101-107.

McSherry W., and Draper, P. (1998). The debates emerging in the literature surrounding the concept of spirituality as applied to nursing. *Journal of Advanced Nursing,* 27(4), 683-691.

May, J.M. (1958). *The ecology of human disease.* Volume 1. New York: M.D. Publications.

Midgley, J., and Livermore, M. (1998). United States of America. In J. Dixon and D. Macarov (Eds.), *Poverty: A persistent global reality* (pp. 229-247). London: Routledge.

Millar, J.S. (1993). *A report on the health of British Columbians: Provincial Health Officer's annual report 1992*. Victoria, BC: Ministry of Health and Ministry Responsible for Seniors.

Miller, G. (2007). *Review and critical synthesis of literature on wellness: BC atlas of wellness*. Victoria, BC: University of Victoria, Faculty of Human and Social Development.

Ministry of Children and Family Development (2006). About fetal alcohol syndrome disorder. *www.mcf.gov.bc.ca/fasd/index.htm*. Accessed December, 2006.

Ministry of Education (2001). *How are we doing? An overview of Aboriginal education results for province of BC, 2001*. Victoria, BC: Author.

Ministry of Education (2004). *Safe, caring and orderly schools: A guide*. Victoria, BC: Author.

Ministry of Education (2006). *Public libraries statistics 2005*. Public Library Services Branch. Victoria, BC: Author.

Ministry of Education and Ministry of Health (2005). *School food sales and policies provincial report*. Victoria, BC: ActNow BC.

Ministry of Environment (2006). *Alive and inseparable. British Columbia's coastal environment: 2006*. Victoria, BC: Ministry of Environment. *www.env.gov.bc.ca/soe/bcce/*. Accessed August, 2007.

Ministry of Health (2005). *Baby's best chance. Parents' handbook of pregnancy and baby care*. 6th edition. Victoria, BC: Author.

Ministry of Health Planning (2003). *A Framework for Core Functions in Public Health*, Working Paper, Draft #3. Victoria, BC: Ministry of Health Planning.

Ministry of Health Services (2004). *British Columbia nutrition survey: Report on energy and nutrition intakes*. Victoria, BC: Author.

Ministry of Health Services (2004a). *BC's tobacco control strategy: Targeting our efforts*. Victoria, BC: Author. *www.tobaccofacts.org/pdf/bc_strategy.pdf*. Accessed June, 2007.

Ministry of Water, Land and Air Protection (2002). *Environmental trends in British Columbia*. Victoria, BC: Author.

Ministry of Water, Land and Air Protection (2004). *Weather climate and the future. BC's plan*. Victoria, BC: Author.

Moberg, D.O. (1984). Subjective measures of spiritual well-being. *Review of Religious Research*, 25(4), 351-364.

Monmonier, M. (2005). Critic, deconstruct thyself: A rejoinder to Koch's nonsense of Snow, *Cartographica*, 40(3), 105-108.

Mookerjee, R., and Beron, K. (2005). Gender, religion and happiness. *Journal of Socio-Economics*, 34(5), 674-685.

Moser, G., and Corroyer, D. (2001). Politeness in the urban environment: Is city life still synonymous with civility? *Environment and Behavior*, 33, 611-625.

Myers, D. (1987). Community-relevant measurement of quality of life: A focus on local trends. *Urban Affairs Quarterly*, 23, 108-125.

Myers, J.E., Sweeney, T.J., and Witmer, M. (2005). A holistic model of wellness. *www.mindgarden.com/products/wells.htm*. Accessed August, 2007.

Myres, A.W. (1988). National initiatives to promote breastfeeding: Canada, 1979-85. In D. Jelliffe and E. Jelliffe (Eds.), *Programmes to promote breastfeeding* (pp. 101-112). Oxford: Oxford University Press.

National Wellness Institute (1983). *Life style assessment questionnaire* (2nd ed.). Stevens Point, WI: National Wellness Institute.

Ng, E., Wilkins, R., Gendron, F., and Berthelot, J-M. (2005). *Dynamics of immigrants' health in Canada: Evidence from the National Population Health Survey*. Ottawa: Statistics Canada.

Nicholls, C.L., Ho, K.K., and Foster, L.T. (1993). *Local Health Area statistical profiles for British Columbia: Maps supplement*. Victoria, BC: Ministry of Health and Ministry Responsible for Seniors

Non-smokers Rights Association (NSRA) (2006). *Compendium of 100% smoke-free public place municpal by-laws*. Toronto: NSRA. *www.nsra-adnf.ca/cms/index.cfm?group_id=1421*. Accessed August, 2007.

Oliphant, L.E. (2001). Toward a uniform definition of wellness: A commentary. *Research Digest*, Series 3, 15.

Oliver, L., and Hayes, M.V. (2005). Neighbourhood socio-economic status and the prevalence of overweight Canadian children and youth. *Canadian Journal of Public Health*, 96(6), 415-420.

Oliver, L., and Hayes, M.V. (2007). Does choice of spatial unit matter for estimating small-area disparities? *Canadian Journal of Public Health*, Supplement on Place and Health, May/June.

Ostry, A. (2005). The early development of nutrition policy in Canada: Impacts on mothers and children. In C. Warsh (Ed.), *Children's health issues in historical perspective* (pp. 191-208). Waterloo, ON: Wilfred Laurier Press.

Ostry, A, Rideout, K., Levy-Milne, R.D., and Martin C. (2005). *Food sales and nutrition policies in British Columbia's schools*. Prepared for the BC Ministry of Health, Healthy Living/Chronic Disease Prevention Branch, Victoria.

Ostry, A. (2006). *Nutrition policy in Canada, 1870-1939*. Vancouver: University of British Columbia Press.

Owen, T.R. (1999). The reliability and validity of a wellness inventory. *American Journal of Health Promotion*, 13, 180-182.

Pacione, M. (1999). The geography of poverty and deprivation. In M. Pacione (Ed.), *Applied geography: Principles and practice* (pp. 400-413). London: Routledge.

Paloutzian, R.F., and Ellison, C.W. (1982). Loneliness, spiritual well-being, and the quality of life. In L.A. Poplau and D. Perlman (Eds.), *Loneliness: A sourcebook of current theory, research, and therapy* (pp. 224-237). New York: Wiley.

Pargament, K.I. (1999). The psychology of religion and spirituality? Yes and No. *International Journal for the Psychology of Religion*, 9(1), 3-16.

ParticipACTION (2004). The mouse that roared: A marketing and health communications success story. *Canadian Journal of Public Health*, 95(Suppl. 2). *www.cpha.ca/shared/cjph/archives/index04.htm#95_sup2*. Accessed April, 2007.

Pavot, W., Diener, E., and Fujita, F. (1990). Extraversion and happiness. *Personality and Individual Differences*, 11, 1299-1306.

Persson, T., and Tabellini, G. (1994). Is inequality harmful for growth. *American Economic Review*, 84(3), 600-621.

Pickett, K.E., and Pearl, M. (2001). Multilevel analyses of neighbourhood socio-economic context and health outcomes: A critical review. *Journal of Epidemiology and Community Health*, 55, 111-122.

Poon, C., Chittenden, M., Saewyc, E., Murphy, A., and McCreary Centre Society (2006). *Promoting healthy bodies: Physical activity, weight, and tobacco use among BC youth*. Vancouver: McCreary Centre Society.

Public Health Agency of Canada (2006). Determinants of health. *www.phac-aspc.gc.ca/media/nr-rp/2006/2006_06bk2_e.html*. Accessed March, 2007.

Public Health Agency of Canada (2007). The sensible guide to healthy pregnancy. Ottawa: Author. *www.healthypregnancy.gc.ca*. Accessed March, 2007.

Pyle, G.F. (1979). *Applied medical geography*. Washington: VH Winston and Sons.

Randall, J.E., and Williams, A.M. (2002). Urban quality of life: An overview. *Canadian Journal of Urban Research*, 10(2), 167-173.

Raphael, D. (Ed.) (2004). *Social determinants of health: Canadian perspectives*. Toronto: Canadian Scholars' Press.

Renger, R.F., Midyett, S.J., Mas, F.G., Erin, T.E., McDermott, H.M., Papenfuss, R.L., Eichling, P.S., Baker, D.H., Johnson, K.A., and Hewitt, M.J. (2000). Optimal living profile: An inventory to assess health and wellness. *American Journal of Health Promotion*, 24(6), 403-412.

Richards, P.S., and Bergin, A.E. (1997). *A spiritual strategy of counseling & psychotherapy*. Washington, DC: American Psychological Association.

Rickhi, B., and Aung, S. (2006). *Wellness is a state of mind, body and spirit*. Complementary and Alternative Health Affiliate of the Canadian Health Network. Ottawa: Public Health Agency of Canada.

Rideout, K., and Ostry, A. (2006). A conceptual model for developing food security indicators for use by regional health authorities. *Canadian Journal of Public Health*, 97(3), 233-236.

Rideout, K., Martin, C., Levy-Milne, R., and Ostry, A. (in press). Food sales and nutrition policies in British Columbia schools. *Canadian Journal of Public Health*.

Robinson, A.H., Morrison, J.L., Muehrcke, P.C., Kimmerling, A.J., and Guptill, S.C. (1995). *Elements of cartography*, 6th Edition. New York: Wiley.

Rogerson, R., Findlay, A., Morris, A., and Paddison, R. (1989a). Variations in quality of life in urban Britain: 1989. *Cities*, 6, 227-233.

Rogerson, R., Findlay, A., Morris, A., and Paddison, R. (1989b). Indicators of quality of life: Some methodological issues. *Environment and Planning A*, 21, 1655-1666.

Ross, N.A., Tremblay, S.S., and Graham, K. (2004). Neighbourhood influences on health in Montreal, Canada. *Social Science and Medicine*, 59, 1485-1494.

Rushton, G. (2002). Public health, GIS, and spatial analytic tools. *Annual Review of Public Health*, (24), 43-56.

Ryan, R.M., and Deci, E.L. (2001). On happiness and human potentials: A review of research on hedonic and eudaemonic well-being. *Annual Review of Psychology*, 52, 141-166.

Ryan, R.M., and Frederick, C.M. (1997). On energy, personality and health: Subjective vitality as a dynamic reflection of well-being. *Journal of Personality*, 65, 529-565.

Ryff, C.D., and Singer, B.H. (1998). The contours of positive human health. *Psychological Inquiry*, 9(1), 1-28.

Ryff, C.D., and Singer, B.H. (2006). Best news yet on the six-factor model of well-being. *Social Science Research*, 35, 1103-1119.

Sackney, L., Noonan, B., and Miller, C.M. (2000). Leadership for educator wellness: An exploratory study. *International Journal of Leadership in Education*, 3(1), 41-56.

Saewyc, E. (2007). Research Director, McCreary Centre Society, Burnaby. Personal communication, February.

Sarason, S.B. (2000). Porgy and Bess and the concept of wellness. In D. Cicchetti, J. Rappaport, I. Sandler, and R.P. Weissberg (Eds.), *Promotion of wellness in children and adolescents* (pp. 427-437). Washington DC: CWLA Press.

Schuster, T.A.L., Dobson, M., Jauregui, M., and Blanks, R.H.I. (2004). Wellness lifestyles I: A theoretical framework linking wellness, health lifestyles, and complementary and alternative medicine. *Journal of Alternative and Complementary Medicine*, 10(2), 349-356.

Seaward, B.L. (1997). *Managing stress: Principles and strategies for health and well-being* (2nd edition). Boston, MA: Jones and Bartlett Publishers.

Seaward, B.L. (2002). *Managing stress: Principles and strategies for health and well-being* (3rd edition). Boston, MA: Jones and Bartlett.

Sechrist, W.C. (1979). Total wellness and holistic health. *Health Education*, 10(5), 27.

Sheldon, K.M., and Elliot, A.J. (1999). Goal striving, need satisfaction, and longitudinal well-being: The self-concordance model. *Journal of Personality and Social Psychology*, 76, 482-497.

Sheldon, K.M., and Kasser, T. (1998). Pursuing personal goals: Skills enable progress, but not all progress is beneficial. *Personality and Social Psychology Bulletin*, 24, 1319-1331.

Shields, M., and Tjepkema, M. (2006). Regional differences in obesity. *Health Reports*, 17(3), 61-67.

Skevington, S.M., Lofty, M., and O'Connell, K.A. (2004). The World Health Organization's WHOQOL-BREF quality of life assessment: Psychometric properties and results of the international field trial. A report from the WHOQOL Group. *Quality of Life Research*, 13, 299-310.

Smith, D.M. (1973). *The geography of social well-being in the United States*. New York: McGraw-Hill.

Smith, M., and Kelly, C. (2006). Wellness tourism. *Tourism Recreation Research*, 31(1), 1-4.

Smith, T., Nelischer, M., and Perkins, N. (1997). Quality of an urban community: A framework for understanding the relationship between quality and physical form. *Landscape and Urban Planning*, 39(2), 229-241.

Snow, J. (1855). *On the mode of communication of cholera*. London: John Churchill.

Statistics Canada (2006). *Low income cut-offs for 2005 and low income measures for 2004*. Income Research Paper Series. Income Statistics Division. Ottawa: Author.

Stephenson, P.H., Elliott, S.J., Foster, L.T., and Harris J. (Eds). *A persistent spirit: Towards understanding Aboriginal health in British Columbia*. Victoria, BC: Canadian Western Geographical Series, Vol. 31.

Strohmaier, R., and Burr, K. (1992). British Columbia: The physical, socioeconomic, and health services network setting. In L.T. Foster and M.C.R. Edgell (Eds.), *The geography of death: Mortality atlas of British Columbia* (pp. 63-165). Victoria, BC: Canadian Western Geographical Series, Vol. 26.

Sun, Y. (2005). *Development of neighbourhood quality of life indicators*. Saskatoon: Community-University Institute for Social Research (CUISR). University of Saskatchewan.

Tait, C.L. (2003). *Fetal alcohol syndrome among Aboriginal people in Canada: Review and analysis of the intergenerational links to residential schools*. Prepared for the Aboriginal Healing Foundation. Ottawa: Aboriginal Healing Foundation.

Teague, M.L. (1987). *Health promotion: Achieving high-level wellness in the later years*. Indianapolis, IN: Benchmark Press.

Tjepkema, M. (2006). Adult obesity. *Health Reports*, 17(3), 11-27.

Toronto Community Foundation (2004). *Toronto's vital signs 2004: The city's annual check-up.* Toronto: Toronto Community Foundation.

Townsend, P., and Davidson, N. (Eds.) (1982). *Inequalities in health: The Black Report.* Harmondsworth, UK: Penguin.

Townshend, I.J. (2001). The contribution of social and experiential community structures to the intra-urban ecology of well-being. *Canadian Journal of Urban Research*, 10(2), 175-215.

Travis, J.W. (1981). *The Wellness Inventory.* Mill Valley, CA: Wellness Associates.

Travis, J.W., and Ryan, R.S. (1988). *Wellness workbook.* Berkeley: Ten Speed Press.

Turcotte, M., and Schellenberg, G. (2007). *A portrait of seniors in Canada, 2006.* Statistics Canada. Ottawa: Ministry of Industry.

US Office of the Surgeon General (2006). The Health Consequences of Involuntary Exposure to Tobacco Smoke: A Report of the Surgeon General. *www.surgeongeneral.gov/library/secondhandsmoke/.* Accessed August, 2007.

van Kamp, I., Leidelmeijer, K., Marsman, G., and de Hollander, A. (2003). Urban environmental quality and human well-being: Towards a conceptual framework and demarcation of concepts; A literature study. *Landscape and Urban Planning*, 65, 5-18.

Veenhoven, R. (2001). World Database of Happiness: Catalogue of happiness in nations (online database). Rotterdam: Erasmus University. *www1.eur.nl/fsw/happiness/index.html.* Accessed August, 2007.

Vital Statistics (2005). Annual report for 2004. Ministry of Health, Victoria. *www.vs.gov.bc.ca/stats/annual/2004/index.html.* Accessed August, 2007.

Vital Statistics (2006). Annual report for 2005. Ministry of Health, Victoria. *www.vs.gov.bc.ca/stats/annual/2005/index.html.* Accessed August, 2007.

Waste, R. (1998). *Independent cities.* Oxford: Oxford University Press.

Watson, D.E., Krueger, H., Mooney, D., and Black, C. (2005). *Planning for renewal: Mapping primary health care in British Columbia.* Vancouver: Centre for Health Services and Policy Research, University of British Columbia. *www.chspr.ubc.ca/Research/primarycaremapping/.* Accessed November, 2005.

Wechsler, H., Brener, N.D., Kuester, S., and Miller, C. (2001). Food service and foods and beverages available at school: Results from the school health policies and programs study. *Journal of School Health*, 71, 313.

Westgate, C.E. (1996). Spiritual wellness and depression. *Journal of Counseling and Development*, 75, 26-35.

Wilson, W. (1967). Correlates of avowed happiness. *Psychological Bulletin, 67, 294-306.*

Witmer, J.M., and Sweeney, T.J. (1992). A holistic model for wellness and prevention over the life span. *Journal of Counseling and Development*, 71, 140-148.

World Health Organization (1986). Ottawa Charter for Health Promotion. First International Conference on Health Promotion. Ottawa: WHO. *www.who.int/hpr/NPH/docs/ottawa_charter_hp.pdf.* Accessed August, 2007.

World Health Organization (2004). Report on health - Global strategy on diet, physical activity and health. *www.who.int/dietphysicalactivity/strategy/eb11344/en/.* Accessed August, 2007.

World Health Organization (2007). Public health mapping and geographic information systems. *www.who.int/health_mapping/en/.* Accessed August, 2007.

WESTERN GEOGRAPHICAL PRESS
Faculty of Social Sciences, Department of Geography, University of Victoria

WESTERN GEOGRAPHICAL SERIES

1 The Geographer and Society (1970)
2 Geographica (1970)
3 Resources, Recreation and Research (1970)
4 Okanagan Water Decisions (1972)
6 Oil Pollution as an International Problem (1973)
7 Handbook of Geographical Games (1973)
9 Modifying the Weather (1973)
10 Themes on Pacific Lands (1974)
11 Calgary: Metropolitan Structure and Influence (1975)
13 Pacific Salmon: Management for People (1977)
14 Specialists and Air Pollution: Occupations and Preoccupations (1977)
15 Edmonton: The Emerging Metropolitan Pattern (1978)
18 Regina: Regional Isolation and Innovative Development (1980)
20 Environmental Aesthetics: Essays in Interpretation (1982)
21 Tourism in Canada: Selected Issues and Options (1983)
23 Reducing Cancer Mortality: A Geographical Perspective (1986)
24 The Future Saskatchewan Small Town (1988)
25 Landscape Evaluation: Approaches and Applications (1989)
26 The Geography of Death: Mortality Atlas of British Columbia, 1985-1989 (1992)
27 Community, Environment and Health: Geographic Perspectives (1992)
28 Trade Opportunities: Saskatchewan/Canada—Shandong/China (1993)
29 The Determinants of Population Health: A Critical Assessment (1994)
30 Land of Genghis Khan: The Rise and Fall of Nation-States in China's Northern Frontiers (1995)

missing volume numbers are out of print

CANADIAN WESTERN GEOGRAPHICAL SERIES
Western Geographical Press; distributed by UBC Press

31 A Persistent Spirit: Towards Understanding Aboriginal Health in BC (1995) out of print
32 Building and Rebuilding Harmony: The Gateway to Victoria's Chinatown (1997)
33 Troubles in the Rainforest: British Columbia's Forest Economy in Transition (1997)
34 The Dragon's Head: Shanghai, China's Emerging Megacity (1998)
35 Too Small to See, Too Big to Ignore: Child Health and Well-being in British Columbia (2002)
36 British Columbia, The Pacific Province: Geographical Essays (2001)
37 Prospects for Development in the Asia-Pacific Area (2000)
38 Demography, Democracy, and Development: Pacific Rim Experiences (2002)
39 The Youth of British Columbia: Their Present and Their Future (2005)
40 The British Columbia Atlas of Child Development (2005)
41 Contemporary Issues in Mental Health: Concepts, Policy, and Practice (2007)
42 The British Columbia Atlas of Wellness (2007)

INTERNATIONAL WESTERN GEOGRAPHICAL SERIES
John Wiley and Sons, Ltd.

Cartographic Design: Theoretical and Practical Perspectives (1996)
Quality Management in Urban Tourism (1997)